The Leukemic Cell

METHODS IN HEMATOLOGY

Volume 2

The Leukemic Cell

EDITED BY

D. *Catovsky* MD, MRCPath

Senior Lecturer in Haematology and Medicine
and Honorary Consultant Physician, MRC Leukaemia Unit,
Royal Postgraduate Medical School, London.

CHURCHILL LIVINGSTONE
EDINBURGH LONDON MELBOURNE AND NEW YORK 1981

CHURCHILL LIVINGSTONE
Medical Division of Longman Group Limited

Distributed in the United States of America by
Churchill Livingstone Inc., 19 West 44th Street,
New York, N.Y. 10036, and by associated companies,
branches and representatives throughout the world.

First published 1981

ISBN 0 443 01911 8

British Library Cataloguing in Publication Data
Catovsky, D
  The leukemic cell. — (Methods in haematology).
  1. Leukemia — Diagnosis
  2. Diagnosis, Laboratory
  I. Title   II. Series
  616.1′55′075   RC643   80.41107

Printed in Great Britain by Butler & Tanner Ltd, Frome and London

Foreword

Hematology, par excellence, is the discipline where laboratory and clinical medicine coalesce. Perhaps it is the accessibility of the blood as an organ that makes this possible. The 'Methods in Hematology' series is intended to bring together technical methods related to a particular blood disorder or group of disorders. The description of an investigation will include not only a full account of how it should be done, but also an account of its clinical and scientific basis, of the principles on which the method is based, the problems that may be encountered in its performance and their resolution, and a discussion of the significance of the result.

The publishers, Churchill Livingstone, are advised on the choice of topics and of editors, by a small board from both Europe and the USA. The editor is invariably a leading scientist in his discipline and the contributors each experts in their respective fields. The intention is generally to omit those methods dealt with adequately in standard accounts of methodology and to include those which may pose special problems, newer but potentially valuable technics and technics that may be useful at a research level while, at the time of writing, not yet used in day-to-day practice.

This second volume in the series is concerned with the characterization of the leukemic cell. Leukemia is a field in which new developments are rapidly translated into day-to-day practice. Even where the tests are not available, a frequent practice is to send blood or marrow to a laboratory where they can be performed. Dr Daniel Catovsky, as a member of the Medical Research Council Leukaemia Unit of the Royal Postgraduate Medical School, London, has been at the sharp end of many of these developments and he has brought together a group of eminent workers from the United States of America, United Kingdom, France, Germany and Australia to contribute to this volume. It is hoped that this book will encourage more hematologists to use these technics and that this in turn will lead to a better understanding of these diseases and provide a sounder basis for their clinical management.

London, 1981

I. Chanarin

Preface

The development of new objective criteria for the diagnosis and classification of leukemia has led to a better characterization of the various forms of the disease, and has facilitated the recognition of new disease entities. It has led, too, to a greater insight into the natural history of leukemia and to improvements in patient management. Indeed, therapy and research in leukemia has served as a model for understanding and treating other neoplastic processes.

Much of this progress has resulted from technological advances which, in the past few years, have permitted a more accurate description of the cellular events in hemopoietic malignancies. It has often been difficult for hematologists to keep abreast with the rapid methodological developments. The aim of this book is to make this task easier by setting out the technics currently available for the study of leukemic cells in sufficient detail to make them of practical value. With few exceptions, methods regarded as useful for diagnosis and cell characterization, and which are essential for further research in this field, have been included.

Hematologists, pathologists, clinicians and other scientists actively involved in leukemia research and practice will find an account of the methods used in leading laboratories in Europe and the USA, not easily found in this form elsewhere. This has been achieved by the high standard of work of all the contributors who have combined simplicity of presentation with depth of knowledge of the frequently complex modern technics.

I wish to acknowledge the invaluable secretarial assistance of Mrs Day Haysome and Miss Sue Masterson, and the cooperation of the staff of Churchill Livingstone. The printing of the illustrations was supported by donations from the Société Chimique Pointet Girard, Upjohn Ltd, Raymond A. Lamb and Mercia Brocades Ltd.

London, 1981   D.C.

Contributors

J. Breton-Gorius PhD
Directeure de Recherche, Unité de Recherche sur les Anémies, Inserm
U.91, Hôpital Mondor, Creteil France.

Rolf Burkhardt MD
Professor of Medicine and Head of Department of Knochenmarkdiagnostik,
University of Munich; Head of Department of Haematomorphology,
Gesellschaft für Strahlen und Umweltforschung mbH, Munich.

Daniel Catovsky MD, MRCPath
Senior Lecturer in Haematology and Medicine and Hon. Consultant
Physician, MRC Leukaemia Unit, Royal Postgraduate Medical School,
London.

Mary Sue Coleman PhD
Assistant Professor, Department of Biochemistry, University of Kentucky,
Lexington, Kentucky, USA.

Gerald R. Crabtree MD
Assistant Professor of Pathology, Dartmouth Medical School, Hanover,
New Hampshire, USA.

Marie-Therèse Daniel MD
Chef de Travaux, Institut de Recherche sur les Leucémies et les Maladies
du Sang, Paris, France.

Georges Flandrin MD
Professor Agrégé, Institut de Recherche sur les Leucémies et les Maladies
du Sang, Paris, France.

Marie-Françoise Gourdin BS
Attachée de Recherche, Unité de Recherche sur les Anémies, Inserm
U.91, Hôpital Henri Mondor, Creteil, France.

John J. Hutton MD
Professor, Departments of Medicine and Biochemistry, University of Texas
Health Sciences Center, San Antonio, Texas, USA.

George Janossy MD, PhD, MRCPath
Senior Lecturer in Immunology, Department of Immunology, Royal Free
Hospital, London.

Donald Metcalf MD, FRACP, FAA
Head, Cancer Research Unit, Walter and Eliza Hall Institute of Medical
Research, Melbourne, Australia.

Allan Munck PhD
Professor of Physiology, Dartmouth Medical School, Hanover, New
Hampshire, USA.

Felix Reyes MD
Maître de Conférence Agregé, Unité de Recherche, Inserm U.91, Hôpital
Henri Mondor, Creteil, France.

Janet D. Rowley MD
Professor, Section of Hematology and Oncology, Department of Medicine,
University of Chicago, Illinois, USA.

Kendal A. Smith MD
Associate Professor of Medicine, Dartmouth Medical School, Hanover, New
Hampshire, USA.

Joseph R. Testa PhD
Research Associate and Assistant Director, Cytogenetics Laboratory,
Section of Hematology and Oncology, Department of Medicine, the
University of Chicago, Chicago, Illinois, USA.

Contents

1
Overview

D. Catovsky

INTRODUCTION

For many years cell morphology on Romanowsky stained films was the mainstay in the diagnosis of the acute and chronic leukemias in their myeloid (AML, CML) and lymphoid (ALL, CLL) forms. We are now aware that, within these broad groups, there are numerous entities which differ in their response to therapy and prognosis. The combination of morphology, chromosome analysis and membrane and enzyme markers, for example, has helped the recognition of blast transformation of CML with typical features of AML or ALL[1-4] (Ch. 5 and 7). Another windfall from a multiparameter analysis of leukemic cells has been the recognition of a good correlation between specific chromosome abnormalities and some forms of leukemia (see below).

The new technics have been particularly helpful in the analysis of morphologically 'undifferentiated' blast cells, which includes a high proportion of cases

Table 1.1 Methods for the study of leukemic cells

Morphology	Light microscopy Ultrastructure (TEM, SEM)[a] Cell volume estimations
Cytochemistry	Light microscopy Ultrastructure (TEM)
Histology	Plastic embedding Immunoperoxidase
Membrane markers	RBC rosetting tests Immunofluorescence Antibodies to antigens and Ig[b]
Enzyme assays	Terminal transferase Adenosine deaminase Hexosaminidase; other enzymes
Culture systems	Clonal growth in agar Permanent cell lines
Chromosomes	Banding technics
Hormone receptors	Glucocorticoids
Cell kinetics	Autoradiography Flow microfluorimetry

[a] TEM: transmission electron microscopy; SEM: scanning electron microscopy.
[b] Ig: immunoglobulins (heavy and light chains).

of ALL, particularly the L2 type of the FAB classification.[5] The most important methods for this purpose, at the present time, are listed in Table 1.1.

What follows is a personal account as to how these research tools have facilitated the analysis of patients in the context of clinical hematology.

MORPHOLOGY

The basis of diagnosis is examination of blood and marrow films; most leukemias are diagnosed with this material. In a proportion of cases the need for extra information derives from the knowledge that some prognostic features may be disclosed by other technics. For example, in ALL, surface marker studies may reveal T-cell features which carry a worse prognosis and perhaps indicate a more aggressive therapeutic approach. In most cases of AML, by using the criteria of the FAB group,[5] the patterns of maturation into granulocytic (M2), monocytic (M4, M5), or erythropoietic (M6) cells can be determined on light microscopy only. In the less mature forms (M1 and M5), cytochemical technics (Ch. 2) are important for correct classification.

One of the forms of AML more readily recognized by morphology is hypergranular promyelocytic leukemia (M3), as described in the original FAB paper.[5] But a variant form of M3, characterized by a paucity of granulation also exists.[6] Typical M3 cells are seen, but in very small numbers, and the main distinguishing feature is the bilobed or reniform nucleus. These patients have the hemorrhagic diathesis regularly present in M3, but, in contrast to the typical M3 cases, the variant form has an extremely high WBC count.

The important contribution of ultrastructural analysis by means of transmission electron microscopy (TEM) is detailed in Chapter 4. In my experience TEM is extremely useful in the recognition of Sézary cells, small and large cleaved cells in follicular lymphoma presenting in leukemic phase, poorly differentiated plasmablasts, and, in some instances, in distinguishing prolymphocytic leukemia (PLL) from CLL.[7]

TEM is of particular value in the diagnosis of double leukemias. We have recently been able to study four patients in whom a lymphoproliferative disorder, CLL, follicular lymphoma or hairy-cell leukemia, was associated with AML in three and a chronic myelomonocytic leukemia in another.

Morphological studies on leukemic cells could be taken a step further by the analysis of cell volume histograms obtained by a Coulter model ZBI, linked to a Channelyzer. This system permits the definition of the modal volume of the leukemic population, the presence of heterogeneity and an objective comparison between cell sizes in different leukemias.[8]

CYTOCHEMISTRY

Cytochemical technics are of value in distinguishing between AML and ALL and the various AML subtypes[9,10] (Ch. 2) and hence in their classification,[5] especially when the maturation features are not obvious in Romanowsky stained films. The peroxidase reaction visualized by TEM (as described in Ch. 4) adds important information in cases of CML in blast crisis by demonstrating enzyme activity in megakaryoblasts, and demonstrates myeloid blasts with small granules not visible by light microscopy as well as basophil promyelocytes.[11]

ACID PHOSPHATASE

By applying the acid phosphatase reaction at ultrastructural level we have been able to demonstrate a small lysosomal granule characteristic of monoblasts. These granules, of 0.05 to 0.2 μm in size, contain acid phosphatase (Fig. 1.1), but lack peroxidase and appear to be one of the earliest features of monocytic differentiation.[12] They are not observed in myeloblasts, where the earliest sign of differentiation is the presence of myeloperoxidase activity in the membranes and primary granules.[12]

Cytochemical reactions for acid phosphatase and alpha-naphthyl acetate esterase have also been helpful in the study of normal and leukemic lymphoid cells.[13] A localized strong paranuclear acid phosphatase reaction is characteristic of human fetal thymocytes[14] and in blast cells in the majority of ALL cases with positive T-lymphocyte markers[15] (Ch. 2). Two recent studies have shown the value of this reaction in diagnosing T-ALL with incomplete or immature

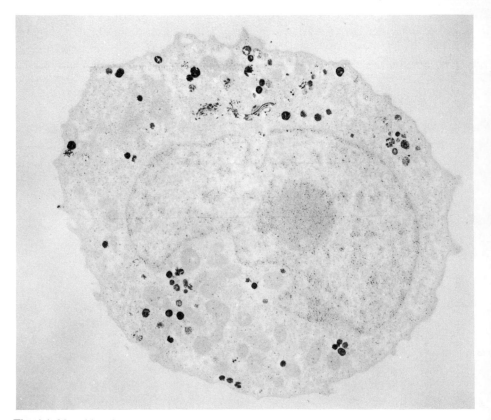

Fig. 1.1 Monoblast from a patient with acute monocytic (M5) leukemia showing acid phosphatase reaction in small cytoplasmic granules and the Golgi membranes (Gomori method,[12] unstained section, ×12 600). The myeloperoxidase reaction was negative in the same case.

membrane phenotype (pre-T) as shown by negative sheep RBC(E)-rosette formation.[16,17] Similar findings were reported in T-lymphoblastic lymphomas of childhood.[18] The acid phosphatase reaction in T-blasts in TEM is seen mainly in the membranes of the Golgi apparatus[13] and differs from that seen in monoblastic leukemia which is in very small granules in the cytoplasm.[12]

Although it is not clear whether there are significant differences in acid phosphatase content between mature B and T lymphocytes, this reaction is useful in characterizing some chronic lymphoid leukemias. CLL of B-cell type is usually negative, whilst most cases of T-CLL and Sézary syndrome show a strong reactivity, which in TEM is confined to lysosomal granules of varying size.[13]

ALPHA-NAPHTHYL ACETATE ESTERASE (ANAE)

There is good correlation between the proportion of peripheral blood lymphocytes with a localized (dot-like) ANAE reaction and the percentage of E-rosettes.[13] Unlike the reaction observed in monocytes, the reaction in lymphocytes is resistant to the inhibition by sodium fluoride. Studies by Grossi et al[19] have suggested that ANAE is positive in the subset of T-lymphocytes with Fc receptors for IgM (Tμ), whilst T-lymphocytes with Fc receptors for IgG (Tγ) are negative. In several of our cases with T-CLL in which Tγ lymphocytes were the predominant population, the ANAE reaction was negative.[13] In contrast, the reaction was consistently positive in the cells of T-prolymphocytic leukemia.

HISTOLOGY

The role of histology in the diagnosis and management of leukemia has lagged behind other technics. A tissue diagnosis is essential in most other tumors including the malignant lymphomas. Not enough attention has been given in the past to the bone marrow structure considering that it is the hemopoietic organ primarily affected in leukemia. Fortunately, considerable advances are taking place at the present time which will hopefully change this situation. New technology such as plastic embedding and semi-thin sections of undecalcified bone marrow, as detailed in Chapter 3, have brought about improved morphological analysis with preservation of the tissue structure.

Immunological methods can be applied to paraffin-embedded or frozen bone marrow sections. By means of the immunoperoxidase reaction, particularly the 'unlabeled antibody peroxidase-antiperoxidase (PAP)' method,[20] antigens, immunoglobulin molecules or enzymes can be localized at tissue level with great sensitivity. One example of this is the demonstration of the ALL antigen[2] in neoplastic cell infiltrates in the testis and the cerebellum.[21] The use of the immunoperoxidase technics at ultrastructural level is described in Chapter 4. Other technological achievements such as the 'labeled antigen' procedure which gives a low background on paraffin-embedded tissue sections, and the immunoenzymatic labeling with alkaline phosphatase which allows the detection of two antigens in the same section by combining with immunoperoxidase, were the subject of a workshop report.[22]

Although less essential for routine diagnosis, the study of the bone marrow structure is critical when aspirates are unsatisfactory due to poor or excessive cellularity or a degree of myelofibrosis. The mode in which the bone marrow is infiltrated is often important in the diagnosis of non-Hodgkin lymphomas.[23] The presence of discrete foci of blast cells could be of value in the study of preleukemic states and may facilitate the diagnosis of blast transformation in some patients with CML.[24] A detailed description of the value of bone marrow histology in the diagnosis and classification of leukemia and related disorders is given in Chapter 3.

One of the most important uses of bone marrow biopsy is in the analysis of specimens taken after intensive cytotoxic therapy in AML, particularly during the early stages. It is often a question of deciding whether treatment should continue (if residual blasts are still prominent) or a momentary halt is indicated (if the picture is that of hypoplasia). In our experience these decisions are difficult with bone marrow aspirates only because in half the instances the material obtained is small in quantity and of low reliability.

The process of bone marrow regeneration following induction therapy in AML is preceded by a phase of 'structured fat' which appears to be required to sustain normal hemopoiesis.[25] In contrast, hemopoietic regeneration after ablative therapy of CML in blast crisis followed by autologous reconstitution with buffy-coat cells[26] takes place earlier than in AML and independently of the presence of fat cells.[25]

MEMBRANE MARKERS

Lymphoid cells may differ substantially in the type and quantity of specific binding sites and antigens present on their membrane (Ch. 5). Lymphocyte populations are extremely heterogeneous and numerous stages in the development of T (thymic) and B (bursal) cells are now recognized.[27,28] They can be defined by the presence or absence of certain markers and the chances of determining the surface phenotype of a given cell increases with the number and reliability of the technics employed.

This information is important for the characterization of leukemic cells derived from B and T lines. The concept that phenotypically immature cells correlate with blast cell morphology is roughly correct for the T-cell lineage.[29] It is also applicable to B-cells although less strictly so because the processes of lymphocyte transformation and modulation which take place in lymph nodes (e.g. in the germinal centers[30]) often result in blast-looking cells which may, however, be immunologically mature.[29] These differentiated B-cells are the targets for neoplastic change in most non-Hodgkin's lymphomas.[23,30]

Because the distinction between acute (blastic) and chronic (mature-looking) lymphoid leukemias is still clinically useful, any classification should take into account the morphology and the surface markers of the cells involved. The wider terms of 'lymphoproliferative' or 'immunoproliferative' are still often used, as they embrace related disorders, bridging the gap between leukemia (blood and bone marrow in the strict sense) and lymphoma (lymph nodes or other tissues primarily involved).

CHRONIC LYMPHOID LEUKEMIAS

These are proliferations of differentiated B- or T-lymphocytes, often reflecting normal counterparts present in the peripheral blood. There is a suggestion that, with more sensitive technics for the detection of membrane immunoglobulins (SmIg), such as the mixed antiglobulin and the direct antiglobulin rosetting tests, most 'null' (non-B, non-T) or third population cells in the peripheral blood could be shown to belong to the B-cell lineage.[28]

There are several subsets within the major B and T populations which are represented by very small percentages in the peripheral blood. Cell typing of the chronic leukemias (see below) has been useful in identifying these relatively rare lymphocyte types; this, in turn, may be of value for the purpose of raising monoclonal antibodies which will facilitate studies of their normal function and distribution (Ch. 5).

Chronic T-cell leukemias

These are characterized by lymphocytes which form E-rosettes, are negative for the enzyme terminal transferase and are always SmIg negative. The existence of rare normal T-cell subsets bearing Ia-like antigenic determinants or complement (C3) receptors[31] can be supported by the demonstration of C3[32, 33] or Ia[34, 35] in E+ leukemic cells.

In an ongoing study aimed at defining the cell populations in these disorders (in collaboration with Drs M. F. Greaves, G. Janossy and M. Pepys and Professor A. V. Hoffbrand) we have identified two T-CLL cases with the phenotype: E + , Fcγ + , Ia + , C3 − [34] which support the findings in normal blood of a subset of Fcγ lymphocytes bearing the Ia-antigen.[36, 37] A similar phenotype, but negative for Ia, was demonstrated in two other T-CLL's, presumably corresponding to a proliferation of the Ia−, Tγ subset.[37] In two other patients we have observed membrane phenotypes which have not yet been identified in normal blood lymphocytes. One of them, with an unusual T-CLL 'lymphoma', was E + , Fcγ − , Fcμ − , Ia +, C3 + and the other, a T-PLL, was similar except that the Ia-antigen was absent.

Further advances in the characterization of T-cells resulted from the studies by Moretta et al[38] showing that two T-lymphocyte subsets which have either helper or suppressor activity can be identified respectively by the presence of Fcμ and Fcγ receptors (Tμ and Tγ lymphocytes possessing distinct morphological and cytochemical features).[20] Studies with these markers have shown that these immunoregulatory T-lymphocytes not only proliferate in some T-cell leukemias,[34, 37] but also that they may be present in abnormal proportions in some B-cell leukemias (see below). In addition to the rosetting technics for the identification of Tγ and Tμ cells (see Ch. 5), these lymphocytes may have a different expression of the TH_2 antigen(s).[40] Thus, leukemias of the TH_2 negative subset (presumably Tμ) have now been reported[41] and one of our T-CLL patients with the Fcγ +, Ia− subset was already found to be TH_2 positive (Dr G. Janossy, personal communication).

Chronic lymphocytic leukemia

B-CLL, the common form of the disease, results from the monoclonal proliferation of B-lymphocytes with weak expression of SmIg, usually IgM $\pm$ IgD, binding of mouse RBC,[29,34] Ia antigen and receptor sites for C3.[27] In a proportion of cases the detection of SmIg is below the threshold of routine immunofluorescence testing, although it might be demonstrated by more sensitive technics. This may be important because B-cells without detectable SmIg, but with receptors for C3 (CR_1 only) have been demonstrated in 2.4 per cent of normal peripheral blood cells[31] and in B-CLL the complement detected is CR_2, without CR_1.[27] As CR_2 is not present in the SmIg-negative B-cells of normal blood, the B-lymphocyte of CLL may thus originate from a separate subset.

Studies with mouse RBC rosetting, the test most consistently positive in this disease,[34] suggest that the B-CLL lymphocyte represents a cell which has stopped at an early stage in the process of B-cell maturation.[27] We have shown a marked difference in the expression of this receptor between peripheral blood (high) and other tissues such as lymph nodes and bone marrow (low), suggesting that it might reflect the recirculation property of some lymphocytes.[42]

The various membrane properties of the B-CLL lymphocyte, which include abnormal cap formation when stained for SmIg and incubated at 37°C,[43] help in the differential diagnosis with other B-lymphoproliferative disorders, namely B-PLL and the leukemic phase of non-Hodgkin's lymphomas.[34,43,44] The difference in SmIg density between B-CLL (low) and the other disorders (high) can now be quantitated accurately by various technics, including rapid flow microfluorimetry[45,46] (see Ch. 5 for uses of the fluorescence activated cell sorter).

Although the percentage of 'normal' T-lymphocytes in B-CLL is low as a rule, relating largely to the height of the WBC, when calculated in absolute numbers they often are increased.[47] This finding, and the possibility of assessing the T-cell subsets with relatively simple rosetting technics[30] has stimulated interest in the role played by the T-cell subsets in this disease.

Kay et al[48] and ourselves[49] have observed a significant and persistent increase in the proportion of Tγ (suppressor) lymphocytes, and, conversely, a decrease in Tμ (helper) cells in B-CLL compared with normal controls. Similarly, a helper defect in purified T-cells from CLL was suggested by functional studies.[50] Our initial observation in 13 patients[49] has now been extended to 40 patients and, in addition, we have evidence suggesting that the higher values of Tγ-lymphocytes are seen in the most advanced stages of the disease, implying that it may be a secondary phenomenon. Nevertheless, the imbalance in the T-cell subsets may be significant in relation to some of the complications commonly seen in B-CLL such as hypogammaglobulinemia and autoimmunity, as it has been documented in other diseases.[51]

Hairy-cell leukemia (HCL)

This condition, despite its relative rarity, has attracted considerable interest, firstly because of the initial conflicting reports on the origin of the hairy cell, and, secondly, because of the lack of information regarding a normal counterpart for the hairy cell within the known leukocyte populations.

Table 1.2 Evidence for the B-cell nature of hairy cells

Monoclonal SmIg with rapid cap formation [34, 54–59]

Synthesis and secretion of Ig and free light chains [56, 58–62]

Monoclonal cytoplasmic Ig in 5% of cases [57, 60]

Small paraprotein spikes in serum and/or light chain proteinuria in approx. 10% [58, 60, 63]

Rosetting with mouse RBC in 30% [34, 54]

Expression of B-lymphocyte antigens shown by anti-B and anti-HCL heteroantisera [64–66]

Presence of HLA-DR (Ia-like) alloantigens [57, 67]

HCL cell line infected with EBV [67]

It is now clear that in the majority of patients, hairy cells bear B-membrane markers. In addition, a few cases with T-cell features and, interestingly, some 'hybrids' with B- and T-cell markers simultaneously, have also been reported. [52, 53] The data demonstrating the B-cell characteristics of HCL are summarized in Table 1.2. All the recent studies showing SmIg on hairy cells have been carried out avoiding the known technical pitfalls discussed in Chapter 5, which were partly responsible for some of the earlier conflicting reports.

As shown in Table 1.3, monoclonal SmIg are readily demonstrated in over 90 per cent of cases. However, and different from most other B-lymphoproliferative disorders, there is a high proportion of cases involving IgG and IgA, often associated with other heavy chains but sharing the same light chain. [34, 56–58] As these Ig classes are associated with the late stages of the B-cell differentiation pathway, they suggest that HCL arises from a 'mature' B-cell, probably not represented in normal peripheral blood but, presumably, a resident of the spleen and/or the bone marrow.

A monocytic origin for the hairy cell, suggested because of its presumptive phagocytic potential, has been discussed elsewhere. [54, 68] The endogenous peroxidase-like activity in hairy cells shown in unfixed material at TEM, described in Chapter 3, remains to be reconciled with the above observations.

Table 1.3 Membrane immunoglobulins in hairy-cell leukemia (HCL)

Author (year)	No. of cases	IgM	IgD	M+D	IgG	G+M+D or G+D	IgA[b]	Poly-clonal	Negative
Burns et al (1978)[56]	15	–	–	1	7	5	2	–	–
Catovsky et al (1979)[34]	26	2	4	4	5	–	9	1	1
Cohen et al ((1979)[59]	6	2	–	–	2	2	–	–	–
Jansen et al (1979)[57]	15	–	–	–	4	2	7	–	2
Rieber et al (1979)[58]	8	1	–	4	2	1	–	–	–
Total (percentage)	70 (100%)	5 (7%)	4 (5.7%)	9 (12.8%)	20 (28.5%)	10 (14%)	18 (25.7%)	1 (1.4%)	3 (4%)

[a] By a rosetting method.

[b] Rarely alone; usually plus one or more heavy chains.

ACUTE LYMPHOBLASTIC LEUKEMIA (ALL)

The most important advances in the field of surface markers in leukemia have taken place in ALL. In the last five years there has been a transition from ALL as a morphological entity to a disorder, where an ever-increasing range of antigens and enzymes (Ch. 5 and 7) have revealed an important heterogeneity, both in immunological and clinical terms, and some basic concepts about its cellular origin.[21]

The clinical significance of the findings in ALL was realized early on[69,70] with the recognition of an atypical form: T-ALL, closely related to lymphoblastic lympoma,[18,23,30,71] and characterized by high WBC counts, an anterio mediastinal mass and a bad prognosis, features which were confirmed in subsequent studies.[72,73] The important discovery by Greaves[2] of the ALL antigen present in the majority of non-B, non-T blasts has helped to identify the most common form (70 per cent of cases) of ALL in childhood (see Ch. 5 for preparation of the anti-ALL serum). A number of other immunological tests, namely, E-rosettes, particularly when stable at $37°C$, SmIg,[75] anti-human thymocyte sera,[2,16] Ia-like antigens,[2] cytoplasmic IgM[76-78] and the enzyme terminal transferase (TdT) (see below and Ch. 7) define the phenotype of the cells in the early stages of lymphoid differentiation (Fig. 5.9). Forms with 'intermediate' membrane pheontypes (e.g. ALL $\pm$ anti-T $+$) are rare, but well recognized.[15,16]

The identification of several ALL subtypes, in addition to T-ALL, has proven clinically useful. Common-ALL (ALL$+$, Ia$+$, TdT$+$) includes the majority of patients with a high chance of cure.[72] About 20 to 30 per cent of common-ALLs have a pre-B phenotype (ALL$+$, Ia$+$, TdT$+$, cyt. IgM$+$)[76-78] but no special clinical features,[78] although in one series four out of six patients presented with tumors.[77]

Null-ALL (ALL $-$, Ia $+$, TdT $+$) may represent a leukemia derived from an earlier precursor cell than common-ALL. Although rare in children (8 per cent of cases) its incidence is greater (28 per cent) in adult-ALL[34] and it may be one of the reasons why adult patients fare significantly worse than children. B-ALL is also rare in children (1 to 2 per cent) but less so in adults (12 per cent) in our experience.[34] In most cases it is associated with L3 (Burkitt-type) blast-cell morphology[75] and may correspond to the leukemic presentation of the sporadic form of Burkitt's lymphoma which, outside Africa, has frequently bone marrow involvement[79] and abdominal masses.[18]

It has been argued[73] that a classification based on the presence of E-rosettes (T) or SmIg (B) or their absence (non-B, non-T) may suffice for clinical purposes. It should be pointed out that non-B, non-T ALL (the largest group) is still clinically heterogeneous and, in addition to common-ALL and its pre-B variant, will include pre-T ALL (E$-$, anti-T$+$)[2,16] which, on clinical and cytochemical grounds, is more akin to T-ALL and lymphoblastic lymphoma,[18] and true null-ALL which appears to fare worse than common-ALL.[72]

The difficulty in diagnosing relapse early enough by morphology only has led to attempts to use immunological markers to identify cells in relapse. This was successful to a limited degree in half the adult cases of ALL[80] but the tests were hampered, in the other half, for a variety of reasons. One of them was minor shifts in membrane phenotypes, now known to occur in approximately 10 per cent of childhood ALLs.[80,81] In contrast to ALL, encouraging data on the use of antisera against leukemia-associated antigens to determine early relapse in AML have recently been reported.[82] This is surprising if one considers earlier studies on myeloid-associated antigens whose expression appeared to be linked to the maturation of granulocytes and monocytes and to be shared by normal and leukemic cells.[83] However, if the studies of Baker et al[82] are confirmed and extended, the observations may have important clinical applications.

ENZYME ASSAYS

This is another field of major progress. In addition to myeloid enzymes, usually detected by cytochemical methods (Ch. 2), there are lymphoid and stem-cell enzymes.[84] The most important, terminal deoxynucleotidyl transferase, is reviewed in Chapter 7. In addition to its presence in thymic cells,[85] TdT has now been demonstrated in the nucleus of an early precursor cell in human bone marrow which has an identical membrane phenotype (TdT+, ALL+, Ia+) as the blasts in common-ALL and cases of CML in 'lymphoid' blast crisis[86] (Fig. 5.9).

Also of increasing interest are enzymes involved in the metabolic pathway of purines, chiefly 5' nucleotidase (5'N), adenosine deaminase (ADA) and purine nucleoside phosphorylase (PNP), which are found either in the external surface of the cell membrane (5'N) or the cytoplasm (ADA and PNP) of lymphoid cells. These enzymes have been found to be associated with the development of immunodeficiency in man.

TERMINAL TRANSFERASE (TdT)

The biochemical assay of TdT, detailed in Chapter 7, and, more recently, the immunofluorescence method[86,87] (Ch. 5), have facilitated the studies of large numbers of leukemia patients. Correlation between both test systems is generally good, but discrepancies, largely due to variable TdT content between cells, do exist (see Fig. 7.2).

The presence of TdT in ALL cells and in blast crisis of CML was first reported by McCaffrey et al.[88] It has subsequently been found to be extremely useful in classifying lymphoid malignancies. With the exception of B-ALL, all forms of ALL are usually positive. Some emphasis has been put on the advantages of this assay to make the distinction between ALL and AML, which is therapeutically so important. However, between 5 and 10 per cent of AML cases may have detectable or moderately raised TdT levels[34,87,89] (see Ch. 7). In our experience, some of these cases are immature forms of AML and others may constitute 'mixtures'; the latter are not uncommon in CML in blast crisis.

The finding of positive TdT levels in AML, although very rare, may have clinical implications. In a case studied by us, 10 to 20 per cent of blast cells were positive with myeloperoxidase using light and electron microscopy, compatible with AML (M1) according to the FAB criteria.[5] However, TdT was raised and 60 per cent of blasts were stained positive in the immunofluorescence test performed by Dr G. Janossy. Based on the 'conventional' diagnosis, therapy for AML was given with no response, whilst the patient later achieved a complete remission following switch to ALL-specific therapy (vincristine and prednisolone). Similarly, a better response to vincristine-prednisolone than to AML-therapy was reported in patients with TdT-positive AML.[89]

TdT estimations have been useful, too, in the diagnosis of non-Hodgkin's malignant lymphomas. A positive TdT has been found in most cases of lymphoblastic lymphoma, whether E-rosette-positive (T) or negative (pre-T),[87,89,90] whilst it is negative in most B-cell lymphomas.[90] One exception to this are two out of 14 children with Burkitt-type lymphoma (L3 morphology and monoclonal SmIg) reported by Bernard et al.[18]

Mature (post-thymic) T-lymphocytes lack TdT, as do most cases of T-CLL, T-PLL and Sézary syndrome.[34,91] It appears, too, that within children with T-lymphoblastic lymphoma, there is a more mature form which lacks TdT.[18] We have studied two children with an anterior mediastinal mass, pleural effusion and no bone marrow involvement, whose blasts were E+, TdT−, acid phosphatase+. It remains to be seen in future cases whether this constitutes a defined entity and, in particular, whether the apparent longer remission durations observed will hold.[18]

ADENOSINE DEAMINASE (ADA)

ADA activity is high in many lymphoid tissues; it is greater in thymocytes than in tonsil cells and it is 10- to 12-fold greater in T- than in B-lymphocytes.[92] It may not be surprising, therefore, that all studies performed on B-CLL have shown extremely low values.[84,92-94] It has been suggested that ADA levels in B-CLL are about half those found in normal B-lymphocytes.[92] Preliminary data on five cases of chronic T-cell leukemias (3 T-CLL; 2 T-PLL) show normal or moderately raised levels (in collaboration with Dr K. Ganeshaguru).

The early studies have also shown high ADA activity in ALL but the enzyme is also raised in AML.[93,95] The ADA activity in ALL is four times higher than in normal lymphocytes; the highest levels were observed in T-ALL rather than in non-B, non-T ALL.[96,97] This is slightly different from TdT which has the highest levels in the latter; both ADA and TdT are low in B-ALL.[97]

Perhaps more important than its value in diagnosis are observations on ADA that have opened the way to therapeutic advances. A potent inhibitor of ADA, 2'-deoxycoformycin, an antibiotic produced by fermentation from *Streptomyces antibioticus*, has been shown to be selectively lymphocytotoxic when injected in mice[98] and subhuman primates.[99] Because of the high ADA levels in ALL, particularly T-ALL (Table 1.4), the clinical implications are obvious. The results of a phase I study in man describing the pharmacology of single i.v. injections of the inhibitor have been published.[100] Selective lymphopenia and some responses in refractory ALL patients have been observed.

The antileukemic and immunosuppressive potential of this new agent is being actively investigated at the present time. Its effects appear to be potentiated when used in combination with adenosine analogs.[99]

PURINE NUCLEOSIDE PHOSPHORYLASE (PNP)

PNP can be demonstrated in the cytosol of lymphoid cells by a biochemical assay or a cytochemical technic by light microscopy and by TEM.[101] Decreased activity has been found in B-CLL,[93,101] in contrast to a single case of T-CLL with positive cells.[101] Only one study has been carried out so far in ALL and the report describes normal values (as in peripheral blood lymphocytes) in non-B, non-T ALL (14 cases), but significantly decreased in T-ALL (8 cases).[102] Whether these differences will be important in diagnosis and will allow useful chemotherapeutic intervention with specific inhibitors is not yet clear.

5′ NUCLEOTIDASE (5′N)

This enzyme was studied in immune deficiency and in CLL. As with ADA and PNP, 5′N plays a role in lymphocyte physiology. Estimations of 5′N in isolated lymphocyte populations suggest a higher activity in B-cells;[103] assays with less purified fractions failed to show differences.[104,105]

As with ADA and PNP, studies in B-CLL showed consistently low enzyme activity,[104–106] whilst normal values were found in T-CLL (Table 1.4).[105] Low

Table 1.4 Enzymes of purine metabolism in normal and leukemic cells[a]

Cells	5′N	ADA	PNP
Lymphocytes	+	+	+
B-	+/++	±	±
T-	+	+	+
B-CLL	−	−	−
T-CLL	+	+/++	+
Thymocytes	−	++	
T-ALL	−	+++	±
Non-B, Non-T ALL	+	++	+
B-ALL		±	
References	103–107	92–97	93,101,102

[a] Activity = −/± decreased; + 'normal' values; ++/+++ increased.

5′N was also found in other B-lymphoproliferative disorders.[105] It is not certain whether the low enzyme activity in the B-CLL cells is due to a fundamental abnormality in the purine metabolism, or reflects the level of these enzymes in immature B-lymphocytes, not represented in normal peripheral blood.

There are significant differences in 5′N levels between non-B, non-T ALL (activity as in normal lymphocytes) and T-ALL (tenfold lower activity).[107] The low activity in T-ALL may reflect the low 5′N activity in thymocytes[104] and it appears to follow the trend observed with PNP, but contrasting with ADA (Table 1.4).

OTHER ENZYMES

Findings with other enzyme assays which are relevant to the leukemic cell are reviewed elsewhere.[84] Of great interest are the studies with a glycosidase: N-acetyl-β-D-glucosaminidase. Quantitative estimations in whole cells have shown a higher activity in B- than in T-lymphocytes, and significantly lower values in B-CLL.[108] This parallels the decreased content of other lysosomal enzymes in B-CLL demonstrated with cytochemical methods (see Ch. 2). The pattern of isoenzyme expression, rather than differences in enzyme content, was analyzed in leukemia by Ellis et al[109] by means of ion-exchange chromatography. An abnormally high peak of an isoenzyme intermediate (Hex. I) was observed only in common-ALL and not in other forms of acute leukemia.[109] There is a good correlation between the presence or absence of Hex. I and the membrane phenotype of the blast cells. The value of this assay in the diagnosis of ALL in relation to other tests is yet to be defined. It may be useful for patient monitoring as it is not found during complete remission.[109]

CHROMOSOME ANALYSIS

New banding technics, described in Chapter 6, have improved dramatically our capacity for detecting karyotype abnormalities in leukemia. They have also allowed the discovery of associations between some chromosome anomalies and specific types of leukemia. It is generally accepted that the abnormalities observed are non-random and that they affect particular chromosomes in a similar way with either loss or gain or structural changes at specific loci.[110] The most consistent findings in human neoplasia are those observed in CML, AML, ALL and non-Hodgkin lymphomas, and will be outlined below (see Ch. 6 for full details).

THE PHILADELPHIA (Ph[1]) CHROMOSOME

In addition to its unique diagnostic value in CML, the Ph[1] chromosome has been used to monitor attempts to eradicate the disease during its chronic phase. In its acute (blastic) phase new chromosome changes occur which are markers of more malignant cell clones.

Of great theoretical interest has been the demonstration of the Ph[1] chromosome in a significant minority of adult patients with ALL.[1,34,111] In some of these cases hematologic features of CML in chronic phase are apparent at diagnosis, but in many they are not. Because of the sensitivity of the 'lymphoid' clone to anti-ALL therapy, a rapid complete remission has often been achieved followed in some by typical CML in chronic phase. This has led to the belief that CML and Ph[1]-positive ALL are part of the same spectrum of hematological abnormalities also described as Ph[1]-positive leukemia.[1]

ABNORMALITIES IN AML

Since the First International Workshop held in Helsinki,[112] it has become apparent that specific chromosome translocations (t) observed in AML relate

directly to some of the morphological types of the disease.[5] This has been defi-
nitely established in the Second International Workshop held recently in
Leuven[113] for M3 and t(15;17) and M2 and t(8;21).

There is increasing evidence that the presence or absence of chromosome
abnormalities in AML is closely linked with prognosis. As the initial remission
rates in AML are now of the order of 70 to 80 per cent using intensive chemotherapy regimens and more effective supportive care, it will be important to
re-examine this point critically and, in particular, to see whether chromosome
analysis could have predictive value in relation to the early or late relapses in
AML or to identify patients with a high probability of cure. The latter may
be of value when considering indications for more radical attempts to treat the
disease such as bone marrow transplantation.

t(15;17)
This translocation (Ch. 6) has been found only in cases of acute promyelocytic
leukemia (M3). Reports from a number of centers and the analysis of a large
series of AML cases in the First and Second Chromosome Workshops[112,113]
demonstrated that this unique translocation is found in 40 to 50 per cent of
M3 cases.

One important finding resulting in part from the discovery of this association
was the recognition of a variant form of M3 (see above), which in all published
cases has been found to be t(15;17).[115,116] As the M3 variant may present real
diagnostic difficulties when examining Romanowsky stained films only,[6] the importance of a specific chromosome aberration associated with it is even greater.
The diagnosis of the M3 variant is also facilitated by the demonstration of very
small cytoplasmic granules at TEM level, which are not readily visible at light
microscopy.[115]

t(8;21)
The morphological analysis of blood and bone marrow films of cases submitted
to the Second International Workshop[113] with this translocation has shown that
in most cases the type of AML was classified as M2, myeloblastic leukemia with
maturation.[5] This 'classical' form of AML has been linked with t(8;21) by previous authors who noted the presence of neutrophil abnormalities and Auer rods
in the myeloblasts.[117-119] The translocation (8;21) is only found in M2 leukemia
but not all M2 cases have this abnormality; its incidence has been estimated
to be around 10 per cent.[113,119]

Although chromosomal abnormalities in AML are associated with bad prognosis, t(8;21) seems to be an exception. All the studies[113,117-119] have shown a
higher response rate and longer survival in cases with t(8;21) than in AML
cases with other chromosome abnormalities, being comparable with that of cases
with a normal karyotype.[113]

MYELODYSPLASTIC SYNDROMES

These include: (1) cases of refractory sideroblastic anemia or cytopenias with
a cellular bone marrow without an increase in blasts, also described as 'preleu-

kemia'; (2) cases with an increase in blasts in the bone marrow, short of the percentages required for a diagnosis of AML (40 to 50 per cent), also described as 'smoldering' or 'oligoblastic' leukemias. The latter have been described in the FAB study[5] as refractory anemia with excess of blasts (RAEB) and, when associated with peripheral blood monocytosis, as chronic myelomonocytic leukemia (CMML). Many hematological features seen in AML, particularly M2, are often found in those patients. Some evolve to AML within short periods of time (6 months to 2 years) whilst in others the disease remains unchanged and they often die of intercurrent complications. Attempts to predict the progression to AML have been carried out by analyzing the degree of blast cell infiltration, the bone marrow karyotype and the clonal growth in agar cultures.

The Second International Chromosome Workshop addressed itself to this question and material from 244 patients was available for analysis. The preliminary information available shows that, as in AML, chromosome abnormalities are found in half the cases.[113] Twice as many (60 per cent) of the deceased patients had an abnormal karyotype compared with those with a normal karyotype (29 per cent). A previous study suggested that the incidence of overt leukemia was greater (77 per cent) in cases with chromosome abnormalities than those without (39 per cent).[100]

Although several of the abnormalities observed in the myelodysplastic syndromes are similar to AML, the incidence of some, affecting chromosomes 5($-5/5q-$) and 7($-7/7q-$), appears to be greater.[113] One of these ($5q-$) has been associated with a hematological syndrome similar to RAEB.[121,122] It would be important to determine in future studies whether AML patients presenting with $5q-$ have a documented preleukemic phase. This abnormality is also more frequent in AML secondary to anti-cancer therapy.[113]

MARKER CHROMOSOME 14q+

Since the original observation by Manolov and Manolova of a marker chromosome 14q+ in Burkitt lymphoma,[123] numerous reports have firmly established 14q+ as the most characteristic finding in lymphoid neoplasias. This abnormality could arise through different mechanisms. In Burkitt lymphoma both endemic (African) and sporadic (American and European), it results from the reciprocal translocation of the end segments of chromosomes 8 and 14, t(8;14).[124] A t(8;14) is also found in B-cell lines derived from that tumor, whether or not they carry the Epstein-Barr virus (EBV).[125] Of great interest are two reports demonstrating the 8;14 translocation in European cases presenting as B-ALL.[124,126] In these cases both the surface markers and the cell morphology were identical to those seen in African Burkitt lymphoma (Table 1.5). The Table also illustrates that, although the presenting blast cell count is often low, the prognosis is uniformly poor. Other cases of B-ALL have been described with the 14q+ chromosome, but either without demonstrating the origin of the translocation[127] or, in one, translocated from the long arm of chromosome 11.[128] A marker 14q+ was also found in cell lines derived from B-ALL.[129]

The chromosome 14q+ has been found too in non-Hodgkin's lymphomas, usually of follicular center origin.[130,131] The accumulated data suggest that the

Table 1.5 Translocation (8;14) in B-ALL

Case No.	Author	Age/sex	Morphology (5)	SmIg	Blast cell count ($\times 10^9/1$)	Survival
1	Mitelman et al[124]	62/M	L3	IgMλ	1.2	2 m
2		10/M	L3	IgMκ	4.1	5 m
3		12/M	L3	IgMλ	1.3	9 m
4	Berger et al[126]	4/M	L3	IgMκ	4.8	–
5		6/M	L3	+	2.1	–
6		76/M	L3	IgMλ	0.1	3 m

presence of this marker is strongly associated with B-cell neoplasias (Ch. 6).[124] It is not yet clear whether the origin of the translocation, which is specifically linked to Burkitt lymphoma and Burkitt-type ALL in the case of t(8;14), relates to the target cell involved, the etiology of the disease or some other mechanisms. The presence of 14q+ may be important in diagnosis if found in otherwise non-specific lymph node lesions.[132,133] Rarely, a marker 14q+ has been found in T-cell leukemia arising in patients with ataxia telangiectasia.[132]

CULTURE SYSTEMS

The most important development in this field has been the possibility of clonal growth, in semisolid culture media, of committed precursor cells of granulocytes and monocytes (CFU-C), eosinophils, megakaryocytes and erythrocytes (BFU-E). The methodology and the main findings related to leukemia are fully discussed in Chapter 8.

In recent years it has also become possible to grow in culture subpopulations of lymphoid cells. These technics are at an early stage of development and it is not yet clear whether they test the growth of early progenitors or of fully committed cells. Finally, an important aspect of culture systems has been the possibility of perpetuating the phenotypic features of leukemia and lymphoma cells by means of the establishment of permanent cell lines. As they can be repeatedly tested and used for immunization and absorption purposes they constitute a valuable research tool.

AGAR CULTURES OF CFU-C

Two clinical applications of this technic in the study of human leukemia will be commented on here.

Dysmyelopoietic syndromes

As mentioned above, these disorders include cases without an increase in bone marrow blasts which may develop AML after short periods, thus constituting a true preleukemic state. In cases which show an increase in blasts the argument remains as to whether they are already a form of leukemia (smoldering or oligo-blastic) or not (RAEB). The clonal growth *in vitro* of bone marrow CFU-C may, by comparison with findings in AML, add information to help predict a leukemic evolution.

An abnormal colony growth of CFU-C was demonstrated by Greenberg and Mara[134] in 72 per cent of patients with preleukemic states, progressive changes prior to the development of AML were detected in some. In that study a very low growth of CFU-C ($\leqslant 2$ colonies/10^5 bone marrow cells) correlated with a short survival (less than 2 years); this could not be predicted by other clinical features.

Two important studies on CFU-C agar cultures in oligoblastic and preleukemic patients were recently published by Spitzer et al[135] and Verma et al.[136] In both groups of patients, those which showed a non-leukemic pattern of growth (low colony formation, normal cluster/colony ratio and normal cell differentiation in the colonies) had a longer survival and lower incidence of progression to AML than those which showed a leukemic growth pattern (excessive number of clusters with or without colonies consisting mainly of blast cells) similar to that observed in AML.[135,156] If these findings are confirmed, it may be possible to distinguish true preleukemia from other refractory anemias. It might be of interest to see whether the growth pattern correlates with the presence of chromosome abnormalities and if both have predictive value independently.

Chronic myeloid leukemia

The number of CFU-C in the bone marrow colonies in CML is greater than normal (Ch. 8.). The characteristic finding in CML than CFU-C numbers in the peripheral blood are significantly higher than in the bone marrow[137] has been exploited by our group for the treatment of CML in blast crisis.[138] Large numbers of CFU-C and, by implication, pluripotent stem cells, are collected from the peripheral blood by repeated leukapheresis early in the chronic phase of the disease. These buffy coats are cyropreserved and used as autografts to speed the hematological recovery following intensive therapy of the blast cell phase which, in some patients, includes total body irradiation.[138] In most patients a second chronic phase was re-established and in some it was of prolonged duration.

LYMPHOID COLONIES

Assays to study the colony growth of various lymphocyte populations are being developed at the present time. Hopefully, they could be applied to the study of lymphoid malignancies in the same way as agar cultures have been employed for the study of myeloproliferative disorders.

T-cell colonies

A number of methods have been published using single or double layer[140,142] technics. The presence of a mitogen, usually phytohemagglutinin, in the system is essential. It is not clear, however, whether these are true clonal assays.

Two interesting points have emerged from our studies using Löwenberg & de Zeeuw's double layer technic.[140] Firstly, good colony formation can be obtained from bone marrow samples, of the same order as peripheral blood, despite the lower initial numbers of T-cells.[141] Secondly, studies with $T\gamma$ and

Tμ cell subsets isolated from peripheral blood T-lymphocytes have suggested that, in this assay system, Tμ cells were largely responsible for colony formation.[142] With a different culture method Claësson et al[143] have also reported that T-colonies originated from a non-Tγ (presumably Tμ) cell fraction. These findings help to interpret our observation of a reduced or absent colony growth by the T-lymphocytes of B-CLL.[144] As mentioned earlier, Tγ cells predominate in the T-cell fractions of B-CLL.[49]

Colony formation in T-CLL, in which the leukemic cells have often the surface pehnotype of Tγ cells, was also found to be reduced or absent.[34,141]

B-cell colonies

Two recent reports have described colony assays for human B-cells. One of them describes the growth of B-lymphocyte colonies from adult blood, cord blood and tonsils.[145] The other, which requires the presence of irradiated T-cells in the system, is apparently suitable for the study of normal and neoplastic B-lymphocytes.[146]

PERMANENT CELL LINES

Human hemopoietic cell lines can be characterized by their morphology, cytochemistry, culture behavior, karyotype, the presence of EBV, their isoenzyme profile and membrane phenotype. Some of these features are essential in proving the true neoplastic derivation of a particular line and can be used for their classification.

Most B-cell lymphoblastoid lines derived from normal lymphocytes and from Burkitt lymphomas[125] carry the EBV genome. Other lymphoma-derived cell lines have also B-cell membrane characteristics (Ch. 5) and, rarely, lack the EBV nuclear antigen. One such EBV-negative cell line was grown in our laboratory from the malignant ascitic fluid of a patient with follicular lymphoma in transformation.[147] As in the original material, a marker chromosome 14q+ was present in all mitoses examined.[131] Some histiocytic lymphoma-derived cell lines have also been described and, recently, the establishment of a permanent cell line from the bone marrow of a patient with malignant histiocytosis has been reported.[148]

Lymphoblastoid cell lines derived from acute leukemias are usually EBV-negative and can be defined by their membrane phenotype. Lines with the phenotype of common-ALL,[149,150] pre-B-ALL,[151] T-ALL[150,152] and B-ALL, 14q+[129] have now been established. For details of the surface markers characteristic of the various ALL-derived cell lines see Greaves and Janossy[2] and Chapter 5 (Table 5.4).

One benefit of the availability of these cell lines, is that they can be used to raise specific antisera to test leukemia cases.[153] For example, an antiserum to the T-lymphoblastoid cell line HSB-2 (absorbed with the B-cell line SB) has been useful in identifying a T-lymphocyte antigen used to diagnose T-ALL cases with negative E-rosettes.[152] Reciprocally, antibodies to line SB, absorbed with HSB-2, were used to detect the Ia-like antigen.[152]

Cells of the Reh line (common-ALL phenotype) have been used in a pro-gram of active immunotherapy.[149] Lymphoblastoid cell lines were also used to test the *in vitro* sensitivity to new cytotoxic modalities. For example, ALL-cell lines were shown to be highly sensitive to growth inhibition by the deoxy-nucleotide thymidine[154] when compared with normal B-cell lines. In contrast, the myeloid line HL-60 (see below) was equal or less sensitive to inhibition by thymidine than normal myeloid stem cells.[155]

There are a few myeloma-derived cell lines which produce light chains *in vitro* or whole immunoglobulin molecules, identical to the original tumor cells. A cell line from a patient with γ-heavy chain disease has helped to study the molecular basis of the disease.[156] An EBV-negative line from a case of T-HCL has also been well characterized. As the original cells, it produces the isoenzyme 5 of acid phosphatase and, unlike other human T-cell lines, it acts as a potent source of colony-stimulating activity.[157] An EBV-positive line from a B-HCL has also been reported.[68]

Myeloid cell lines are less easy to establish than lymphoid ones, and are, therefore, less common. The first and better known, K562, was reported by Lozzio and Lozzio,[158] and originated from a case of Ph^1-positive CML in blast transformation. Although initially regarded as being constituted by granulocytic precursors, it has recently been shown to have erythroid features. Cells of this line have now been shown to express on their surface a unique RBC sialoglycoprotein: glycophorin[159] present in erythroid precursors and mature RBC in man. Red cell differentiation can be further achieved with appropriate inducers, e.g. sodium butyrate.[160] Studies with antibodies to glycophorin have now been extended to the study of undifferentiated leukemias in order to identify cases with early erythroid differentiation.[161]

A myeloid line, HL-60, derived from a case of acute promyelocytic leukemia has also been well characterized.[162] Blast cells of this line can be induced to differentiate by low mol.wt. compounds, e.g. dimethyl sulfoxide, to granulocytes with phagocytic properties and responsive to chemotactic stimuli.[162] Two other cell lines derived from patients with AML have been reported.[163,164]

Suitable culture manipulations in cell lines have also been valuable in blurring the sometimes rigid distinctions between lymphoid and myeloid features. This was shown, for example, with some EBV-positive human B-lymphoblastoid cell lines which, following exposure to butyric acid, can express 'myeloid' enzymes, namely alkaline phosphatase, naphthol AS-D chloracetate esterase and lysozyme.[165] There is no doubt that new and exciting findings will be forthcoming with the present battery of well characterized cell lines and that new lines representing less well known stages of hemopoietic cell differentiation will evolve and increase our potential for manipulating the leukemic cell *in vitro*.

GLUCOCORTICOID RECEPTORS

Specific intracellular receptor sites for glucocorticoids are essential for a response to these hormones. The rationale for measuring these receptors and full details of the various assay systems are given in Chapter 9.

Early studies have been geared to leukemias known to respond to prednisolone: ALL and CLL,[166,167] and have shown that the presence of receptors correlates well with the sensitivity *in vitro* and *in vivo* to these agents. In ALL, the number of receptors is high in non-B, non-T ALL and low in T-ALL, and this correlates with remission duration.[166] Findings in cases with intermediate levels suggests that the number of receptors may have clinical significance independently of cell type, WBC and age.[166]

Results of further studies, in particular in non-Hodgkin's lymphoma's and CML in blast transformation are awaited with interest as they may have important implications for the treatment of these patients.

CELL KINETICS

The conventional technics for the study of cell kinetics are autoradiography, to assess the incorporation of tritiated thymidine (3HT) during DNA synthesis, and the enumeration of mitotic figures, which determine respectively the labeling (LI) and mitotic (M) indices.[168,169]

Cells in the G_0 and G_1 phases of the cell cycle have diploid (2N) DNA content, cells in G_2 and M have tetraploid (4N) DNA content and S phase cells have intermediate values. It is now possible to measure the DNA content of individual cells using fluorescent dyes such as acridine orange, ethidium bromide and propidium iodide. The development in recent years of pulse cytophotometers permits the analysis of these cells in suspension at high flow rates across a laser beam. The new instruments, such as the fluorescence activated cell sorter (see Ch. 5) or the cytofluorograph, can examine large numbers of cells in a very short time. This contrasts with the long periods necessary for the development of autoradiographs. Thus, when treatment depends on kinetic data, the speed in obtaining the result is an important practical consideration.

An original method, combining Coulter volume and DNA content by flow cytometry, has recently been proposed for the dynamic analysis of mixed cell populations in human lymphomas.[170] With that approach, paired cell-by-cell measurements can be used to help in distinguishing large aneuploid tumor cells, often with greater proliferative activity, from smaller diploid cells which are usually non-proliferating.[170]

Information from animal models suggested that chemotherapy was more effective in rapidly proliferating tumours. It was soon realized, however, that human leukemia differs from animal models in that the cells are not in rapid and uncontrolled proliferation and that a large percentage of them may not be in cycle. Leukemic cells, in fact, divide more slowly than their normal counterparts, and their population expands by accumulation and lack of differentiation.[168,169] Because of this they are not all susceptible to phase-specific drugs such as cytosine arabinoside and 6-thioguanine. This led to attempts to synchronize cells into the cell cycle in order to make them more susceptible to such agents. Results of efforts in this direction have not been uniformly rewarding.

Autoradiographic studies in acute leukemia indicated that the morphological heterogeneity observed within the same case was directly related to cells being in different phases of the cell cycle. Large blasts with fine chromatin were proliferating whilst smaller cells with more condensed chromatin were in a resting stage. There is no information in ALL about possible kinetic differences between the morphological types L1 and L2, proposed in the FAB classification.[5] On the other hand, it has been shown that the L3 (Burkitt) type has the greatest proliferative activity within ALL[171] and this is usually apparent from the examination of the bone marrow.[5]

Cell kinetic studies in ALL and non-Hodgkin's lymphoma in childhood have recently been reviewed.[169, 171] Murphy et al[171] demonstrated a significantly higher LI (mean: 42 per cent of bone marrow blasts) in non-Hodgkin's lymphoma, the majority being of B-cell type, than in common-ALL (mean: 4.8 per cent). The LI in T-ALL had intermediate values (mean: 11.6 per cent). They concluded that the cell surface phenotype was the main factor determining the growth fraction of those lymphoid tumors and that the kinetic data had prognostic implications. B-cell lymphomas are highly sensitive to initial chemotherapy, but they relapse early and have the shortest survival. In contrast, common-ALL has the lowest LI and longest survival; T-ALL has intermediate prognosis and intermediate LI values.[171] Because of these close correlations it will be important to establish in the near future whether the kinetic characteristics of the leukemia have independent prognostic value.[171] This could be possible by analysis of the kinetic data within a group with similar membrane phenotype, e.g. common-ALL. One such study could look for differences between childhood and adult ALL, known to differ significantly in prognosis, particularly as the typically smaller cell, L1[5] predominates in children and the large one, L2, is more frequent in adults.

Cell kinetics studies in AML have not shown a consistent relationship between increase in LI and response to therapy and prognosis. More information is obviously needed in AML as new chemotherapeutic agents become available and as the higher standard of supportive care permits the better identification of non-responsive cases by decreasing the proportion of deaths from intercurrent causes.

CONCLUSIONS

This overview has aimed at stressing the growing areas regarding cell characterization and improved diagnosis in human leukemia. The remaining chapters will give all the specific detailed information necessary for most of the new technical developments to be applied extensively to patient management. Progress in this field has resulted always from the balanced combination of laboratory and clinical research. This approach should be the key to good hematology practice today, and has inspired the preparation of this volume throughout.

REFERENCES

1 Catovsky D 1979 Ph¹-positive acute leukaemia and chronic granulocytic leukaemia: one or two diseases? British Journal of Haematology 42: 493–498
2 Greaves M F, Janossy G 1978 Patterns of gene expression and the cellular origins of human leukaemias. Biochimica et Biophysica Acta 56: 193–230
3 Greaves M F, Verbi W, Reeves B R, Hoffbrand A V, Drysdale H C, Jones L, Sacker L S, Samaratunga I 1979 'Pre-B' phenotypes in blast crisis of Ph¹-positive CML: evidence for a pluripotential stem cell 'target'. Leukaemia Research 3: 181–191

4 Vogler L B, Crist W M, Vinson P C, Sarrif A, Brattain M G, Coleman M S 1979 Philadelphia-chromosome-positive pre-B-cell leukemia presenting as blast crisis of chronic myelogenous leukemia. Blood 54: 1164–1170

5 Bennett J M, Catovsky D, Daniel M T, Flandrin G, Galton D A G, Gralnick H R, Sultan C (1976) Proposals for the classification of the acute leukaemias. (FAB Co-operative Group). British Journal of Haematology 33: 451–458

6 Bennet J M, Catovsky D, Daniel M T, Flandrin G, Galton D A G, Gralnick H R, Sultan C 1980 A variant form of hypergranular promyelocytic leukaemia (M3). British Journal of Haematology 44: 169–170

7 Costello C, Catovsky D, O'Brien M, Galton D A G 1980 Prolymphocytic leukaemia. British Journal of Haematology 44: 389–394

8 Costello C, Wardle J, Catovsky D, Lewis S M 1980 Cell volume studies in B-cell leukaemia. British Journal of Haematology 45: 209–214

9 Hayhoe F G J, Quaglino D, Doll R 1964 The cytology and cytochemistry of acute leukaemias. Her Majesty's Stationery Office, London

10 Schmalzl F, Braunsteiner H 1971 The application of cytochemical methods to the study of acute leukemia. Acta Haematologica 45: 209–217

11 Marie J P, Vernant J P, Dreyfus B, Breton-Gorius J 1979 Ultrastructural localization of peroxidases in 'undifferentiated' blasts during the blast crisis of chronic granulocytic leukaemia. British Journal of Haematology 43: 549–558

12 O'Brien M, Catovsky D, Costello C 1980 Ultrastructural cytochemistry of leukaemic cells: characterization of the early small granules of monoblasts. British Journal of Haematology 45: 201–208

13 Catovsky D, Costello C 1980 Cytochemistry of normal and leukaemic lymphocytes: a review. Basic and Applied Histochemistry, 23: 255–270

14 Stein H, Müller-Hermelink, H K 1977 Simultaneous presence of receptors for complement and sheep red blood cells on human fetal thymocytes. British Journal of Haematology 36: 225–230

15 Catovsky D, Cherchi M, Greaves M F, Pain C, Janossy G, Kay H E M 1978 The acid phosphatase reaction in acute lymphoblastic leukaemia. Lancet i: 749–751

16 Thiel E, Rodt H, Netzel B, Huhn D, Hoffbrand A V, Thierfelder S 1979 Characterization of seven subgroups of acute lymphoblastic leukemia (ALL) in 200 patients by multimarker analysis. Fifth Meeting of the International Society of Hematology, European and African Division, Abstracts II, Hamburg, p 33

17 McKenna R W, Brynes R K, Nesbit M E, Bloomfield C D, Kersey J H, Spanjers E, Brunning R D 1979 Cytochemical profiles in acute lymphoblastic leukemia. Blood 54 (suppl 1): 197a

18 Bernard A, Boumsell L, Bayle C, Richard Y, Coppin H, Penit C, Rouget P, Micheau C, Clausse B, Gerard-Marchant R, Dausset J, Lemerle J 1979 Subsets of malignant lymphomas in children related to the cell phenotype. Blood 54: 1058–1068

19 Grossi C E, Webb S R, Zicca A, Lydyard P M, Moretta L, Mingari M C, Cooper M D 1978 Morphological and histochemical analysis of two human T-cell subpopulations bearing receptors for IgM or IgG. Journal of Experimental Medicine 147: 1405–1417

20 Sternberger L A 1979 Immunocytochemistry, 2nd edn. Wiley, New York, Ch 5, p 104–169

21 Hoffmann-Fezer G, Thierfelder S, Pielsticker K, Rodt H 1979 Immunohistochemical demonstration of cell surface antigens on tissue sections of lymphomas. Leukemia Research 3: 297–304

22 Seligmann M, Knapp W 1978 Workshop report on Immunohaematology. In: Knapp W, Holubar K, Wick G (eds) Immunofluorescence and Related Staining Techniques. Elsevier, Amsterdam, p 277–291

23 Lennert K 1978 Malignant Lymphomas other than Hodgkin's Disease. Springer-Verlag, Berlin

24 Islam A, Catovsky D, Goldman J M, Galton D A G 1979 Value of long-core biopsy in detection of discrete bone-marrow lesions. Lancet i: 878

25 Islam A, Catovsky D, Galton D A G 1980 Histological study of bone marrow regeneration following chemotherapy for acute myeloid leukaemia and chronic granulocytic leukaemia in blast transformation. British Journal of Haematology 45: 535–540

26 Goldman J M, Johnson S A, Islam A, Catovsky D, Galton D A G 1980 Haematological reconstitution after autografting for chronic granulocytic leukaemia in transformation: the influence of previous splenectomy. British Journal of Haematology 45:

27 Ross G D 1979 Identification of human lymphocyte subpopulations by surface marker analysis. Blood 53: 799–811

28 Haegert D G, Coombs R R A 1979 Do human B and null lymphocytes form a single immunoglobulin-bearing population? Lancet ii: 1051–1053

29 Catovsky D, Cherchi M, Galton D A G, Hoffbrand A V, Ganeshaguru K 1978 Cell differentiation in B- and T-lymphoproliferative disorders. In: Clarkson B, Marks P A, Till J (eds) Cold Spring Harbor Conferences on Cell Proliferation. Cold Spring Harbor, New York, vol 5, p 811–822

30 Lukes R J, Collins R D 1974 Immunologic characterization of human malignant lymphomas. Cancer 34: 1488–1503

31 Ross G D, Winchester R J, Rabellino E M, Hoffman T 1978 Surface markers of complement receptor lymphocytes. Journal of Clinical Investigation 62: 1086–1092

32 Shevach E, Edelson R, Frank M, Lutzner M, Green I 1974 A human leukemia with both B and T cell surface receptors. Proceedings of the National Academy of Sciences (USA) 71: 863–866

33 Toben H R, Smith R G 1977 T lymphocytes bearing complement receptors in a patient with chronic lymphocytic leukaemia. Clinical and Experimental Immunology 27: 292–302

34 Catovsky D, Pittman S, O'Brien M, Cherchi M, Costello C, Foa R, Pearse E, Hoffbrand A V, Janossy G, Ganeshaguru K, Greaves M F 1979 Multiparameter studies in lymphoid leukemias. American Journal of Clinical Pathology 72: 736–745

35 Fu S M, Chiorazzi N, Wang C Y, Montazeri G, Kunkel H G, Ko H S, Gottlieb A B 1978 Ia-bearing T lymphocytes in man. Journal of Experimental Medicine 148: 1423–1428

36 Samarut C, Gebuhrer L, Brochier J, Betnel H, Revillard J-P 1977 Presence of 'Ia-like' antigens on human T lymphocytes bearing receptors for IgG. European Journal of Immunology 7: 908–910

37 Greaves M F, Verbi W, Festenstein H, Papasteriadis C, Jaraquemada D, Hayward A 1979 'Ia-like' antigens on human T cells. European Journal of Immunology 9: 356–362

38 Moretta L, Webb S R, Grossi C E, Lydyard P M, Cooper M D 1977 Functional analysis of two human T cell subpopulations: Help and suppression of B cell response by T cells bearing receptors for IgM (Tμ) or IgG (Tγ). Journal of Experimental Medicine 146: 184–200

39 Hoffman R, Kopel S, Hsu S D, Dainiak N, Zanjani E D 1978 T cell chronic lymphocytic leukemia: Presence in bone marrow and peripheral blood of cells that suppress erythropoiesis in vitro. Blood 52: 255–260

40 Evans R L, Lazarus H, Penta A C, Schlossman S F 1978 Two functionally distinct subpopulations of human T cells that collaborate in the generation of cytotoxic cells responsible for cell mediated lympholysis. Journal of Immunology 120: 1423–1428

41 Reinherz E L, Nadler L M, Rosenthal D S, Moloney W C, Schlossman S F 1979 T-cell-subset characterization of human T-CLL. Blood 53: 1066–1075

42 Cherchi M, Catovsky D 1980 Mouse RBC rosettes in chronic lymphocytic leukaemia: different expression in blood and tissues. Clinical and Experimental Immunology 38: 411–415

43 Cohen H J 1978 B-cell lymphosarcoma cell leukemia: dynamics of surface membrane immunoglobulin. Annals of Internal Medicine 88: 317–322

44 Aisenberg A C, Wilkes B 1976 Lymphosarcoma cell leukemia: The contribution of cell surface study to diagnosis. Blood 48: 707–715

45 Dighiero G, Follezou J Y, Roisin J P, Ternynck T, Binet J L 1976 Comparison of normal and chronic lymphocytic leukemia lymphocyte surface IG determinants using peroxidase-labelled antibodies. II. Blood 48: 559–566

46 Slease R B, Wistar R Jr, Scher I 1979 Surface immunoglobulin density on human peripheral blood mononuclear cells. Blood 54: 72–87

47 Foa R, Catovsky D, Brozovic M, Marsh G, Ooyirilangkumaran T, Cherchi M, Galton D A G 1979 Clinical staging and immunological findings in chronic lymphocytic leukemia. Cancer 44: 483–487

48 Kay N E, Johnson J D, Stanek R, Douglas S D 1979 T-cell subpopulations in chronic lymphocytic leukemia: abnormalities in distribution and in in vitro receptor maturation. Blood 54: 540–544

49 Lauria F, Foa R, Catovsky D 1980 Increase in Tγ lymphocytes in B-cell chronic lymphocytic leukaemia. Scandinavian Journal of Haematology 24: 187–190

50 Chiorazzi N, Fu S M, Ghodrat M, Kunkel H G, Rai K, Gee T 1979 T cell helper defect in patients with chronic lymphocytic leukemia. Journal of Immunology 122: 1087–1090

51 Waldmann T A, Blaese R M, Broder S, Krakauer R S 1978 Disorders of suppressor immunoregulatory cells in the pathogenesis of immunodeficiency and antoimmunity. Annals of Internal Medicine 88: 226–238

52 Cawley J C, Burns G F, Nash T A, Higgy K E, Child J A, Roberts B E 1978 Hairy-cell leukemia with T-cell features. Blood 51: 61–69

53 Jansen J, Schuit H R E, Schreuder G M Th, Muller H P, Meijer C J L M 1979 Distinct subtype within the spectrum of hairy cell leukemia. Blood 54: 459–467

54 Catovsky D 1977 Hairy-cell leukaemia and prolymphocytic leukaemia. Clinics in Haematology 6: 245–268

55 Zidar B L, Winkelstein A, Whiteside T L, Shadduck R K, Zeigler Z, Smith W I, Rabin B S, Krause J R, Lee R E 1977 Hairy cell leukaemia: seven cases with probable B-lymphocytic origin. British Journal of Haematology 37: 455–465

56 Burns G F, Cawley J C, Worman C P, Karpas A, Barker C R, Goldstone A H, Hayhoe F G J 1978 Multiple heavy chain isotypes on the surface of the cells of hairy cell leukemia. Blood 52: 1132–1147

57 Jansen J, Schuit H R E, van Zwet Th L, Meijer C J L M, Hijmans W 1979 Hairy-cell leukaemia: a B-lymphocytic disorder. British Journal of Haematology 42: 21–33

58 Rieber E P, Hadam M R, Linke R P, Saal J G, Riethmuller G, Von Heyden H W, Waller H D 1979 Hairy cell leukaemia: surface markers and functional capacities of the leukaemic cells analysed in eight patients. British Journal of Haematology 42: 175–197

59 Cohen H J, George E R, Kremer W B 1979 Hairy cell leukemia: cellular characteristics including surface immunoglobulin dynamics and biosynthesis. Blood 53: 764–775

60 Golde D W, Stevens R H, Quan S G, Saxon A 1977 Immunoglobulin synthesis in hairy cell leukaemia. British Journal of Haematology 35: 359–365

61 Utsinger P D, Yount W J, Fuller C R, Logue M J, Orringer E P 1977 Hairy cell leukemia: B-lymphocyte and phagocytic properties. Blood 49: 19–27

62 Gordon J, Smith J L 1978 Free immunoglobulin light chain synthesis by neoplastic cells in leukaemic reticuloendotheliosis. Clinical and Experimental Immunology 31: 244–250

63 Yoon J M 1979 Light chain proteinuria in non-plasma cell neoplasmas. Blood 54 (suppl. 1): 216a

64 Kitani T 1977 Characterization of an anti-hairy cell serum. In: Seno S, Takaku F, Irino S (eds) Topics in Haematology. Excerpta Medica, Amsterdam, p 882–884

65 Stuart A E, Dewar A E 1979 Properties of anti-hairy cell serum. British Journal of Haematology 41: 163–168

66 Espinouse D, Touraine J L, Schmitt D, Revol L 1980 Specific anti-hairy cell and anti-B-cell antisera: characterization of surface antigens and origin of hairy cells. Clinical and Experimental Immunology 39: 756–767

67 Lemon S M, Pagano J S, Utsinger P D, Sinkovics J G 1979 Cultured 'hairy cells' infected with Epstein-Barr virus: evidence for B-lymphocyte origin. Annals of Internal Medicine 90: 54–55

68 Jansen J, Meijer C J L M, Van der Valk P, Bruyn W C, Leijh P C J, Ottolander G J, Van Furth R 1979 Phagocytic potential of hairy cells. Scandinavian Journal of Haematology 23: 69–79

69 Catovsky D, Goldman J M, Okos A, Frisch B, Galton D A G 1974 T-lymphoblastic leukaemia: a distinct variant of acute leukaemia. British Medical Journal 2: 643–646

70 Sen L, Borella L 1975 Clinical importance of lymphoblasts with T markers in childhood acute leukemia. New England Journal of Medicine 292: 828–832

71 Jaffe E S, Berard C W 1978 Lymphoblastic lymphoma, a term rekindled with new precision. Annals of Internal Medicine 89: 415–417

72 Chessells J M, Hardisty R M, Rapson N T, Greaves M F 1977 Acute lymphoblastic leukaemia in children: classification and prognosis. Lancet ii: 1307–1309

73 Kumar S, Carr T F, Evans D I K, Morris-Jones P, Hann I M 1979 Prognostic significance of cell surface markers in childhood acute lymphoblastic leukaemia. Clinical and Laboratory Haematology 1: 121–128

74 Borella L, Sen L 1975 E-receptors on blasts from untreated acute lymphocytic leukemia: comparison of temperature dependence of E rosettes formed by normal and leukemic lymphoid cells. Journal of Immunology 114: 187–190

75 Flandrin G, Brouet J C, Daniel M T, Preud'homme J L 1975 Acute leukemia with Burkitt's tumor cells: a study of six cases with special reference to lymphocyte surface markers. Blood 45: 183–188

76 Vogler L B, Crist W M, Lawton A R, Bockman D E, Pearl E R, Cooper M D 1978 Pre-B-cell leukemia. New England Journal of Medicine 298: 872–878

77 Brouet J C, Preud'homme J L, Penit C, Valensi F, Rouget P, Seligmann M 1979 Acute lymphoblastic leukemia with pre-B-cell characteristics. Blood 54: 269–273

78 Crist W M, Vogler L B, Sarrif A, Pullen J, Bartolucci Falleta J, Humphrey B, Van Eys J,

Cooper M 1979 Clinical and laboratory characterization of pre-B cell leukemia in children. Blood 54: 183a

79 Levine P H, Cho B R, Connelly R R, Berard C W, O'Conor G T, Dorfman R F, Easton J M, De Vita V T 1975 The American Burkitt Lymphoma Registry: A progress report. Annals of Internal Medicine 83: 31–36

80 Greaves M F, Paxton A, Janossy G, Pain C, Johnson S, Bell R, Lister T A 1980 Acute lymphoblastic leukaemia associated antigen. III. Alterations in expression during treatment and in relapse. Leukaemia Research 4: 1–14

81 Borella L, Casper J T, Lauer S J 1979 Shifts in expression of cell membrane phenotypes in childhood lymphoid malignancies at relapse. Blood 54: 64–71

82 Baker M A, Falk J A, Carter W H, Taub R N, The Toronto Leukaemia Study Group 1979 Early diagnosis of relapse in acute myeloblastic leukemia. Serologic detection of leukemia-associated antigens in human marrow. New England Journal of Medicine 301: 1353–1357

83 Roberts Marion M, Greaves M G 1978 Maturation linked expression of a myeloid cell surface antigen. British Journal of Haematology 38: 439–452

84 Catovsky D 1980 Leucocyte enzymes in leukaemia. In: Roath S (ed) Topical Reviews in Haematology. J. Wright & Sons Ltd, Medical Publishers, Bristol, vol 1, p 157–185

85 Chang L M S 1971 Development of terminal deoxynucleotidyl transferase activity in embryonic calf thymus gland. Biochemical and Biophysical Research Communications 44: 124–131

86 Janossy G, Bollum F J, Bradstock K F, McMichael A, Rapson N, Greaves M F 1979 Terminal transferase-positive human bone marrow cells exhibit the antigenic phenotype of common acute lymphoblastic leukemia. Journal of Immunology 123: 1521–1529

87 Kung P C, Long J C, McCaffrey R P, Ratcliff R L, Harrison T A, Baltimore D 1978 Terminal deoxynucleotidyl transferase in the diagnosis of leukemia and malignant lymphoma. American Journal of Medicine 64: 788–794

88 McCaffrey R, Harrison T A, Parkman R, Baltimore D 1975 Terminal deoxynucleotidyl transferase activity in human leukemic cells and in normal thymocytes. New England Journal of Medicine 292: 775–780

89 Mertelsmann R, Koziner B, Filippa D A, Moore M A S, Beck J D, Clarkson B D 1979 Prognostic significance of terminal deoxynucleotidyl transferase activities (TdT) in human leukemias and lymphomas. Fifth Meeting of the International Society of Hematology – European and African Division – Abstracts II, p 26, Hamburg

90 Habeshaw J A, Catley P F, Stansfield A G, Ganeshaguru K, Hoffbrand A V 1979 Terminal deoxynucleotidyl transferase activity in lymphoma. British Journal of Cancer 39: 566–569

91 Penit C, Brouet J-C, Rouget P 1977 Terminal deoxynucleotidyl transferase in acute lymphoblastic leukemias and chronic T-cell proliferations. Leukemia Research 1: 345–350

92 Huang A T, Logue G L, Engelbrecht H L 1976 Two biochemical markers in lymphocyte subpopulations. British Journal of Haematology 34: 631–638

93 Scholar E M, Calabresi P 1973 Identification of the enzymatic pathways of nucleotide metabolism in human lymphocytes and leukemia cells. Cancer Research 33: 94–103

94 Ludwig H, Kuzmits R, Pietschmann H, Müller M M 1979 Enzymes of the purine interconversion system in chronic lymphatic leukemia: decreased purine nucleoside phosphorylase and adenosine deaminase activity. Blut 39: 309–315

95 Smyth J F, Harrap K R 1975 Adenosine deaminase activity in leukaemia. British Journal of Cancer 31: 544–549

96 Smyth J F, Poplack D G, Holiman B J, Leventhal B G, Yabro G 1978 Correlation of adenosine deaminase activity with cell surface markers in acute lymphoblastic leukemia. Journal of Clinical Investigation 62: 710–712

97 Coleman M S, Greenwood M G, Hutton J J, Holland P, Lampkin B, Krill C, Kastelic J E 1978 Adenosine deaminase, terminal deoxynucleotidyl transferase (TdT) and cell surface markers in childhood acute leukemia. Blood 52: 1125–1131

98 Smyth J F, Young R C, Young D M 1978 In vivo toxicity to lymphoid tissue by 2'-deoxycoformycin. Cancer Chemotherapy and Pharmacology 1: 49–51

99 Rogler-Brown T, Cummings F J, Parks Jr R E, Calabresi P 1979 Hematologic effects of deoxycoformycin alone or in combination with adenosine analogs in rhesus monkeys. Blood 54 (suppl 1): 91a

100 Smyth J F, Chassin M M, Paine R M, Jackman A L, Harrap K R, Adamson R H, Johns D G 1980 The clinical pharmacology of the adenosine deaminase inhibitor 2'-deoxycoformycin Journal of Clinical Investigation

101 Borgers M, Verhaegen H, De Brabander M, De Cree J, De Cock W, Thoné F, Geuens G

1978 Purine nucleoside phosphorylase in chronic lymphocytic leukemia (CLL). Blood 52: 886–895

102 Blatt J, Reaman G H, Levin N, Poplack D G 1979 Nucleoside phosphorylase as a marker in human T cell acute lymphoblastic leukemia. Blood 54 (suppl 1): 180a

103 Rowe M, De Gast C G, Platts-Mills T A E, Asherson G L, Webster A D, Johnson S M 1979 5'-Nucleotidase of B and T lymphocytes isolated from human peripheral blood. Clinical and Experimental Immunology 36: 97–101

104 Quagliata F, Faig D, Conklyn M, Silber R 1974 Studies on the lymphocyte 5'-Nucleotidase in chronic lymphocytic leukemia, infectious mononucleosis, normal subpopulations and phytohemagglutinin-stimulated cells. Cancer Research 34: 3197–3202

105 Kramers M T C, Catovsky D, Foa R, Cherchi M, Galton D A G 1976 5' Nucleotidase activity in leukaemic lymphocytes. Biomedicine 25: 362–365

106 Silber R, Conklyn M, Grusky G, Zucker-Franklin D 1975 Human lymphocytes: 5'-Nucleotidase-positive and -negative subpopulations. Journal of Clinical Investigation 56: 1324–1327

107 Reaman G H, Levin N, Muchmore A, Holiman B J, Poplack D G 1979 Diminished lymphoblast 5'nucleotidase activity in acute lymphoblastic leukemia with T-cell characteristics. New England Journal of Medicine 300: 1374–1377

108 Crockard A D, Lewis M H R, Bridges J M 1979 N-acetyl-β-D-glucosaminidase activity in normal and chronic lymphocytic leukaemic lymphocytes. Clinica Chimica Acta 93: 151–156

109 Ellis R B, Rapson N T, Patrick A D, Greaves M F 1978 Expression of hexosaminidase isoenzymes in childhood leukemia. New England Journal of Medicine 298: 476–480

110 Mitelman F, Levan G 1978 Clustering of aberrations to specific chromosomes in human neoplasms III. Hereditas 89: 207–237

111 Bloomfield C D, Lindquist L L, Brunning R D, Yunis J J, Coccia P F 1978 The Philadelphia chromosome in acute leukemia. Virchows Archives B 29: 81–91

112 First International Workshop on Chromosomes in Leukaemia 1978 Chromosomes in acute non-lymphocytic leukaemia. British Journal of Haematology 39: 311–316

113 Rowley J 1980 General report of the Second International Workshop on Chromosomes in Leukaemia. Cancer Genetics and Cytogenetics (in press)

114 Golomb H M, Vardiman J W, Rowley J D, Testa J R, Mintz U 1978 Correlation of clinical findings with quinacrine-banded chromosomes in 90 adults with acute non-lymphocytic leukemia. New England Journal of Medicine 299: 613–619

115 Golomb H M, Testa J R, Vardiman J W, Butler A E, Rowley J D 1979 Cytogenetic and ultrastructural features of de novo acute promyelocytic leukemia. The University of Chicago experience (1973–1978). Cancer Genetics and Cytogenetics 1: 69–78

116 Berger R, Bernheim A, Daniel M T, Valensi F, Flandrin G, Bernard J 1979 Translocation t(15;17), leucemie aiguë promyelocytaire et non promyélocytaire. Nouvelle Revue Francaise d'Hematologie 21: 117–131

117 Sakurai M, Sandberg A A 1976 Chromosomes and causation of human cancer and leukemia. XI. Cancer 37: 285–299

118 Kamada N, Okada K, Oguma N, Tanaka R, Mikami M, Uchino H 1976 C-G translocation in acute myelocytic leukemia with low neutrophil alkaline phosphatase activity. Cancer 37: 2380–2387

119 Trujillo J M, Cork A, Ahearn M J, Youness E L, McCredie K B 1979 Hematologic and cytologic characterization of 8/21 translocation acute granulocytic leukemia. Blood 53: 695–706

120 Nowell P, Finan J 1978 Chromosome studies in preleukemic states. IV. Myeloproliferative versus cytopenic disorders. Cancer 42: 2254–2261

121 Sokal G, Michaux J L, Van Den Berghe H, Cordier A, Rodhain J, Ferrant A, Moriau M, De Bruyere M, Sonnet J 1975 A new hematologic syndrome with a distinct karyotype: the 5q- chromosome. Blood 46: 519–533

122 Kaffe S, Hsu L Y F, Hoffman R, Hirschhorn K 1978 Association of 5q- and refractory anemia. American Journal of Hematology 4: 269–272

123 Manolov G, Manolova Y 1972 Marker band in one chromosome 14 from Burkitt lymphomas. Nature 237: 33–34

124 Mitelman F, Andersson-Anvret M, Brandt L, Catovsky D, Klein G, Manolov G, Manolova Y, Mark-Vendel E, Nilsson P G 1979 Reciprocal 8;14 translocation in EBV-negative B-cell acute lymphocytic leukemia with Burkitt-type cells. International Journal of Cancer 24: 27–33

125 McCaw B K, Epstein A L, Kaplan H S, Hecht F. 1977 Chromosome 14 translocation in

African and North American Burkitt's lymphoma. International Journal of Cancer 19: 482–486

126 Berger R, Bernheim A, Brouet J C, Daniel M T, Flandrin G 1979 t(8;14) translocation in a Burkitt's type of lymphoblastic leukaemia (L3). British Journal of Haematology 43: 87–90

127 Slater R M, Philip P, Badsberg E, Behrendt H, Hansen N E, van Heerde P 1979 A 14q+ chromosome in a B-cell acute lymphocytic leukemia and in a leukemic non-endemic Burkitt lymphoma. International Journal of Cancer 23: 639–647

128 Roth D G, Cimino M C, Variakojis D, Golomb H M, Rowley J D 1979 B cell acute lymphoblastic leukemia (ALL) with a 14q+ chromosome abnormality. Blood 53: 235–243

129 Minowada J, Oshimura M, Tsubota T, Higby D J, Sandberg A A 1977 Cytogenetic and immunoglobulin markers of human leukemic B-cell lines. Cancer Research 37: 3096–3099

130 Fukuhara S 1978 Significance of 14q translocations in non-Hodgkin lymphomas. Virchows Archives of B Cell Pathology 29: 99–106

131 Catovsky D, Pittman S, Lewis D, Pearse E 1977 Marker chromosome 14q+ in follicular lymphoma in transformation. The Lancet ii: 934

132 Pierre R V 1978 Cytogenetics in malignant lymphoma. Virchows Archives B 29: 107–112

133 Mitelman F, Klein G, Andersson-Anvret M, Forsby N, Johansson B 1979 14q+ marker chromosome in an EBV-genome-negative lymph node without signs of malignancy in a patient with EBV-genome-positive nasopharyngeal carcinoma. International Journal of Cancer 23: 32–36

134 Greenberg P L, Mara B 1979 The preleukemic syndrome. Correlation of in vitro parameters of granulopoiesis with clinical features. American Journal of Medicine 66: 951–958

135 Spitzer G, Verma D S, Dicke KA, Smith T, McCredie K B 1979 Subgroups of oligoleukemia as identified by in vitro agar culture. Leukemia Research 3: 29–39

136 Verma D S, Spitzer G, Dicke K A, McCredie K B 1979 In vitro agar culture patterns in preleukemia and their clinical significance. Leukemia Research 3: 41–49

137 Goldman J M, Th'ng K H, Lowenthal R M 1974 In vitro colony-forming cells and colony stimulating activity in chronic granulocytic leukaemia. British Journal of Cancer 30: 1–12

138 Goldman J M, Catovsky D, Hows J, Spiers A S D, Galton D A G 1979 Cryopreserved peripheral blood cells functioning as autografts in patients with chronic granulocytic leukaemia in transformation. British Medical Journal 1: 1310–1313

139 Claësson M H, Rodger M B, Johnson G R, Whittingham S, Metcalf D 1977 Colony formation by human T-lymphocytes in agar medium. Clinical and Experimental Immunology 28: 526–534

140 Löwenberg B, de Zeeuw H M C 1979 A method for cloning T-lymphocytic precursors in agar. American Journal of Hematology 6: 35–43

141 Foa R, Catovsky D 1979 T-lymphocyte colonies in normal blood, bone marrow and lymphoproliferative disorders. Clinical and Experimental Immunology 36: 488–495

142 Foa R, Lauria F, Catovsky D 1980 Evidence that T-colony formation is a property of $T\mu$ (helper) lymphocytes. Clinical and Experimental Immunology 42: 152–155

143 Claësson M H, Andersen V, Sonderstrup-Hansen G 1978 Colony formation by subpopulations of human T-lymphocytes. I. Effects of phytohaemagglutinin and lymphocytosis-promoting factor from Bordetella pertussis. Clinical and Experimental Immunology 34: 364–373

144 Foa R, Catovsky D, Lauria F, Galton D A G 1980 Reduced T-colony forming capacity by T-lymphocytes from B-chronic lymphocytic leukemia. British Journal of Haematology (in press)

145 Radnay J, Goldman I, Rozenszajn L A 1979 Growth of human B-lymphocyte colonies in vitro. Nature 278: 351–353

146 Izaguirre C, Minden M, McCulloch E A 1979 A colony assay for normal and malignant B-lymphocyte progenitors. Blood 54: 172a

147 Goldman J M, Th'ng K H, Catovsky D, Pittman S., O'Brien M 1978 A continuous cell line from a patient with follicular lymphoma in transformation. Experimental Hematology 6 (suppl 3): 28

148 Kadin M E, Holt L, Najfeld V 1979 Malignant histiocytosis: establishment and characterization of a permanent cell line. Blood 54 (suppl 1): 173a

149 Rosenfeld C, Goutner A, Choquet C, Venuat A M, Kayibanda B, Pico J L, Greaves M F 1977 Phenotypic characterisation of a unique non-T, non-B acute lymphoblastic leukaemia cell line. Nature 267: 841–843

150 Schneider U, Schwenk H U 1977 Characterisation of T and non-T cell lines established from children with acute lymphoblastic leukemia and non-Hodgkin-lymphoma after

leukemic transformation. In: Thierfelder S, Rodt H, Thiel E (eds) Immunological Diagnosis of Leukemias and Lymphomas. Springer-Verlag, Berlin, p 265–269

151 Minowada J, Koshiba H, Janossy G, Greaves M F, Bollum F J 1979 A Philadelphia chromosome positive human leukaemia cell line (NALM-1) with pre-B characteristics. Leukemia Research 3: 261–266

152 Kaplan J, Ravindranath Y, Peterson W D Jr 1977 T and B lymphocyte antigen-positive null cell leukemias. Blood 49: 371–378

153 Billing R, Clark B, Guidera K, Minowada J 1978 Heteroantiserum against acute lymphocytic leukemia raised to the lymphoblastoid cell line NALM-1. International Journal of Cancer 22: 694–699

154 Fox R M, Piddington S K, Tripp E H, Dudman N P, Tattersall M H N 1979 Thymidine sensitive of cultured leukaemic lymphocytes. Lancet ii: 391–393

155 Akman S, Ross D, Rosen H, Salinger C, Bachur N, Andrews P, Chou E, Wiernik P 1979 Effects of thymidine on leukemia and normal human blood cell growth in vitro. Experimental Hematology 7 (suppl 6): 136

156 Buxbaum J N, Alexander A, Olivier O 1978 Gamma heavy chain disease in man: synthesis of a deleted γ_3 immunoglobulin by lymphoid cells in short and long term tissue culture. Clinical and Experimental Immunology 32: 489–497

157 Golde D W, Quan S G, Cline M J 1978 Human T lymphocyte cell line producing colony-stimulating activity. Blood 52: 1068–1072

158 Lozzio C B, Lozzio B B 1975 Human chronic myelogenous leukemia cell-line with positive Philadelphia chromosome. Blood 45: 321–334

159 Andersson L C, Nilsson K, Gahmberg C G 1979 K 562 – A human erythroleukemic cell line. International Journal of Cancer 23: 143–147

160 Andersson L C, Jokinen M, Gahmberg C G 1979 Induction of erythroid differentiation in the human leukaemia cell line K 562. Nature 278: 364–365

161 Andersson L C, Gahmberg C G, Teerenhovi L, Vuopio P 1979 Glycophorin as a cell surface marker of early erythroid differentiation in acute leukemia. International Journal of Cancer 23: 717–720

162 Gallagher R, Collins S, Trujillo J, McCredie K, Ahearn M, Tsai S, Metzgar R, Aulakh G, Ting R, Ruscetti F, Gallo R 1979 Characterization of the continuous differentiating myeloid cell line (HL-60) from a patient with acute promyelocytic leukemia. Blood 53: 713–733

163 Karpas A, Khalid G, Burns G, Hayhoe F G H 1978 Continuous culture of malignant leukaemic cells from human acute myelomonocytic leukaemia. Cytological, cytochemical, cytogenetic and immunological studies. British Journal of Cancer 37: 308–315

164 Kauffer H P, Golde D W 1978 Acute myelogenous leukemia: a human cell line responsive to colony stimulating activity. Science 200: 1153–1154

165 Greenberger J S, Karpas A, Gans P J, Neumann H, Moloney W C 1978 Increased myeloid-associated enzymes in Epstein-Barr virus nuclear antigen-positive human cell lines exposed to butyric acid in vitro. Blood 51: 1073–1085

166 Lippman M E, Yarbro G K, Leventhal B G 1978 Clinical implications of glucocorticoid receptors in human leukemia. Cancer Research 38: 4251–4256

167 Crabtree G R, Smith K A, Munck A 1978 Glucocorticoid receptors and sensitivity of isolated human leukemia and lymphoma cells. Cancer Research 38: 4268–4272

168 Killman S-A 1968 Acute leukemia: The kinetics of leukemia blast cells in man. Series Haematologica I 3: 38–102

169 Mauer A M, Murphy S B 1979 Kinetic studies of cells in childhood leukemias. American Journal of Clinical Pathology 72: 753–755

170 Shackney S E, Skramstad K 1979 A dynamic interpretation of multiparameter studies in the lymphomas. American Journal of Clinical Pathology 72: 756–764

171 Murphy S B, Melvin S L, Mauer A M 1979 Correlation of tumor cell kinetic studies with surface marker results in childhood non-Hodgkin's lymphoma. Cancer Research 39: 1534–1538

2

Cytochemistry in the Classification of Leukemias

Georges Flandrin   Marie-Thérèse Daniel

Cytochemical methods are important for the accurate identification of leukemic cells, particularly in the acute types, and hence for determining treatment and evaluating prognosis. Hayhoe et al[1] combined cytochemistry with the classical morphological criteria (Romanovsky staining). Using four methods, Sudan black B, peroxidase, leukocyte alkaline phosphatase and PAS, they suggested that it was possible to determine four different types:[2] acute lymphoblastic leukemia (ALL); acute myeloblastic leukemia (AML); myelomonocytic leukemia and erythremic myelosis.

Loeffler[3,4] also used four cytochemical technics in order to classify acute leukemia but without taking into consideration cell morphology. He identified the following types of acute leukemia: peroxidase type; esterase and peroxidase; esterase type; PAS type and undifferentiated type (when all reactions were negative).

Bennett et al[5] proposed a classification (FAB) based on morphology and supplemented in certain cases with cytochemistry (peroxidase and NASDA). In the FAB classification, the myeloid leukemias were divided into six groups (M1 to M6) on the basis of differentiation and degree of maturation. A further subclassification has been proposed for the non-myeloid leukemias (lymphoblastic)[6] but with the exception of the rare leukemia with Burkitt's cells[7,5] these classifications of ALL did not correlate with the immunological cell markers. T-cell ALL could be distinguished, however, because of its cytochemical positivity with the acid phosphatase reaction.[8,9]

In the chronic leukemias cytochemistry has been of lesser value in classification. Absent or very low leukocyte alkaline phosphatase levels are usual in chronic myelogenous leukemia.[10]

In lymphoproliferative disorders it has been shown[11,8] that the lymphocytes of chronic lymphocytic leukemia have an increased glycogen (PAS) content, but this finding is not of diagnostic or prognostic significance. Recent findings with various lysosomal acid hydrolases (acid phosphatase, beta-glucuronidase and esterases) have stimulated interesting studies as part of an effort in the cytochemical characterization of T- and B-lymphocytes.[12–16]

METHODS

ALKALINE PHOSPHATASE (MODIFIED FROM KAPLOW[17,1])

Reagents
1. *Fixative*: methanol-formol (9:1) stored at 4°C
2. *Buffer A* (propanediol solution):
     2-amino-2 methyl 1,3-propanediol 10.5 g
     Distilled H_2O to make 500 ml
3. *Buffer B*:
     Buffer A   12.5 ml
     N 10 HCl   2.5 ml
     H_2O to make   50 ml
4. Alpha-naphthyl acid phosphate, sodium salt
5. Fast Garnet GBC salt
6. Harris' hematoxylin.

Method
1. Air-dried, thinly spread peripheral blood films are fixed after 3 h in cold fixative for 30 s and rinsed briefly in running water
2. The incubating medium is prepared as follows immediately before use:
     Buffer solution B   50 ml
     Alpha-naphthyl phosphate   50 mg
     Fast Garnet GBC salt   50 mg
3. Incubate slides 10 min at room temperature in filtered medium (use ash-free, wide-pore filter)
4. Rinse in running water
5. Counterstain in Harris' hematoxylin 10 min
6. Mount in glycerin jelly.

The cytochemical reaction product is brown; nuclei are stained blue.

PERIODIC ACID—SCHIFF (PAS) (MODIFIED FROM MacMANUS[1])

Reagents
1. *Fixative*: methanol-formol (9:1) stored at 4°C
2. Periodic acid solution prepared by dissolving 1 g in 100 ml distilled water. The solution can be stored for several months in a dark bottle
3. Schiff's reagent is purchased commercially but it can be prepared[1]
4. Sodium metabisulfite solution 10 g in 100 ml distilled water
5. 1 N hydrochloric acid (HCl)
6. Mayer's solution.

Method
1. Air-dried, thinly spread peripheral blood or bone marrow films are fixed in cold fixative for 10 min and rinsed in running water
2. Immerse in periodic acid solution for 10 min, wash again and dry
3. Immerse in Schiff's basic fuchsin in the dark for 30 min

4. Rinse 3 times in the following solution:

Metabisulfite   6 ml
HCl   5 ml
Distilled H_2O to make   100 ml

5. Wash with tap water. Dry in air
6. Counterstain with Mayer's hemalum for 10 min. Rinse in running water for 10 min
7. Mount in Eukitt (Vitromed-Basel).

The cytochemical reaction product is red; nuclei are stained blue.

MYELOPEROXIDASE

The technic used is a modification of the Graham-Knoll peroxidase method.[18]

Reagents
1. *Solution A* (stored in the dark):
   0.25 g if benzidine base in 100 ml 95° ethanol
2. *Solution B*:
   0.25 g sodium nitroprusside in 100 ml distilled water
3. *Solution C*:
   100 ml solution A + 2 ml solution B
4. *Diluted H_2O_2*
   3 per cent H_2O_2 0.1 ml
   Distilled H_2O to make   50 ml
5. Giemsa solution at 10 per cent in Sörensen buffer pH 6.4.

Method
1. *Fixation*: cover films with solution C for 3 min. Shake off excess fixative
2. Incubate for 5 min in the following solution:
   Solution C   50 ml
   H_2O_2 solution   50 ml prepared and filtered immediately before use
3. Wash with Sörensen buffer pH 6.4
4. Counterstain with filtered buffered Giemsa
5. Wash with tap water and dry
6. Mount in Eukitt.

The cytochemical reaction product is blue-green. Alternative technics avoiding the use of benzidine are available.[19,20,21]

SUDAN BLACK B (AFTER SHENAN AND STOREY[1])

Reagents
1. Sudan black B 0.3 g in 100 ml absolute ethanol
2. *Buffer*: dissolve 16 g crystalline phenol in 30 ml absolute ethanol. Add to 100 ml distilled water in which 0.3 g hydrated disodium hydrogen phosphate ($Na_2HPO_2 + 12 H_2O$) has been dissolved

3. *Working stain*: add 40 ml buffer to 60 ml Sudan black B solution and filter by suction. Keeps 2 to 3 months.

Method
1. Fix air-dried films in formalin vapor 5 to 10 min
2. Wash in running tap water 10 min
3. Immerse in working stain 1 h
4. Wash off with 70 per cent ethanol
5. Wash with tap water 2 min
6. Blot dry and counterstain with Leishman or May-Grünwald Giemsa.

The cytochemical reaction product is black; nuclei are stained blue.

ESTERASES

NAPHTHOL AS-D ACETATE ESTERASE (NASDA) (AFTER LÖFFLER[22] AND SCHMALZL[23])

Reagents
1. *Fixative*: 40 per cent formalin
2. 0.1 mol/l phosphate buffer pH 6.9
3. Propylene-glycol 1–2
4. Naphthol AS-D acetate solution
    Naphthol AS-D acetate   11 mg
    Acetone   2 ml
5. Fast blue BB salt.

Method
1. Fix air-dried peripheral blood or bone marrow films with formalin vapor at room temperature 5 min
2. Wash with tap water and dry
3. Immerse slides for 70 min at room temperature in the following solution prepared and filtered just before use:
    Phosphate buffer   100 ml
    Propylene-glycol   2 ml
    Naphthol AS-D acetate solution   1.9 ml
    (add the substrate solution dropwise and slowly shaking the buffer propylene-glycol mixture)
    Fast blue BB   200 mg
4. Wash in running water briefly; dry in air
5. Counterstain with the Feulgen reaction
6. Mount in glycerin jelly.

The cytochemical reaction product is blue; the nuclei are stained red.
For the inhibition of NASDA, add 1.5 mg/ml of sodium fluoride (NaF) to the buffer.

ACID ALPHA-NAPHTHYL ACETATE ESTERASE (ANAE)

This method from Mueller et al[14] has a long incubation time in acid medium.

Reagents

1. *Fixative*: cold Baker's formol-calcium pH 6.7. (Kulenkampff et al[15] recommend fixing the film whilst wet in 2.5 per cent glutaraldehyde/saline pH 7.2 for 10 min at 4°C)
2. *Solution A*: 1 g pararosanilin acridin-free dissolved in 20 ml distilled water to which 5 ml HCl is added. This is stored in the dark at 4°C
3. *Solution B*: freshly prepared sodium nitrite solution ($NaNO_2$) 4 per cent in distilled water
4. 0.067 mol/l phosphate buffer pH 5
5. Alpha-naphthyl acetate
6. Acetone
7. 2 mol/l NaOH
8. Methyl green 1 per cent as counterstain.

Method

1. Fix air-dried films at 4°C for 10 min and wash in distilled water 20 min
2. Incubate for 3 h at room temperature in the following freshly prepared and filtered solution:
   2.4 ml of hexazonium pararosanilin (mix 1.2 ml of solution A and 1.2 ml of solution B and shake for a few seconds)
   40 ml of phosphate buffer
   10 mg of alpha-naphthyl acetate on 0.4 ml acetone. The mixture is adjusted to pH 5.8 using 2 mol/l NaOH
3. Wash in distilled water for 10 min
4. Counterstain with methyl green
5. Mount in glycerin jelly.

The cytochemical reaction product is brown.

ALPHA-NAPHTHYL BUTYRATE ESTERASE (FROM LI ET AL[24] MODIFIED BY HIGGY ET AL[16])

Reagents

1. Formalin
2. 0.1 mol/l phosphate buffer pH 8
3. Alpha-naphthyl butyrate
4. Fast Garnet GBC salt
5. Harris' hematoxylin.

Method

1. Fix air-dried films in formalin vapor for 4 min
2. Wash briefly in distilled water and dry

3. Incubate at room temperature for 15 to 30 min in the following medium:
   10 ml phosphate buffer
   0.025 ml solution of 0.01 ml of alpha-naphthyl butyrate in 0.5 ml acetone
   3 mg fast Garnet GBC salt
4. Wash briefly in distilled water
5. Counterstain 10 min in hematoxylin
6. Wash in running water 10 min
7. Mount in glycerin jelly.

The cytochemical reaction product is brown.

CHLOROACETATE ESTERASE (FROM MOLONEY ET AL[25])

Reagents
1. *Fixative*: methanol-formalin (9:1)
2. 0.1 mol/l Michaelis buffer pH 7.4:
   0.1 mol/l Veronal   60 ml
   0.1 mol/l HCl   40 ml
3. Propylene-glycol
4. Naphthol AS-D (NASD) chloroacetate solution:
   NASD chloroacetate   40 mg
   Acetone   3.2 ml

Method
1. Fix films for 3 min. Rinse in tap water; dry in air
2. Immerse slides for 30 min in the following solution, which is prepared and
   filtered just before use:
   Buffer   40 ml
   Distilled water   40 ml
   Propylene-glycol   2 ml
   NASD chloroacetate solution   3.2 ml
   (add the substrate solution dropwise and slowly shaking the buffer propylene-glycol mixture)
   Fast Garnet GBC   80 mg
3. Rinse and dry in air
4. Counterstain with Harris' hematoxylin for 10 min
5. Rinse in running water for 10 min
6. Mount in glycerin jelly.

The cytochemical reaction product is red; nuclei are stained blue.
Double esterase staining involves using first the NASDA procedure with fast
blue BB as coupler, followed by NASD chloroacetate with pararosanilin as
coupler. The reaction in monocytic cells is blue and in granulocytic cells red.

ACID PHOSPHATASE (MODIFIED FROM GOLDBERG AND BARKA[26])

Reagents

1. *Fixative*: 60 per cent aqueous acetone
2. *Solution A*:
    1 ml pararosanilin 4 per cent in HCl
    1 g pararosanilin acridin-free dissolved in 20 ml distilled water to which is added 5 ml concentrated HCl. This is stored in the dark at 4°C
    1.5 ml freshly prepared solution of $NaNO_2$ 4 per cent in distilled water
3. *Solution B*: Michaelis buffer pH 5 90 ml
4. *Solution C*: 30 mg naphthol AS-BI phosphate in 3 ml of n-n-dimethyl formamide
5. Harris' hematoxylin.

Method

1. Fix films for 30 min
2. Rinse in tap water; dry in air
3. The working solution is prepared and filtered just before use:
    Solution A 2.5 ml, 60 s after solution A has been prepared add solution B 90 ml
    Solution C 3 ml. Readjust pH to 5 with 1 mol/l NaOH
4. Incubate films at 37°C for 90 min
5. Rinse in abundant tap water
6. Counterstain with Harris' hematoxylin for 10 min (or with methyl green)
7. Wash in tap water for 10 min
8. Mount in glycerin jelly.

The reaction product is dark red; nuclei are stained blue (or green).

Inhibition with tartaric acid
Working solution   90 ml
L (+) tartaric acid   675 mg
Adjust to pH 5 with 1 mol/l NaOH.

BETA-GLUCURONIDASE (MODIFIED FROM HAYASHI[27] AND LORBARCHER[28])

Reagents

1. *Fixative*: methanol-formalin (7:3) stored at 4°C
2. *Solution A*:
    1.5 ml pararosanilin 4 per cent in HCl
    1 g pararosanilin acridin-free dissolved in 20 ml distilled water to which is added 5 ml concentrated HCl. This is stored in the dark at 4°C
    2 ml freshly prepared solution of $NaNO_2$ 4 per cent in distilled water.
3. *Solution B*: acetate buffer pH 5.2
4. *Solution C*: sodium bicarbonate ($NaHCO_3$) 420 mg in 100 ml H_2O (store at 4°C)

5. *Solution D*: 4 mg of naphthol AS-BI-B-D glucuronic acid in 0.6 ml of solution C+solution B to 50 ml.

Method

1. Fix films for 45 to 60 min at 4°C (for marrow films, rinse in acetone to dissolve fat)
2. Rinse in tap water
3. Dry for 30 min
4. Freeze slides for 1 h at −20°C
5. Keep at 4°C until incubation
6. Immerse slides for 1 h at 37°C in the working solution, prepared and filtered just before use as follows:
   3.5 ml solution A
   50 ml solution D
   Adjust to pH 5.2 with 1 mol/l NaOH; add distilled water to make 100 ml
7. Rinse in distilled water
8. Counterstain with Harris' hematoxylin
9. Rinse in tap water for 10 min
10. Mount in glycerin jelly.

The cytochemical reaction product is red.

OIL RED O[29]

Reagents

1. *Fixative*: 40 per cent formalin
2. 2-propanol (50 per cent diluted in distilled H_2O)
3. Oil red O.

Method

1. Fix in formalin vapor 15 min; rinse gently in running water
2. Rinse in 2-propanol
3. Immerse films for 30 min in the following solution:
   30 ml oil red O solution at 0.2 per cent in 2-propanol
   20 ml distilled H_2O. (Cover up; do not filter)
4. Rinse with 2-propanol to shake off excess staining
5. Rinse in distilled water
6. Counterstain in Harris' hematoxylin 10 min
7. Rinse in running water 10 min
8. Mount in glycerin jelly.

The cytochemical reaction product is orange.

ACUTE NON-LYMPHOCYTIC (MYELOID) LEUKEMIA (ANLL)

Acute myeloblastic leukemia (Figs 2.1 to 2.4)

Myeloperoxidase reaction and/or Sudan black B staining
Myeloperoxidase is an enzyme localized exclusively in the azurophil granules

of both granulocytic and monocytic series. Despite uncertainties concerning the specificity of Sudan black B reactions, a positive Sudan reaction is closely related to peroxidase reactivity, that is, both are usually positive in the same samples. More than 5 per cent and usually the majority of blast cells are positive in acute myeloblastic leukemia (AML), with a strongly localized or heavy overall reaction.[1,30] This type of positivity should be distinguished from the more finely granular type found in monoblastic leukemia.[31] Although myeloperoxidase is located in the azurophil granules, positivity may be seen in the cytoplasm of undifferentiated cells totally devoid of granules.[2,30] This cytoplasmic staining in the absence of granules probably represents myeloperoxidase reaction in the perinuclear space, endoplasmic reticulum and Golgi apparatus as demonstrated by ultrastructural cytochemistry.[32,33] Because azurophil granules are almost always present in AML this reaction is usually not essential for its diagnosis. There are, however, a few cases of poorly differentiated AML (among the M1 class of the FAB classification) where the blast cells have little or no granulation. In those cases the striking peroxidase positively establishes the diagnosis of AML and rules out ALL. The myeloperoxidase reaction is then more often useful in M1 than in the M2 class of the FAB classification. The other finding when using the myeloperoxidase reaction in AML is loss of the enzyme in some mature cells of the granulocytic series.[34] Another feature with this enzyme reaction is observed in 'hypergranular' promyelocytic leukemia (M3 in the FAB classification).[5,30,35] In these cases myeloperoxidase is always strongly positive in all blast cells with the reaction product covering up the whole cytoplasm and very often the nucleus too.

Naphthol AS-D chloroacetate esterase
This esterase is positive in the granulocytic series, its reactivity increasing with cell maturity. Thus this reaction is less sensitive than myeloperoxidase for the diagnosis of AML. Some of the more immature AML (among the M1 group) may be totally negative for NASD chloroacetate esterase. In particular this reaction was of no help in patients where the May-Grünwald Giemsa failed to show azurophil granules but the myeloperoxidase reaction was positive. In those cases the NASD chloroacetate reaction was negative.[30]

In 'hypergranular' promyelocytic leukemia (M3), the NASD chloroacetate esterase is strongly positive, more intensely so than in all other types of AML.[30]

PAS reaction
Many blast cells in AML are PAS negative; some others may show a faint cytoplasmic tinge, with or without fine superimposed granules.[1] The 'typical' single coarse-granular pattern of ALL is very unusual in AML (see below).

Acid phosphatase
Acid phosphatase activity in AML is ordinarily greater than in ALL, but seems to be variable and is without sufficient specificity to help in its diagnosis or subclassification. The acid phosphatase reaction in AML is usually diffusely positive in the cytoplasm, with or without superimposed granules, while in ALL

it is granular. The positive versus negative acid phosphatase subclassification is relevant only in the context of ALL.[5]

Naphthol AS-D acetate esterase
This reaction may be positive in variable degree in AML depending on cell maturation. Acute promyelocytic leukemia (M3) shows the more positive reaction.[30] In AML the esterase reaction is unaffected by exposure to NaF in contrast to monocytic leukemia.

Acute monocytic leukemia

Naphthol AS-D acetate esterase
Acute monocytic leukemia (AMoL) is characterised by a strong NASDA activity, inhibited by NaF (Figs 2.5 and 2.6).[23, 31, 36] In the absence of NaF, this reaction is very strong and uniform in the majority of cells. In some cases the reaction is weaker, but it always decreases dramatically after exposure to NaF. This reaction is consistently positive in 'pure' AMoL. A negative result in AMoL is rare.[30]

No major differences in esterase activity exist between the two subclasses of M5, undifferentiated (monoblastic) or differentiated (monocytic) of the FAB classification.[5] This esterase technic allows a better distinction between AMoL and AML to be made, especially in the less differentiated cases (M1).

Alpha-naphthyl acetate as substrate. Others have preferred to use this substrate instead of NASDA.[2] This reaction is strongly positive in AMoL and negative in AML and ALL.

Naphthol AS-D chloroacetate esterase
This reaction is always negative in AMoL but positive in the granulocytic series. However, this is of little practical value in distinguishing AMoL from AML

Figs 2.1–2.16 Magnification of the photomicrographs × 580.

Figs 2.1–2.4 Bone marrow films of a case of myeloblastic leukemia without maturation.

Fig. 2.1 May–Grünwald Giemsa stain showing undifferentiated blast cells without azurophil granulations.

Fig. 2.2 *Myeloperoxidase* in the same case with the majority of blast cells positive (myeloblasts).

Fig. 2.3 *Sudan black B* in the same case, showing an equivalent positive result.

Fig. 2.4 *NASD chloroacetate esterase* in the same case showing complete negativity of the blast cells with the exception of a 'normal' promyelocyte (in this field as a positive control for the reaction).

Figs 2.5 and 2.6 Bone marrow films of a case of acute monocytic leukemia.

Fig. 2.5 *NASDA esterase* reaction showing a strong positivity in all blast cells.

Fig. 2.6 In the same case, exposure to *sodium fluoride* results in a dramatic inhibition of the NASDA reaction.

Figs 2.7 and 2.8 Bone marrow films of a case of acute myelomonocytic leukemia with a prominent abnormal eosinophilic component.

Fig. 2.7 May-Grünwald Giemsa stain showing a majority of eosinophilic cells.

Fig. 2.8 In the same case, *NASD chloroacetate esterase* positivity in abnormal eosinophils.

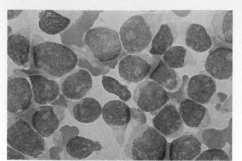

Fig 2.1

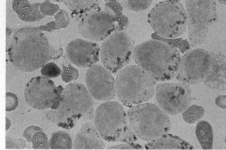

Fig 2.2

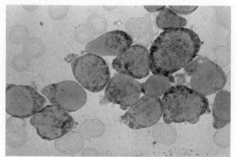

Fig 2.3

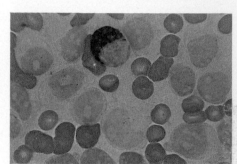

Fig 2.4

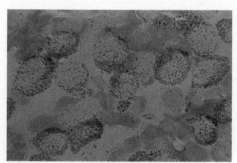

Fig 2.5

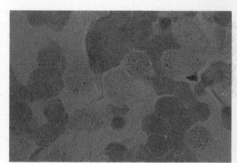

Fig 2.6

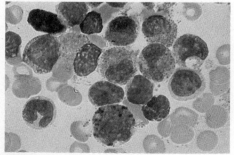

Fig 2.7

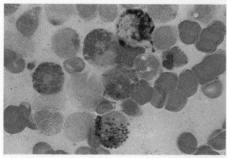

Fig 2.8

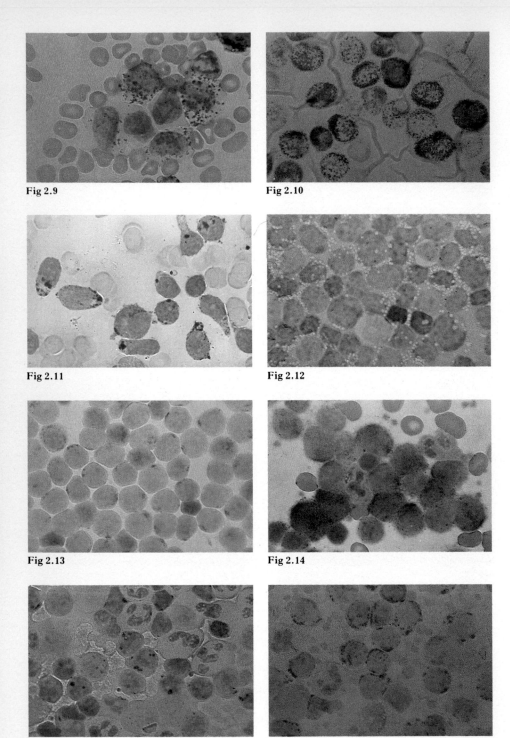

Fig 2.9

Fig 2.10

Fig 2.11

Fig 2.12

Fig 2.13

Fig 2.14

Fig 2.15

Fig 2.16

because, as mentioned earlier, NASD chloroacetate esterase is negative in the less differentiated AML (M1) which are the only cases which require to be distinguished from AMoL.[30]

PAS reaction

This reaction is rather variable in AMoL. Some blast cells are entirely negative, others give a reaction like normal monocytes, showing fine granulation against a background of diffuse cytoplasmic staining. In other cases some cells are strongly positive with coarse granules or blocks of PAS positivity.[1,30,31] This reaction is of no help in the diagnosis of AMoL.

Myeloperoxidase and/or Sudan black B

Very variable results are seen in AMoL with these methods.[1,2,30,31] In some cases the reaction is totally negative in all blast cells, in others the majority of cells are positive and in others only a few cells are positive, with variable degrees of reaction. The pattern of myeloperoxidase reaction in monocytic cells differs, however, from those observed in granulocytic precursors. The positivity is more finely granular and discretely scattered than in AML.[1] The myeloperoxidase reaction of cells of monoblastic (M5 undifferentiated) and monocytic (M5 differentiated) leukemias differ from the reaction of cells of the normal monocytic series. Normal immature monocytes are more strongly positive than mature monocytes; the latter may even be negative. In AMoL the undifferentiated type (or monoblastic) is often but not always, peroxidase negative, probably reflecting in the negative cases a myeloperoxidase deficiency. In the differentiated type (or monocytic) both features can be observed with peroxidase positive cells often predominating.[30]

Fig. 2.9 Peripheral blood in a case of acute monocytic leukemia. *Myeloperoxidase* positive reaction with a typically 'monocytic' pattern with small scattered granules.

Fig. 2.10 Peripheral blood buffy-coat preparation of a case of myelomonocytic leukemia. Double reaction with *NASDA esterase* (blue positivity) and *NASD chloroacetate esterase* (red positivity). The strongly blue reacting cells are typically monocytic, the red-colored cells are maturing granulocytic cells. The cells with only a faint blue positivity remain questionable—granulocytic blast cells or weakly positive monocytic cells?

Fig. 2.11 Bone marrow film in a case of ALL. *PAS* reaction showing a block pattern of positivity, typical of the PAS-type of ALL.

Fig. 2.12 Bone marrow film in a case of L3, ALL (Burkitt's type) with an *Oil red O* positive reaction, corresponding to the vacuoles seen with the May-Grünwald Giemsa stain.

Fig. 2.13 Peripheral blood buffy-coat preparation of a patient with T-ALL. *Acid phosphatase* reaction with the typical clump of positivity in the Golgi zone.

Fig. 2.14 Peripheral blood buffy-coat preparation of a patient with hairy-cell leukemia. *Acid phosphatase* reaction showing a strongly diffuse and granular positivity.

Fig. 2.15 Peripheral blood buffy-coat preparation of a case of Sézary syndrome. *Beta-glucuronidase* reaction showing a strong granular positivity in the Sézary cells.

Fig. 2.16 Peripheral blood buffy-coat preparation of a case of T-CLL. *Beta-glucuronidase* reaction showing strong positivity with numerous scattered granules. In this patient, azurophil granules were present in the majority of lymphocytes on May-Grünwald Giemsa stained smears.

Acid phosphatase
This reaction is usually strongly positive with a diffuse and granular pattern but, since it can sometimes also be strongly positive in AML as well as AMoL, it may not represent a distinctive feature of AMoL.[5]

Acute myelomonocytic leukemia (Figs 2.7 and 2.8)
In acute myelomonocytic leukemia (AMML), M4 of the FAB classification, both granulocytic and monocytic differentiation are present in varying degrees in the bone marrow and peripheral blood.[5] Doubts were raised whether it is possible to distinguish AMML from 'pure' monocytic leukemia (AMoL, or M5).[2] We consider[5] that, when the proportion of monocytes and promonocytes exceeds 20 per cent of the bone marrow cells, AMML can be separated from AML. On the other hand, when the percentage of monocytic cells is high, AMML can be distinguished from AMoL only when the granulocytic blast cells exceed 10 to 20 per cent. The cytochemical reactions (NASDA and myeloperoxidase) are often helpful in making this distinction too (Fig. 2.9). However, in some patients even with these cytochemical reactions a sharp distinction between cell lines may be difficult because intermediate staining reactions occur in both series.

The double staining method, especially when using on the same slide NASDA esterase with a blue coupler (Fast Blue BB) and chloroacetate esterase with a red coupler (Pararosanilin), may be of value in attempting to separate monocytic and granulocytic cells (Fig. 2.10).

Comparison of bone marrow and peripheral blood is often of great importance in diagnosing AMML. Monocytic differentiation is often more obvious in the peripheral blood than in the bone marrow. In contrast, the bone marrow appearance if taken alone may often suggest a diagnosis of AML rather than AMoL.

Auer rods
Auer rods are considered abnormal lysosomes with a spindle shape and peculiar crystalline features on electronmicroscopy. They share the reactivity of other azurophil granules of both granulocytic and monocytic series, both conditions where Auer rods can be found. Auer rods are positive for peroxidase, Sudan black B, acid phosphatase and chloroacetate esterase.[37]

Erythroleukemia
As in myelomonocytic leukemia the criteria defining erythroleukemia (M6 of the FAB classification)[5] are variable. In the FAB classification it depends on the number and the abnormalities of the erythroblasts which are present with other blast cells (usually myeloblasts).

Erythroblasts may show heavy PAS positivity, generally granular in early erythroblasts and diffuse in later ones.[1] The presence or absence of PAS positivity in erythroblasts may also be seen in erythroleukemia.[30] In the blast cells, the cytochemical results are those expected for each type. Most often they are myeloblasts with typical myeloperoxidase positivity, sometimes possibly monocytic precursors or rarely undifferentiated blasts, with no distinguishing cytochemical features.

Megakaryocytes

No special reactivity can be demonstrated with light microscopy cytochemistry on the megakaryocytic series.[38]

The PAS positivity of normal mature megakaryocytes can be found also in the megakaryoblasts of some acute leukemias. The PAS reaction may, however, be negative and cannot therefore be considered as a reliable marker.[39] Weak non-specific esterase activity is often present in megakaryocytic precursors but it is not specific; the NASDA reaction is moderately inhibited by NaF. This lack of a specific cytochemical profile for the megakaryocytic line is usually of no practical importance since these cells only represent a small percentage of those encountered in ANLL (M2, M4, M6) and in refractory anemia with excess of blasts, and therefore do not influence the classification. In the very rare cases of acute leukemia with predominant megakaryoblastic differentiation the precise identification of these blast cells is difficult or even impossible with light microscopy only.[38, 39] A specific marker is present at ultrastructural level and helps in detecting the megakaryocytic origin of such otherwise undifferentiated blasts[38–41] (Ch. 4).

Eosinophilic leukemia

Rare cases of acute myelomonocytic leukemias with a high content of abnormal eosinophils in the bone marrow have been identified.[42–46] These acute leukemias consistently give a positive NASD chloroacetate reaction in the eosinophilic granules, a reaction which is not seen in normal eosinophils.

Basophilic leukemia

Basophilic leukemia is most often a variant of chronic myeloid leukemia (CML) with a high percentage of basophils. This special feature is most often characteristic of the acute phase of CML.

The basophilic cells can easily be identified by their metachromatic granules after toluidine blue or other appropriate staining. True acute basophilic leukemia seems to be exceptionally rare.[47]

Leukocyte alkaline phosphatase (LAP) in acute leukemia

The alkaline phosphatase content of mature granulocytes in acute leukemia is of no practical value.[1, 2] LAP is never low but usually normal or raised in ALL. In ANLL (AML, AMoL, erythroleukemia), on the other hand, the reaction is usually low.

ACUTE LYMPHOBLASTIC LEUKEMIA (ALL)

Cytochemistry has greatly facilitated the separation of ALL from the other types of acute leukemia.[1, 2, 30]

Myeloperoxidase reaction (or alternatively Sudan black staining)
This is negative in ALL and positive in AML. This cytochemical reaction is a more sensitive index of myeloid maturation than the presence of azurophil granules and is of value particularly in distinguishing poorly differentiated AML

(M1 of the FAB classification) from ALL. A complete peroxidase negativity is the best practical criterion for diagnosing ALL.[30]

PAS reaction

Although the PAS reaction has not proved to be very helpful in separating different types of acute leukemia there are marked differences in quantity and distribution of positively reacting material in the various leukemias and even within the same type.[37] Special attention has been paid to the PAS reaction in ALL. The frequency of PAS positivity varies in different published series, positive in most cases[1,2] or only in 60 per cent of cases.[30] Lymphoblasts show great variability in PAS reaction: in positive cases at least a few, and commonly many, of the blast cells are positive. When present, PAS positivity is not diffuse but is seen as coarse granules or blocks against a negative cytoplasmic background (Fig. 2.11).[1] It is this pattern of reaction rather than the percentage of positive blast cells that is of diagnostic importance. This 'typical' coarse granular positivity is present in about half the cases of ALL and seems to be characteristic of the disease. All the cases with a high percentage of PAS-positive blast cells belong to this group.[30] In the few other positive cases the PAS has a fine, regular scattered granular pattern, similar to the positivity which can be observed in ANLL. The presence of PAS-negative cases and the absence of specificity of the type with faint positivity makes the PAS reaction of little help for the diagnosis of ALL.[30,37] A correlation has been found between PAS reactivity in ALL and cytological subclasses based on cell size, with less positivity in the large cell type[30] as well as less PAS material in cases with high leukocyte counts.[48] Among patients with ALL, those of 'PAS-positive type' have a significantly better prognosis than the PAS-negative cases.[4,49] Patients with the PAS-negative type often correspond with those having a positive acid phosphatase reaction[3] in whom the prognosis is worse.[50]

Oil red O

Coarse lipid droplets were demonstrated in the cytoplasmic vacuoles of ALL Burkitt's type (L3 of the FAB classification) (Fig. 2.12). This peculiar feature is similar to those observed in the African Burkitt's tumor.[51,52] These Burkitt's tumor cells are usually devoid of PAS material.[7] In other cases of ALL both Oil red O-positive and PAS-positive material are often present. Cases with Oil red O-positive and PAS-negative cells are rarely observed.[53] This last cytochemical pattern cannot be considered, however, specific of Burkitt's cell type.[53]

Acid phosphatase

A significant advance in the understanding of ALL has been the characterization in terms of B and T surface markers (Ch. 5). Three main types have been recognized. (1) A small proportion of patients (about 2 per cent of ALL) have a monoclonal B-cell proliferation. These patients have the special cytological feature referred to as acute leukemia with 'Burkitt tumor cells'[5,7] (L3 of the FAB classification). (2) In 30 per cent of ALL the blasts have T-cell surface features. (3) In the majority of ALL, the blast cells do not express B- or T-cell markers.[9,50]

With the exception of the correlation between Burkitt's cell type and monoclonal B-cell markers[7] no other clear differences have been recognized by cytology[5] or electronmicroscopy.[54] In contrast some cytochemical reactions have shown significant differences between T and non T-ALL:[8,50] the acid phosphatase reaction is positive in blast cells of the great majority (about 90 per cent)[9] of T derived ALL with a typical localization in a small paranuclear area (Fig. 2.13). In contrast, in the majority of non T-ALL (about 90 per cent)[9] this acid phosphatase reaction was absent or weak and present in a smaller proportion of blast cells.

A weak or negative PAS reaction is often associated with acid phosphatase positive ALL[4] and T-ALL.[8,50] Beta-glucuronidase, another lysosomal enzyme, does not show any obvious difference in positivity between T or non T-ALL subclasses.[9] ANAE when carried out by the method described here is a discriminative marker for T-lymphocytes[14] and shows a weak positive reaction in T-ALL.[15]

LYMPHOPROLIFERATIVE DISORDERS

Chronic lymphocytic leukemia

Lysosomal acid hydrolases: acid phosphatase and beta-glucuronidase
Cytochemical studies of peripheral blood lymphocytes from patients with chronic lymphocytic leukemia (CLL) with high lymphocyte counts have shown decreased activities of these two lysosomal enzymes as compared with normal lymphocytes.[55] This diminution of acid hydrolases in CLL is, however, not constant and a few cases showed beta-glucuronidase and acid phosphatase scores higher than normal.[56,57] Acid phosphatase and beta-glucuronidase activities have been determined cytochemically in B-, T- and non T-lymphocyte subpopulations from normal human peripheral blood.[12] The beta-glucuronidase reaction pattern in lymphocytes, when positive, is granular with two types of positivity: either a single large block or multiple small granules. In normal subjects more than 90 per cent of the T-cells are positive with the two types of reaction represented in equal proportions of cells. B-cells have a more variable positive reaction (10 to 75 per cent) with only the multiple small granule-type of positivity. The acid phosphatase reaction in lymphocytes is remarkably uniform among the cells, in contrast to the findings with beta-glucuronidase. Extrapolation of results obtained with normal peripheral blood T- and B-cells to cells in CLL can be misleading. Since the great majority of cases of CLL are B-cell neoplasms[58] the low activity of beta-glucuronidase and acid phosphatase is a common feature in B-CLL.[56] However, in about 15 per cent of immunologically characterized B-CLL[59] the beta-glucuronidase reaction is positive in the great majority of cells with a single large block of positivity.

In all the cases of T-CLL studied we have observed strong beta-glucuronidase and acid phosphatase reactions in almost all the lymphocytes; the former with either a single large block or the type of positivity with multiple small granules. The latter type of reaction is present in those T-CLL cases with large atypical lymphocytes and numerous large azurophil granules visible on Giemsa staining.[59] This last subtype of T-lymphocyte may be similar to the subclass of large lymphocytes bearing a receptor for IgG and containing azurophil granules present in normal peripheral blood.[13] Although the acid phosphatase and beta-glucuronidase reactions cannot be used as distinctive markers for normal T- or B-lymphoid cells,[12] it is noteworthy that all T-CLLs,[57] circulating Sézary cells, and other T-cell proliferations are positive for beta-glucuronidase (Figs 2.15 and 2.16).[56,60]

Esterases

The cytochemical reactions for non-specific esterase have been shown recently to represent a better criterion than the lysosomal acid hydrolases for defining subpopulations of T- and B-lymphocytes. This finding was first made with alpha-naphthyl acetate (ANAE) as substrate at acid pH.[14] In mouse lymph nodes more than 94 per cent of lymphocytes in the paracortical (thymus dependent) area are positive with a dot-like reaction. In contrast, in the follicular cortex (occupied predominantly by B-cells) less than 7 per cent of lymphocytes are esterase positive. ANAE activity has been investigated in T- and B-human lymphocytes and in leukemic cells.[15] The vast majority of T-lymphocytes showed a localized intense reaction. In the few cases of B-CLL studied, the lymphocytes were essentially negative. In common-ALL (non-T, non-B) ANAE was negative and was positive in T-ALL (see ALL).

Alpha-naphthyl butyrate esterase at pH 8 gives similar results as ANAE and therefore could also be used as a discriminative marker for mature T-lymphocytes.[16]

PAS reaction in CLL

It has been shown that the lymphocytes of CLL have an increased glycogen content.[11] A PAS-positive reaction has been reported in cells of B-prolymphocytic leukemia[8] and less commonly in T-prolymphocytic leukemia. This reaction may be present or absent in Sézary cells.[60] The PAS features in lymphoproliferative disorders show a great variability tending to make its interpretation difficult and are not of practical diagnostic value.[37]

Hairy-cell leukemia (HCL)

HCL is an uncommon leukemia which is still often misdiagnosed as CLL or lymphosarcoma.[61,62] There are some cytochemically distinctive features that can be used as diagnostic aids.

Acid phosphatase

This reaction is stronger in HCL cells than in lymphosarcoma or CLL lymphocytes. With the addition of tartrate, the enzyme activity is equally intense or even stronger.[63-65] The tartrate resistant acid phosphatase (TRAP) has been claimed to be specific for HCL. This enzyme activity indicates the presence of the isoenzyme 5 as shown by Li et al.[66]

However, the TRAP reaction was observed to be positive by Catovsky et al[8] in some cases of B-prolymphocytic leukemia. Further, Higgy et al[16] found that

TRAP activity could be weak or even absent in a proportion of cases of HCL and often partially or even completely inhibited by tartrate.[16]

Esterases

Different esterase activities have been noted in HCL with different substrates such as ANAE.[67] Recently Kass[68] and Higgy et al[16] emphasized the diagnostic value of esterase activity in HCL with alpha-naphthyl butyrate as substrate. They found a distinctive reaction pattern with a mixture of scattered fine granules together, in some instances, with coarser granules localized in a crescent configuration. This hairy-cell positivity remains unchanged after NaF exposure[16] but Kass[68] reported it to be fluoride sensitive.

Beta-glucuronidase is usually negative in HCL[62] in contrast with its important acid phosphatase activity. This dissociation between these two reactions is in striking contrast to the findings in mature lymphocytes of CLL, where the results with both acid hydrolases are similar.[56,57]

MYELOPROLIFERATIVE DISORDERS

Chronic myeloid leukemia (CML)

Leukocyte alkaline phosphatase (LAP)

LAP was found to be markedly depressed in CML.[69-71] Absent or low LAP levels are characteristic although not pathognomonic of CML. However, an elevated LAP may be seen in CML during remission, bacterial infection, blast crisis and pregnancy.[10]

A high LAP is usually associated with leukemoid reactions and with myeloproliferative disorders other than CML such as polycythemia rubra vera and myelofibrosis with myeloid metaplasia.

However, in no instance is a LAP level alone of diagnostic value since other causes of a low LAP have been found: paroxysmal nocturnal hemoglobinuria; viral infections; infectious mononucleosis and idiopathic thrombocytopenic purpura.[10]

Blast crisis of CML

The blast crisis of CML is characterized by the presence of blast cells which show very variable morphological and cytochemical characteristics. Attempts have been made to classify these diverse patterns of the acute phase of CML. The most noticeable cytochemical change is the appearance of myeloid precursors containing PAS material.[72,73] Frequently mixed features are observed with myeloblasts, monoblasts with their own specific cytochemical reactions[74] and megakaryocyte precursors.[75]

In some blast crises the cells have a lymphoblastic cytological appearance with PAS positivity and peroxidase negativity. In this very undifferentiated form of blast crisis it has been suggested that the cells are lymphoid in nature[76,77] (Ch. 5).

Acknowledgment

The figures in this chapter are reproduced by courtesy of Société Chimique Pointet Girard—Réactifs RAL.

REFERENCES

1 Hayhoe F G J, Quaglino D, Doll R 1964 Cytology and cytochemistry of acute leukemias. MRC Special Report, Series no 304, HMSO, London
2 Hayhoe F G J, Cawley J C 1972 Acute leukemia: cellular morphology, cytochemistry and fine structure. Clinics in Haematology. W B Saunders and Co, London
3 Löffler H 1973 Indications and limits of cytochemistry in acute leukaemias. Recent Results in Cancer Research 43: 57–62
4 Löffler H 1973 Biochemical properties of leukemic blast cells revealed by cytochemical methods: their relation to prognosis. Advances in the Biosciences 14: 163–173
5 Bennett J M, Catovsky D, Daniel M T, Flandrin G, Galton D A G, Gralnick H R, Sultan C 1976 Proposals for the classification of the acute leukemia. British Journal of Haematology 33: 451–458
6 Mathe G, Pouillard P, Sterescu M, Amiel J L, Schwarzenberg L, Schneider M 1971 Subdivision of classical varieties of acute leukemia. Correlation with prognosis. European Journal of Clinical and Biological Research 16: 554
7 Flandrin G, Brouet J C, Daniel M T, Preud'homme J L 1975 Acute leukemia with Burkitt's tumor cells: a study of six cases with special reference to lymphocyte surface markers. Blood 15: 183–188
8 Catovsky D, Galetto J, Okos A, Miliani E, Galton D A G 1974 Cytochemical profile of B and T leukaemic lymphocytes with special reference to acute lymphoblastic leukaemia. Journal of Clinical Pathology 27: 767–771
9 Brouet J C, Valensi F, Daniel M T, Flandrin G, Preud'homme J L, Seligmann M 1976 Immunological classification of acute lymphoblastic leukaemia. British Journal of Haematology 33: 319–328
10 Okun D B, Tanaka K R 1978 Leukocyte alkaline phosphate. American Journal of Hematology 4: 293–299
11 Astaldi G, Verga L 1957 Glycogen content of the cells of lymphatic leukaemia. Acta Haematologica 17: 129–135
12 Barr R D, Perry S 1976 Lysosomal acid hydrolases in human lymphocyte subpopulations. British Journal of Haematology 32: 565–572
13 Grossi C E, Webb S R, Zicca A, Lydyard P M, Moretta L, Mingari M C, Cooper M A 1978 Morphological and histochemical analyses of two human T-cells subpopulations bearing receptor for IgM or IgG. Journal of Experimental Medicine 147: 1405–1417
14 Mueller J, Brun Del Re G, Buerki H, Keller H U, Hess M W, Cottier H 1975 Non specific acid esterase activity: a criterion for differentiation of T and B lymphocytes in mouse lymph nodes. European Journal of Immunology 5: 270–274
15 Kulenkampff J, Janossy G, Greaves M F 1977 Acid esterase in human lymphoid cells and leukaemic blasts: a marker for T-lymphocytes. British Journal of Haematology 36: 231–240
16 Higgy K E, Burns G F, Hayhoe F G J 1977 Discrimination of B, T and null lymphocytes by esterase cytochemistry. Scandinavian Journal of Haematology 18: 437–448
17 Kaplow L S 1955 A histochemical procedure for localizing and evaluating leukocyte alkaline phosphatase activity in smears of blood and bone marrow. Blood 10: 1023–1029
18 Kaplow L S 1965 Simplified myeloperoxidase stain using benzidine dihydrochloride. Blood 26: 215–219
19 Kaplow L S 1975 Substitute for benzidine in myeloperoxidase stains. American Journal of Clinical Pathology 63: 451
20 Schaefer H E, Fischer R 1968 Der Peroxydasenachweis an Ausstrichpräparaten sowie an Gewebsschnitten nach Entkalkung und Paraffineinbettung. Klinische Wochenschrift 46: 1228–1230
21 Piette C, Piette M 1978 Caractérisation de la myéloperoxydase par une méthode n'utilisant pas la Benzidine. Feuillets de Biologie 19: 41–43
22 Löffler H 1961 Zytochemischer Nachweis von unspezifischer Esterase in Austricher. Klinische Wochenschrift 39: 1220–1227
23 Schmalzl F, Braunsteiner H 1968 Zur Diagnose Monozytärer Leukämien mit Zytochemischen Methoden. Acta Haematologica 40: 121–133
24 Li C Y, Lam K W, Yam L T 1973 Esterases in human leucocytes. Journal of Histochemistry and Cytochemistry 21: 1–12
25 Moloney W C, McPherson K, Fliegelman L 1960 Esterase activity in leukocytes demonstrated by the use of naphthol AS-D chloroacetate substrate. Journal of Histochemistry and Cytochemistry 8: 200–207

26 Goldberg A F, Barka T 1962 Acid phosphatase activity in human blood cells. Nature (London) 195: 297
27 Hayashi M, Nakajima Y, Fishman W H 1964 The cytologic demonstration of bêta-glucuronide employing naphthol AS-BI glucuronide and hexazonium pararosanilin; a preliminary report. Journal of Histochemistry and Cytochemistry 12: 293–297
28 Lorbacher P, Yam L T, Mitus W J 1967 Cytochemical demonstration of bêta-glucuronidase activity in blood and bone marrow cells. Journal of Histochemistry and Cytochemistry 15: 680–687
29 Pearse A G E 1960 Histochemistry theoretical and applied, 2nd edn. Little Brown, Boston
30 Flandrin G, Daniel M T 1973 Practical value of cytochemical studies for the classification of acute leukemias. Recent Results in Cancer Research 43: 43–56
31 Daniel M T, Flandrin G, Lejeune F, Liso P, Lortholary P 1971 Les estérases spécifiques monocytaires. Utilisation dans la classification des leucémies aiguës. Nouvelle Revue Française d'Hématologie 11: 233–240
32 Bessis M, Maigné J 1970 Le diagnostic des variétés des peroxydases au microscope électronique, son intérêt, ses limites. European Journal of Clinical and Biological Research 15: 691–698
33 Breton-Gorius J, Guichard T 1969 Étude au microscope électronique de la localisation des peroxydases dans les cellules de la moelle osseuse humaine. Nouvelle Revue Française d'Hématologie 9: 678–687
34 Catovsky D, Galton D A G, Robinson J 1972 Myeloperoxidase deficient neutrophils in AML. Scandinavian Journal of Haematology 9: 142–148
35 Bernard J, Weil M, Boiron M, Jacquillat C, Flandrin G, Gemon M F 1973 Acute promyelocytic leukemia: results of treatment by Daunorubicin. Blood 41: 489–496
36 Shaw M T, Nordquist R E 1975 Pure monocytic or histiomonocytic leukemia, a revised concept. Cancer 35: 208–214
37 Scott C S 1978 Cytochemical applications in haematology, with particular reference to acute leukaemias: a review. Medical Laboratory Sciences 35: 111–136
38 Breton-Gorius J, Guichard J 1972 Ultrastructural localization of peroxidase activity in human platelets and megakaryocytes. American Journal of Pathology 66: 277–294
39 Flandrin G, Daniel M T, Valensi F, Schaison G, Breton-Gorius J 1977 Leucémie aiguë à mégacaryoblastes. Etude clinique et morphologique de 11 observations. Actualités hématologiques Masson edit. Paris 11: 200–212
40 Breton-Gorius J, Dreyfus B, Sultan C, Basch A, D'Oliviera J G 1972 Identification of circulating micromegakaryocytes in a case of refractory anemia: an electron microscopic cytochemical study. Blood 40: 453–463
41 Breton-Gorius J, Daniel M T, Flandrin G, Kinet-Denoel G 1973 Fine structure and peroxidase activity of circulating micromegakaryoblasts and platelets in a case of acute myelofibrosis. British Journal of Haematology 25: 331–339
42 Löffler H 1969 Zytochemische Klassifizierung der Akuten Leukosen in Chemo und Immunotherapie der Leukosen und malignen lymphoma Ed. Stacher Wien. Bohmann
43 Leder L D 1970 Akute myelo-monocytäre Leukämie mit atypischen Naphtol AS-D chloroacetate-Esterase positiven Eosinophilen. Acta Haematologica Basel 44: 52–62
44 Schaefer H E, Hellriegel K P, Hennekeuser H H, Hübner G, Zach J, Fischer R, Gross R 1973 Eosinophilenleukämie, eine unreifzellige Myelose mit chloroacetatesterase positiven Eosinophilie. Blut 26: 7–19
45 Flandrin G, Daniel M T 1974 Données actuelles sur la classification cytologique des leucémies aiguës. Bulletin du Cancer 61: 291–308
46 Liso V, Troccoli G, Specchia G, Magno M 1977 Cytochemical 'normal' and 'abnormal' eosinophiles in acute leukemia. American Journal of Hematology 2: 123–131
47 Quattrin N 1973 Leucémies aiguës à basophiles. Nouvelle Revue Française d'Hématologie 13: 745–754
48 Humphrey G B, Nesbit M E, Brunning R D 1974 Prognostic value of the PAS reaction in acute lymphoblastic leukemia. American Journal of Clinical Pathology 61: 393–397
49 Queiser W, Dietrich M, Finke J, Kubanek B, Neu G, Olischläger A, Heimpel H 1972 Vergleich Zwichen Cytologischer und cytochemischen Klassifizierung bei 47 fallen von akuter leukämie. Klinische Wochenschrift 50: 498–503
50 Catovsky D, Goldman J M, Okos A, Frisch B, Galton D A G 1974 T-Lymphoblastic leukaemia, a distinct variant of acute leukaemia. British Medical Journal ii: 634–636
51 Berard C, O'Connor G T, Thomas L B, Torloni H 1969 Histopathological definition of Burkitt's tumor. WHO Bulletin 40: 601

52 Wright D H 1963 Cytology and histochemistry of the Burkitt lymphoma. British Journal of Cancer 17: 50
53 Bennett J M, Dutcher J F 1969 The Cytochemistry of Acute Leukemias, observations on glycogen and neutral fat in bone marrow aspirates. Blood 33: 341–347
54 Pangalis G A, Nathwani B N, Rappaport H, Rosen R B 1979 Acute lymphoblastic leukemia. The significance of nuclear convolutions. Cancer 43: 551–557
55 Douglas S D, Cohnen E, Konig E, Brittinger E 1973 Lymphocyte lysosomes and lysosomal enzymes in chronic lymphocytic leukemia. Blood 32: 935–944
56 Flandrin G, Daniel M T 1974 Bêta-glucuronidase in Sézary cells. Scandinavian Journal of Haematology 12: 23–31
57 Brouet J C, Flandrin G, Sasportes M, Preud'homme J L, Seligmann M 1975 Chronic lymphocytic leukaemia of T-cell origin. Immunological and clinical evaluation in eleven patients. Lancet ii: 890–893
58 Preud'homme J L, Seligmann M 1972 Surface-bound immunoglobulins: a cell marker in human lymphoproliferative diseases. Blood 40: 777–794
59 Flandrin G Bêta-glucuronidase in B and T-CLL (unpublished observations)
60 Flandrin G, Brouet J C 1974 The Sézary cell, cytologic, cytochemical and immunologic studies. Mayo Clinic Proceedings 49: 575–583
61 Catovsky D 1977 Hairy cell leukaemia and prolymphocytic leukaemia. Clinics in Haematology 6: 245–268
62 Flandrin G, Daniel M T, Fourcade M, Chelloul N 1973 Leucémie à 'Tricholeucocytes' (Hairy cell leukaemia). Etude clinique et cytologique de 55 observations. Nouvelle Revue Française d'Hématologie 13: 609–640
63 Yam L T, Li C Y, Lam K W 1971 Tartrate-resistant acid phosphatase isoenzyme in the reticulum cells of leukemic reticulo-endotheliosis. New England Journal of Medicine 284: 357–360
64 Yam L T, Li C Y, Finkel H E 1972 Leukemic reticulo-endotheliosis. The role of tartrate-resistant acid phosphatase in diagnosis and splenectomy in treatment. Archives of Internal Medicine 130: 248–256
65 Katayama I, Li C Y, Yam L T 1971 Histochemical study of acid phosphatase iso-enzyme in leukemic reticulo-endotheliosis. Cancer 29: 157–164
66 Li C Y, Yam L T, Lam K W 1970 Studies of acid phosphatase isoenzymes in human leukocytes. Demonstration of iso-enzymes cell specificity. Journal of Histochemistry and Cytochemistry 18: 901–910
67 Li C Y, Lam K W, Yam L T 1973 Esterase in human leukocytes. Journal of Histochemistry and Cytochemistry 21: 1–12
68 Kass L 1977 Non specific esterase activity in 'Hairy cells'. Acta Haematologica 58: 103–107
69 Wachstein M 1946 Alkaline phosphatase activity in normal and abnormal human blood and bone marrow cells. Journal of Laboratory and Clinical Medicine 31: 1–17
70 Valentine W N, Beck W Q, Folette J H, Mills H, Lawrence J S 1952 Biochemical studies in chronic myelocytic leukemia, polycythemia vera and other idiopathic myeloproliferative disorders. Blood 7: 959–977
71 Tanaka K R, Valentine W N, Fredicks R E 1960 Diseases or clinical conditions associated with low alkaline phosphatase. New England Journal of Medicine 262: 912–918
72 Pederson B 1973 Periodic acid Schiff positive myeloblasts in chronic myelogenous leukaemia. Relation to karyotype evolution. Scandinavian Journal of Haematology 11: 112–121
73 Hammouda F, Quaglino D, Hayhoe F G J 1964 Blastic crisis in chronic granulocytic leukaemia. Cytological, cytochemical and autoradiographic studies of four cases. British Medical Journal i: 1275–1281
74 Castoldi E L, Grusovin E D, Scapoli E L 1975 Consecutive cytochemical staining for the analysis of the blastic population of the acute phase of chronic myeloid leukemia. Biomedecine 23: 12–16
75 Breton-Gorius J, Reyes F, Vernant J P, Tulliez M, Dreyfus B 1978 The blast crisis of chronic granulocytic leukaemia: megakaryoblastic nature of cells as revealed by the presence of platelet-peroxidase—a cytochemical ultrastructural study. British Journal of Haematology 39: 295–304
76 Hutton J J, Coleman M S 1976 Terminal deoxynucleotidyl transferase measurements in the differential diagnosis of adult leukemias. British Journal of Haematology 34: 447–456
77 Janossy G, Greaves M F, Revesz T, Lister T A, Roberts M, Durrant J, Kirk B, Catovsky D, Beard M E J 1976 Blast crisis of chronic myeloid leukaemia (CML). II Cell surface marker analysis of 'lymphoid' and myeloid cases. British Journal of Haematology 34: 179–192

3

Bone Marrow Histology

Rolf Burkhardt

INTRODUCTION

After the heydays of histomorphology, cytology and biochemistry, research in leukemia is now focused on the fields of cytogenesis and cytokinetics. Morphology can keep pace with these trends only to the extent of its ability to advance to the macromolecular scale, and by employing marker technics. However, the slogan of 'hematology without the microscope'[1] remains only an attractive antithesis as long as therapy and cure depend on diagnoses based on both visual and intellectual comprehension. And though the pathological aspects of leukemia are used mainly as diagnostic criteria, they are indeed integral components of the disease process, constituting its structural framework. Therefore, the aim of structural research is to arrive at both a nosological and a pathogenic diagnosis. The purpose of this chapter is to contribute to the attainment of this goal in the field of the leukemias.

   During the past 20 years there have been two major technical improvements in the histopathology of the human bone marrow: the introduction of biopsy of the iliac crest as a routine clinical procedure[2-5] and the production of semithin sections of undecalcified osseous specimens.[5-8] These have broadened the aspects of structural research in the following areas:

1. Quantitation of the parenchymal, stromal, fatty, and osseous tissues
2. Identification of the composition and quality of these tissues with their natural architecture undisturbed
3. Recognition of the structural alterations and their interrelationships in many different conditions.

Thereby several important features have been added to the morphological diagnosis of the leukemias:

1. Composition, localization, extent, and type of spread of the leukemic process
2. Changes in the parenchymal, stromal, fatty, and osseous components as direct or indirect consequences of the leukemia, e.g. immune reactions, angiogenesis, 'myelogenous' osteopathy, siderosis, sideropenia, protein deposits, fibrosis, atrophy and necrosis.

Recognition of these features may assist in the following diagnostic steps:

1. Differential diagnosis and staging
2. Diagnosis of preleukemia and identification of subgroups and complications

3. Prognostic evaluation and monitoring of therapy
4. Recognition of incidental and concomitant conditions, such as tuberculosis, sarcoidosis, osteoporosis, osteomalacia, hyperparathyroidism, Paget's disease, arteriosclerosis, arteritis, and possibly an additional neoplasm.

METHODS

HISTOBIOPSY

Site

In general, the ilium is representative of osseous structure and red marrow as found in the vertebra and sternum, and will reflect deviations due to generalized disease processes.[9,6,10] Moreover, biopsies from this region carry the least risk to the patient and can be performed in children from 1 year of age onwards. In bedridden patients, there is less likelihood of decubitus and contamination after biopsies from the anterior than from the posterior iliac crest. Should bleeding occur it causes less discomfort, and there is no danger of irritation of the sciatic nerves. In our outpatients' clinic, the biopsies are taken routinely from the anterior iliac crest; approximately 6000 have been performed to date. Moreover, our laboratory has processed an additional 12 000 biopsies sent to us from the surrounding districts. We have been unable to detect morphological differences between biopsies taken from the anterior or the posterior ilium. From the point of view of both patient and operator, the anterior iliac crest may be considered the site of preference. As the anterior crest is slightly broader than the posterior, it is always used for taking drill biopsies, i.e. myelotomy.

Technics

There are three technics currently employed to obtain biopsy specimens:

1. Aspiration with subsequent sections of fragments and clots as well as smears[11-13]
2. Needle biopsy: usually longitudinal puncture, with the Jamshidi needle, of the posterior or anterior iliac crest, and sections of the decalcified paraffin embedded specimens[14]
3. Trephine biopsy of the anterior iliac crest, either transverse[15] or longitudinal.[5] The specimens are then either decalcified and embedded in paraffin, or embedded in plastic (methacrylate) without decalcification.[6]

The advantages and disadvantages of the first two technics (aspiration and puncture biopsies) as well as their modifications have been extensively described and reviewed elsewhere.[6,16,13] Only the third, the myelotomy or drill biopsy, will be described in detail here. We prefer the drill biopsy for the following reasons: (1) Performed with sufficient care and skill the discomfort to the patient is hardly, if at all, greater than that caused by needle biopsy. (2) Though the performance of a drill biopsy is somewhat more time consuming, the yield is greater (Fig. 3.1). Note that the surface area of one section from a myelotomy specimen corresponds roughly to that of three needle biopsies. This ratio becomes even greater if the surface area of the needle biopsies is reduced by

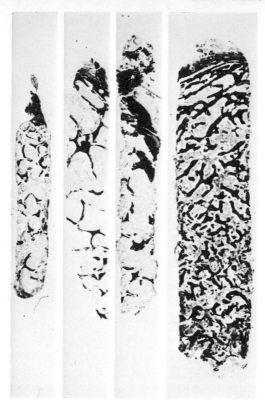

Fig. 3.1 Comparative sections from iliac crest biopsies. Three Jamshidi-needle biopsies, left; myelotomy, right. ($\times 50$)

pressure artifacts due to especially hard or soft bones; such pressure effects are minimized by drilling. (3) One section of a large area gives more reliable information about the structural composition than two or three disconnected sections. (4) The patient is less likely to object to a repeat biopsy after a single, rather than multiple interventions.

MYELOTOMY OR DRILL BIOPSY

Instruments

The appliance comprises a drill plus a set of instruments (manufactured by Institut Dr R. Straumann A.G., CH-4437 Waldenburg, Switzerland). The electromechanical drive makes the drilling a relatively fast, non-traumatic and safe procedure. The set of instruments (Figs 3.2 and 3.3) includes a scalpel (1) for incision of the skin; a funnel (2) for exposing the periosteal surface and to act as a guide and brake for the drill and the other instruments; a hollow punch (3) for the preparation of the periosteum; drills (4) for the trepanation; and a pair of tongs (5) to extract the biopsy. The pincers are used to find the correct location for the funnel, to insert the hemostyptic pellets, and to clip the wound. The instruments are housed in a stainless steel container, which can be sterilized. The drill can be sterilized as a whole after removal of the motor. This has a

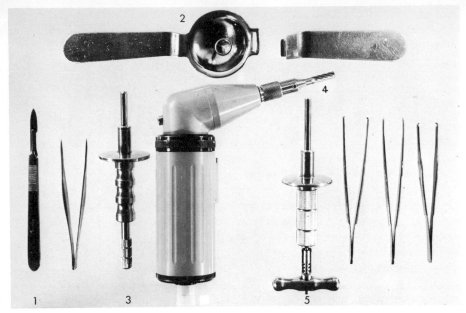

Fig. 3.2 The instrument set for myelotomy, ready for use (see text).

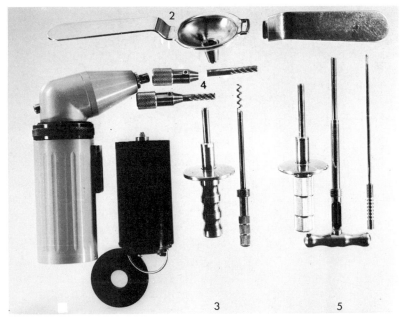

Fig. 3.3 The instruments for myelotomy, dismantled (see text).

power of 14 W and a voltage of 40 V. It is operated at a speed of 2800 r/min, which is reduced by a mechanical gear to 465 r/min to avoid artifacts due to heating and crushing. The drills are made of stainless steel. They have an internal diameter of 4 mm at the cutting edge, widening upwards in a cone-like fashion to prevent crushing of the specimen during operation of the drill. The cutting edges are directed outwards to deflect the debris caused by drilling. To facilitate sharpening and exchange, the cutting edges can be detached from the socket on which they are mounted, and which connects them to the spindle of the motor.

Procedure for myelotomy (Fig. 3.4)

The patient lies on his (her) back on a firm bed. The pelvis is firmly supported at the side of the intervention. Sedation is given beforehand if required. Local anesthesia is performed after disinfection of the skin; the iliac crest and its medial and lateral surfaces are infiltrated with about 10 to 20 ml of 1 per cent lignocaine-solution. When the area is anesthesized an incision of 1 to 1.5 cm is made approximately 3 cm above the anterior superior iliac spine, parallel to the lateral crestal margin. The subcutaneous soft tissues are carefully dissected with the scalpel until the periosteal surface is reached. Then the funnel is introduced through the incision and positioned on the middle of the crest, guided by the pincers, and the sharp serrated edges of the funnel are firmly anchored to the surface of the bone by manual pressure. The punch, with the scraper inside it, is introduced into the funnel, and with a few swift rotary motions the connective tissue is loosened from the surface of the bone and removed by a swab after withdrawal of the punch. Then the drill is applied through the funnel which allows it to penetrate to a depth of about 20 mm into the bone. Normally this can be done without pressure. The drill must be carefully guided when

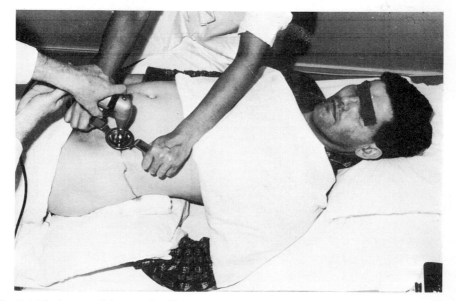

Fig. 3.4 Myelotomy of the anterior iliac crest.

the bone is unusually soft. To avoid heating, e.g. when there is osteosclerosis, the drilling may be discontinuous. The time of actual drilling is $\pm$ 10 s. When the correct depth has been reached, the drill is withdrawn while still rotating. Then the tongs are gently inserted over the drilled specimen and closed by rotation of the outer shell. To avoid crushing the contents, the handle should not be rotated. The tongs, with the specimen inside, are then extracted with a brisk pull. The tongs are opened and the tissue is pushed out with a plunger. The specimen, i.e. the cylinder or the core, is immediately immersed in the fixative. Alternatively it may be cut into two longitudinal halves by a simple device (Fig. 3.5).[17] One half is fixed for embedding into methacrylate, the other is used

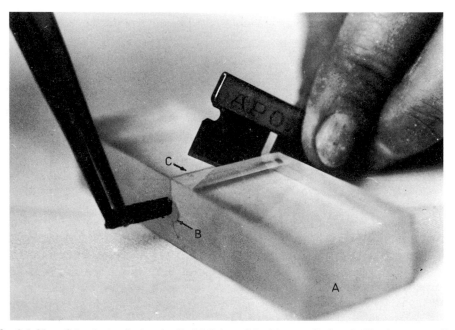

Fig. 3.5 Use of the device for longitudinal halving of the biopsy cylinder. A, Plastic support. B, Longitudinal hole for insertion of cylinder. C, Slit-like aperture for the razor to halve the biopsy without undue pressure.

for electronmicroscopy and histochemistry. For all cytological investigations, bone marrow is also obtained by aspiration from the biopsy site and films are prepared.

Two or three hemostyptic pellets (Topostasin, Hoffmann-La Roche A.G., Basel, Switzerland) are inserted into the biopsy site and the funnel is removed. The wound is closed either by a clip or one suture, covered by a sterile dressing, and protected by adhesive plaster. After 3 days the suture or clip is removed. When the condition of the patient permits, the biopsy is performed in the out-patients' clinic. The patient is advised to stay in bed for 24 h and to rest at home for 1 day after that. To alleviate postoperative pain analgesics may be required. If there is a hemorrhagic diathesis, elastic bandages, about 15 cm wide, are applied around the pelvic girdle immediately after the biopsy. When the risk of infection is high or when, exceptionally, the biopsy is to be taken from unusual sites, the procedure may be performed in an operating theater.

Subcutaneous hemorrhages, secondary wound healing due to infections, and the need for secondary surgical revision of the wound were extremely rare in our experience. Therefore the myelotomy can be considered as a comparatively safe procedure, since it was performed in all patients who would otherwise have been eligible for sternal puncture (including cases with thrombocytopenia and pancytopenia). The risk of bleeding is highest in cases of polycythemia and osteomyelosclerosis.

Indications

Myelotomy is contraindicated: (1) when the patient's condition does not allow any intervention and (2) in patients with hemophilia. Myelotomy is indicated in all cases of leukemia; in particular, at the time of the initial diagnosis and before therapy is given. Therapy may be monitored by means of aspirations, needle biopsy or myelotomy, as required and as the patient's condition permits.

HISTOLOGICAL METHODS

A modification of the technic of Boellaard and Hirsch[18] developed in our laboratory is used.[5-7] The specimen is fixed in a mixture of formaldehyde 40 per cent and absolute methanol with addition of buffer solution: formaldehyde 40 per cent 50 ml, methanol absolute 96 ml, glucose phosphate pH 7.4 0.4 ml. Then it is dehydrated in absolute methanol, six changes in 24 h. The significant advantage of this fixative consists of the speedy and homogeneous fixation with the exact degree of denaturation which is required for the subsequent embedding in plastic.[7,8] Following dehydration, the specimen is transferred into a mixture of methyl-methacrylic acid monomer and nonylphenol-polyglycoletheracetate (Plastoid N[R], Röhm Pharma GmbH, Darmstadt, Germany) an additive which improves the homogeneity of the polymerization in a tissue rich in fat, and the physical condition necessary for the cutting, without causing hygroscopy. The polymerization is catalyzed by benzoyl-peroxyde. This substance is explosive. It has to be dried very carefully and in small amounts before use. These three are the components of the embedding mixture which has to be prepared freshly before use: Methyl-methacrylic acid monomer, destablized 100.0 ml, Plastoid N 25.0 ml, Benzoyl peroxide 3.5 g. After evaporation the polymerization is initiated in a water bath at 46°C for 50 min, then finished at a temperature of 34°C for about 24 h. Six days are required from the biopsy to the stained sections. The volumetric changes of splenic tissue handled in this way are ±5 per cent of its fresh state, measured in two dimensions.[19] Decalcification of bone is unnecessary because of the hornlike quality of the plastic embedding medium. A heavy duty microtome is required for cutting the sections. Serial sections of 3 μm are cut and stained with gallaminblue-Giemsa, with PAS-, with Berlin-blue and according to Gomori or Ladewig. Details of these methods have been reported previously.[6,7] By comparison of the sections at light- and electronmicroscopic level it has been shown that good cellular preservation is combined with the extensive areas of observation afforded by lightmicroscopy.

GENERAL PATHOLOGY OF LEUKEMIA IN BONE MARROW BIOPSIES

Localization, spread, and relationship to the vascular system

As part of the axial skeleton, the bone marrow in the iliac crest is regularly involved in leukemia. We have seen only one case of leukemia without marrow involvement in this region in over 1500 leukemic patients studied. On the other hand, in 227 cases with evidence of acute leukemia in the iliac crest biopsy, the clinical and hematological picture was not diagnostic of leukemia.

To recognize the different types of leukemic spread in the bone marrow it is necessary to study the early stages of its development. The less developed, and the more undifferentiated the leukemic process, the more prominent are

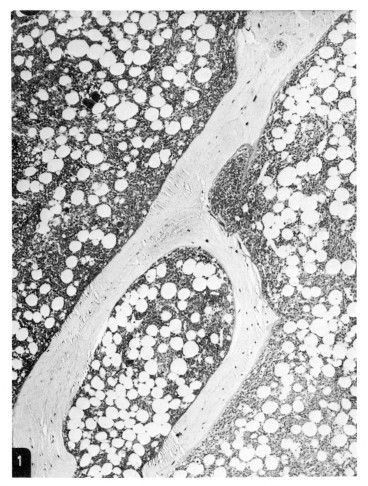

Fig. 3.6 Myelomonocytic leukemia, peritrabecular localisation. (Gallaminblue-Giemsa × 38)

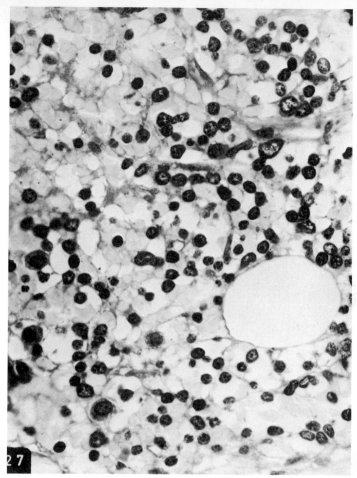

Fig. 3.7 Early stage of childhood acute lymphoblastic leukemia. Note the interstitial localization of the blast cells, the absence of normal hematopoiesis and the disintegration of the sinusoidal capillaries. (Gallaminblue-Giemsa ×375)

the isolated clusters of malignant cells in sections of bone marrow biopsies. In the myeloid leukemias, these clusters are found primarily in the peritrabecular marrow and in the vicinity of arterioles and arterial capillaries, so that character-istic cuff-like infiltrations of these areas are formed as the disease progresses. This applies especially to myelomonocytic leukemia (Fig. 3.6). However, in childhood acute leukemia, the infiltrations are diffuse, without a characteristic localization (Fig. 3.7). In the immature erythroblastic and megakaryoblastic forms of leukemia in adults, mantle-shaped infiltrations are found around the marrow sinusoids, in some of which immature megakaryocytes have replaced the endothelial cells. Within the sinusoidal lumen groups of megakaryo- and erythroblasts showing many mitotic figures may be found. A similar picture of intrasinusoidal proliferation of malignant cells may be found in metastatic carcinoma.

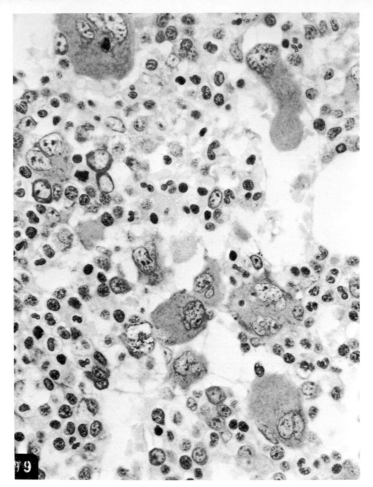

Fig. 3.8 Polycythemia: perisinusoidal origin of erythroblasts and megakaryocytes. The megakaryocytes, varying in size and shape, are grouped mainly along the endothelial borders of the sinusoids, together with erythroblasts. (Gallaminblue-Giemsa ×375)

In contrast with this, differentiated myeloid leukemias show a diffuse infiltration with cells at all stages of maturation. This complicates the histological distinction between the early stages of these leukemias and myeloid hyperplasia. In chronic myeloid leukemia (CML) characteristic cellular proliferations are located in the peritrabecular and percapillary regions of the marrow with a gradient of immature to mature cells directed to the central intertrabecular marrow spaces. A distinct but similar pattern of cellular production is found in polycythemia: i.e. erythropoiesis and megakaryocytopoiesis close to the sinusoids (Fig. 3.8), and granulopoiesis in peritrabecular and perivascular regions of arterial capillaries and arterioles. In certain forms of chronic lymphatic leukemia (CLL), the infiltrations also occur close to the sinusoids; in the majority of the malignant lymphomas and in plasmocytomas, the cells are concentrated initially in the peritravecular regions.[20,21] In rare cases of plasma-cell leukemia and malignant lymphoma, the leukemic clusters are found almost exclusively within the sinusoids, suggesting their immigration from extramedullary sites.[21]

It has been demonstrated that these topographical correlations between leukemic infiltrations and the stromal compartment resemble those of normal hematopoiesis. As previously reported both normal and hyperplastic erythropoiesis and megakaryocytopoiesis take place in the vicinity of the marrow sinusoids;[22,23] while granulopoiesis is found in peritrabecular and pericapillary zones.[24,25] In addition, observations have been made which indicate that these relationships may well be based on some functional cooperation, either concerning nutritive supply or, rather, the dependance of common inductive factors. In CML there may be a 10-fold increase in the number of arterial capillaries, which accompany the leukemic infiltration. In polycythemia rubra vera all vascular compartments, and especially the sinusoids, are increased in number.[26-28] A study of serial sections of biopsies from cases of megakaryocytic leukemia suggests a direct origin of megakaryoblasts from the endothelial cells of the sinusoids.[29]

Summary and conclusion
There are indications that certain bone marrow regions are consistently involved in the majority of leukemias. In CML, and in polycythemia rubra vera the cellular hyperplasia is accompanied by the simultaneous proliferation of components of the capillary circulation. There are close microanatomical relationships between normal as well as leukemic hematopoiesis on one side and the endothelial cells of the sinusoids and arterial capillaries on the other. This relationship provides additional significance to the so-called 'milieu' or hematopoietic microenvironment.[30,31] The leukemias can also be regarded initially as neoplasias of fixed tissues requiring a special vascular stroma. As more histobioptic data are accumulated, their evaluation is likely to prove of considerable prognostic and therapeutic significance.

Preleukemia, aleukemia, immune reaction and relapse
The denomination of preleukemia include cases of aregenerative anemia either with an aplastic or hyperplastic bone marrow that later are recognized as leukemia, usually of the acute myeloid type (AML).[32-34] Gralnick et al[35] have discussed especially the differential diagnosis of myelodysplastic syndromes and preleukemia. The question arises as to whether there are characteristic hematologic anomalies with an increased statistical chance of developing leukemia. We have studied 59 myelotomies from 28 patients suffering from 'preleukemia'. All 28 later developed leukemia as demonstrated in the peripheral blood and in follow-up biopsies. The leukemias were classified as follows: AML in 14 cases, acute promyelocytic in 5, acute myelomonocytic in 4, megakaryoblastic myelosis in 2, undifferentiated leukemia in 2 and the mixed type of AML in 1 case. Sixteen patients were over 60 years of age; 7 were between 20 years and 59 years; and 5 were less than 10 years old. The interval between the diagnosis of 'preleukemia' and the manifestation of leukemia was 2 to 14 m. Figures 3.9 and 3.10 show the development of preleukemia into myeloblastic leukemia. A comparison of

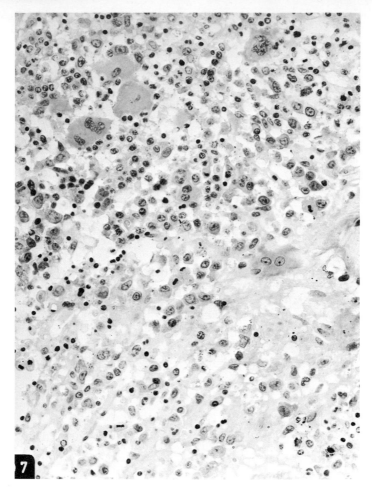

Fig. 3.9 Preleukemic stage. Edematous changes, endothelial disintegration, plasmacytic infiltration and lack of mature granulocytes. (Gallaminblue-Giemsa × 190)

the biopsies from these cases with 86 biopsies from patients in the early stages of leukemia, has failed to establish reliable criteria to distinguish between these two groups. Therefore, preleukemia may be considered as the oligosymptomatic, aleukemic phase of acute leukemia, more readily detectable by histobiopsy than by examination of aspirates, buffy coats or peripheral blood. In both groups we found a considerable decrease in myelopoiesis with a corresponding increase in fatty tissue, together with infiltration of lymphocytes and plasma cells. This bone marrow picture differs from that in aplastic anemia by the presence of scattered foci of leukemic blast cells, located especially in the endosteal and perivascular regions. Such foci can easily be overlooked. Figures 3.11 and 3.12 give examples of this situation in a case of AML. The early stages of leukemia are consistently characterized by features similar to these of an immune reactive marrow aplasia. This gives the impression that the agent which caused the leukemia may at the same time have blocked the normal cellular proliferation, rather than a factor released by the leukemic cells. Once the

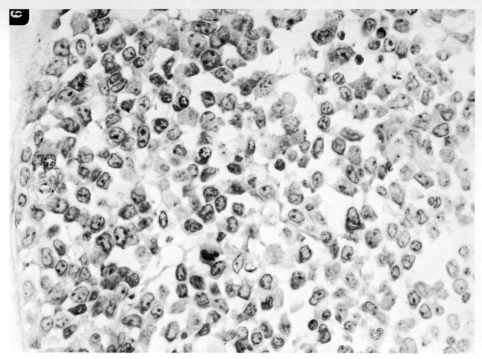

Fig. 3.10 Acute myeloblastic leukemia, fully developed. Note homogeneous marrow infiltration with slightly pleomorphic myeloblasts. Same patient as in Figure 3.9, 4 months later.

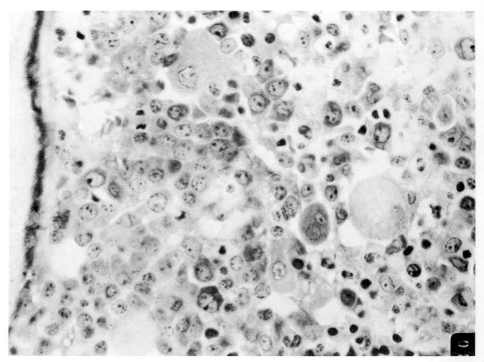

Fig. 3.11 Acute leukemia, initial stage. The peritrabecular localization of blast cells is seen on the left side of the picture. (Gallaminblue-Giemsa ×375)

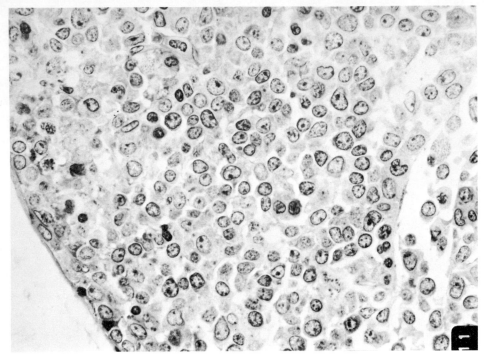

Fig. 3.12 Acute leukemia; same patient as Figure 3.11, repeat biopsy 8 months later. Note that the peritrabecular areas now show a homogeneous infiltration of myeloblasts.

leukemic cells have replaced the normal myelopoiesis, an empty marrow is only observed as a consequence of cytostatic treatment: in this case it closely resembles preleukemic aplasia. The possibility of recognizing small leukemic foci in the biopsy sections constitutes one major indication for histo-biopsy; another is to monitor treatment and to confirm remission.

From our experience, 86 per cent of the pancytopenic syndromes which occur in the course of acute leukemia (aleukemic phase) are due to replacement of the hematopoietic tissue by the leukemic cells. In this group the diagnosis is only established by histobiopsy. A massive leukemic infiltration of the bone marrow may be accompanied by inflammatory cells such as lymphocytes, plasma cells, mast cells, macrophages and eosinophils together with necrotic leukemic cells in variable frequency and degree. Moreover, the role of these elements in the (possible) immunologic response to the leukemic process is unknown.

Myelofibrosis (MF) and osteomyelosclerosis (OMS)

Inflammatory reactions in the bone marrow have frequently been described in cases of MF occurring in the course of chronic leukemias of mixed cellular type. It has long been recognized that the complication of a myeloproliferative disorder with tuberculosis may significantly accelerate the development of myelofibrosis.[36, 37] We have observed a correlation between various stromal components and MF and OMS (Table 3.1).[37] In addition characteristic vascular changes have also been observed (Table 3.2). There are significant

Table 3.1 Stromal changes of the bone marrow in myelofibrosis and osteomyelosclerosis

Histological features	Myelofibrosis $n = 100^a$	Osteomyelosclerosis $n = 100^a$
Marked increase of (semiquantitatively):		
Collagenous fibers	28	63
Eosinophilic granulocytes	39	21
Plasma cells	33	29
Lymphocytes	24	21
Histiocytes with siderin	13	18
Tissue mast cells (counts per 100 mm²)^b	420	737

^{a} n = total number of cases investigated.
^{b} Normal: 160 : 150 (25 biopsies).

Table 3.2 Vascular changes of the bone marrow in myelofibrosis and osteomyelosclerosis

Vascular compartment	Cross sections/100 mm² (averages)		
	Myelofibrosis $n = 100$	Osteomyelosclerosis $n = 104$	Normal controls $n = 30$
Arteries	36	51	24
Arterioles	145	222	58
Arterial capillaries	544	946	253
Sinus	1156	2603	2939

differences between these cases and the normal: there is an increase in the arterial compartment and a decrease in the number of the sinuses.

It seems justified, therefore, to attribute a pathogenic, fibrogenic, effect to the inflammatory reactions, directed against products of the myeloproliferation. The arterial hypervascularization may also be stimulated by the basic myeloproliferation, as well as by the inflammation. However, the most prominent feature of the different leukemic processes that may develop into myelofibrosis is the increase in megakaryocytes, with an average count of 4739/100 mm² compared to the normal of 759/100 mm². Significant correlations between bone marrow fibrosis and other features have been found for necrotic megakaryocytes, edema and mast cells in the group of MF, and for capillaries and plasma cells in OMS. In 41 biopsies from 18 cases of CML, and 169 biopsies from 58 cases of polycythemia (two to seven biopsies in the course of 2 to 15 years), a statistically significant correlation was observed between the degree of fibrosis and the increase in the number of atypical megakaryocytes. There was no correlation between fibrosis, duration of the disease or treatment with ^{32}P. Figures 3.13 and 3.14 illustrate the development of myelofibrosis in CML.

Summary
Myelofibrosis and osteomyelosclerosis are special forms of a stromal reaction common to all leukemias with megakaryocytic proliferation. The pathogenesis is complex. Most probably megakaryocytes and necrotic and inflammatory

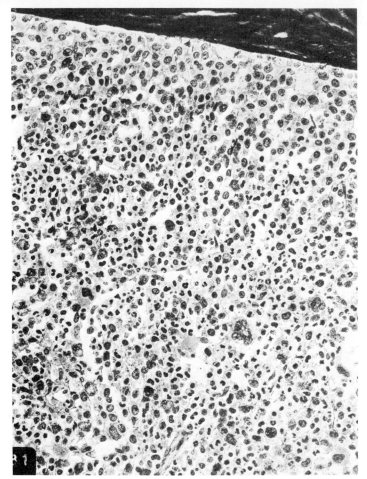

Fig. 3.13 Chronic myeloid leukemia; later developing myelofibrosis. (Gomori stain × 190)

changes in the stroma are involved. Myelofibrosis and osteomyelosclerosis are diagnosed on the basis of biopsy sections which enable the distinction to be made between the aplastic anemia picture of leukemic disorders and MF or OMS.

Myelogenous osteopathy

Since the bone depends on the marrow for its nutrition, it is to be expected that the leukemic marrow changes will affect the skeleton and especially the trabecular bone. Acute leukemia in infancy leads to anomalies of growth, to osteoporosis, and to spontaneous fractures. Osteoporosis is also found in adults, mainly in CML and in polycythemia. These aberrations could be regarded as 'consumptive osteopathies': the angiogenic stroma having been usurped by the leukemic growth.[25, 38, 39] Other types of myelogenous osteodysplasias such as osteosclerosis and paraneoplastic osteodystrophy are rarely seen in the leukemias.

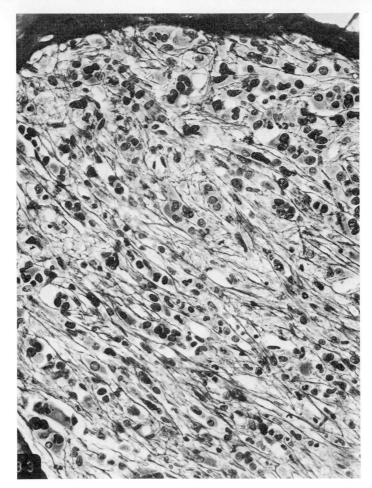

Fig. 3.14 Chronic myeloid leukemia, now myelofibrosis. The fiber bundles are arranged mainly along the capillaries; they are separated by strands of immature and atypical megakaryocytes. Same patient as in Figure 3.13, 1 year later.

The histological diagnosis of a 'myelogenous osteopathy' in leukemia carries a diagnostic and, in some cases, a therapeutic significance. It contributes to the understanding of the stromal changes of leukemia, which have not yet been clarified.

SPECIAL PATHOLOGY

ACUTE LEUKEMIAS (AL)

The accepted classifications of the undifferentiated leukemias, usually called 'acute', are based on cytological criteria.[35, 40–45] Whilst the separation of myeloid and lymphoid types is recognized as of prognostic and therapeutic importance, the relevance of the recognition of subtypes is still under discussion. Interesting results have been published by Mathé et al.[46,47] It is expected that the recognition of additional features demonstrated with enzymatic, genetic, kinetic, and immunological methods will contribute to a better understanding of the pathogenesis.

It has long been considered that bone marrow biopsy in acute leukemias should be confined to cases with an aleukemic blood picture and when attempts at marrow aspiration have been unsuccessful.[48] These indications could now well be extended to include other problems in the pathology of the leukemias, for example the acute leukemias in childhood and adult age known to have a different prognosis. Moreover, in many cases, bone marrow aspirates may not give representative and reproducible results. Consequently there are divergent views in the literature on a number of potentially significant parameters, especially those which require quantitation. Biopsies could provide additional information on (1) the extent as well as the prognostic significance of bone marrow

Table 3.3 Acute leukemia—histobiopsy, clinical signs and cytopenia

Diagnosis from histobiopsy	Number of cases	Cases with positive histobiopsy and insignificant clinical signs of leukemia (%)*	Erroneous histobioptic diagnosis (%)	Cases with pancytopenia	Histobiopsy	
					Hypocellular (%)	Hypercellular (%)
AML including promyelocytic leukemia	180	82	2	125	11	89
ALL = acute lymphoblastic leukemia	20	40	0	4	0	100
AMML = acute myelomonocytic leukemia	38	73	2	27	29	71
AEL = acute erythroblastic and megakaryoblastic leukemia	13	61	15	12	16	84
ALL = acute undifferentiated leukemia	47	74	0	32	18	82
Total	298			200		

*No leukemic blood picture or organ enlargement.

lymphocytosis in the childhood ALL.[49–51] (2) The evaluation of remissions in leukemia; Oshima[52] has stated that there must be fewer than $5000/mm^3$ leukemic cells in films of bone marrow aspirates for restitution of normal hematopoiesis to occur. Generally the absence of leukemic cells in smears of marrow aspirates is accepted as the main criterion for complete remission. But this may not reflect the true situation in the bone marrow. (3) Progressive eosinopenia of the marrow is thought to be an unfavourable prognostic sign.[53] (4) No correlation with prognosis or the course of the disease is attributed to myelofibrosis in ALL by Haan et al.[54] (5) Nor has the morphological classification of the adult forms of AML led to reliable criteria for the choice of specific therapeutic modalities.[55]

Thus it would be advantageous to utilize biopsies on a wider scale; especially when quantitative or structural problems have to be studied. The following histological features may readily be investigated in every biopsy, and may then form the basis for comparative evaluations:

1. Quantitation of the hemoblastic infiltration with respect to erythropoiesis, granulopoiesis, megakaryocytes, and fatty tissue
2. Qualitative evaluation of the cellular type of the leukemic infiltration, its composition, localization and boundaries, its relationship to the capillary system, to the components of the stromal reaction, including fibrous and osseous elements, inflammatory cells, and necrosis.

Our observations in AL are based on biopsies from 298 cases including 29 cases who underwent repeat biopsies during the course of the disease (Table 3.3). The data presented in this table demonstrate the diagnostic significance of the biopsies, especially in the uncharacteristic cases, and also show the relative frequency of a hypercellular marrow combined with a peripheral cytopenia. In AL marrow fibrosis is not involved in the cytopenia. In AML, mostly in adults, there is a high incidence of significant histological results. ALL in children has the highest rate of positive diagnosis and of hypercellular marrows. The results

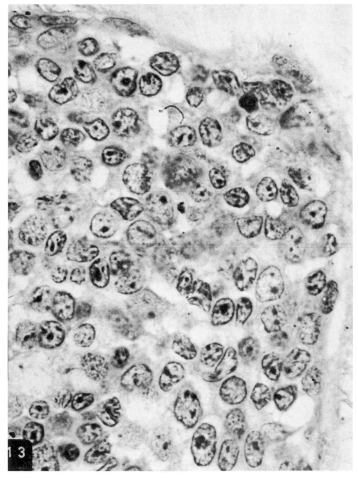

Fig. 3.15 Acute leukemia, undifferentiated type. Dense marrow infiltration with small blast cells, many with indented nuclei. (Gallaminblue–Giemsa × 750)

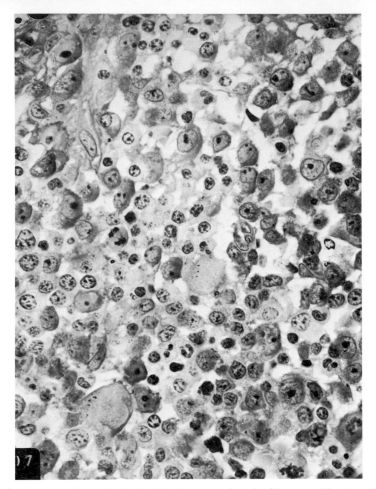

Fig. 3.16 Acute erythroblastic leukemia. Massive atypical erythroblastic proliferation with numerous mitoses and multinucleated forms, mainly located around the marrow capillaries. (Gallaminblue-Giemsa × 345)

in AMML indicate its prolonged course. In AEL histobiopsy is not necessarily diagnostic. The number of undifferentiated leukemias in our series is comparatively low, suggesting that histobiopsy contributes to a more precise classification in AL. Figures 3.15 to 3.17 give examples of the cytomorphologic characteristics of some AL, including unusual forms.

We have investigated 18 cases of AL in remission, as judged by hematological criteria. In biopsies from 6 of the cases a complete remission was confirmed, but in 12 cases the remission proved to be only partial. Kawada[56] has reported that in 7 cases of AML in complete clinical remission, blastic islands were found in the biopsy sections. Therefore it is advisable to perform at least one biopsy after the induction of remission in AL. The indication for histobiopsy in AL include:

1. Differential diagnosis of early aleukemic and aplastic stages from other neo-

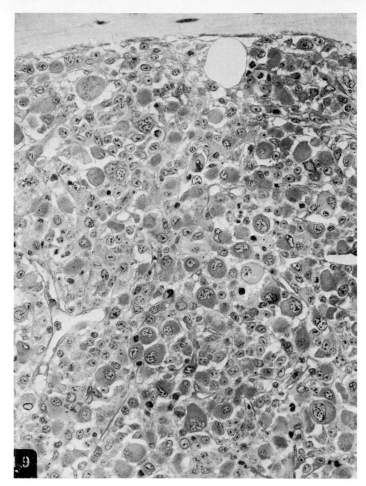

Fig. 3.17 Acute megakaryoblastic leukemia (transformation of CML). The marrow is replaced with megakaryoblasts and immature megakaryocytes; hyperplasia of capillaries. (Gallaminblue-Giemsa × 190)

plasia, such as small cell carcinoma, Ewing's sarcoma, neuroblastoma and Hodgkin's disease
2. Differential diagnosis of the non-leukemic types of erythroblastosis, megakaryoblastosis, and megakaryocytic myelosis
3. Diagnosis in cases when aspiration has failed
4. Confirmation of therapeutic remission and relapse.

Figures 3.18 and 3.19 illustrate the histologic confirmation of incomplete and of complete remission in AML and ALL respectively.

Summary
Histobiopsy provides morphological criteria which supplement the cytological evaluation of the acute leukemias. It also provides a reflection of the extent of the leukemic infiltration in the bone marrow and of the residual hematopoiesis.

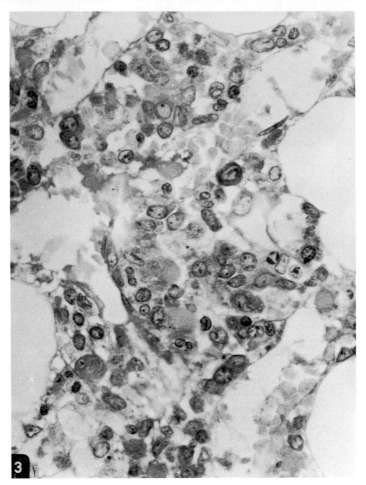

Fig. 3.18 Acute myeloblastic leukemia; incomplete remission after therapy. Hematopoiesis largely diminished. Myeloblastic foci close to capillaries, 6 months after initiation of therapy. (Gallaminblue-Giemsa ×375)

Biopsy sections show the cause—proliferative, fibrotic or aplastic—for a dry tap. Histobiopsy may reveal the presence of secondary diseases and provide reliable criteria for monitoring remission as well as relapse of the disease.

DIFFERENTIATED CHRONIC LEUKEMIAS

The histopathologist hesitates to use the common distinction of acute and chronic leukemias because of the discordance between the maturity and differentiation of the leukemic cells and the course of the disease. This is especially true for the so-called juvenile types of CML, the promyelocytic and the eosinophilic leukemias. Because of the rich morphological variations attributable to different stages of cellular development and maturity, the differentiated leukemias offer numerous starting points for structural descriptions. Using only morphological parameters of clinical significance we arrived at the classification

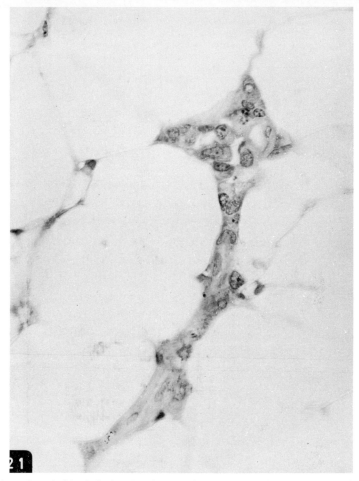

Fig. 3.19 Acute lymphoblastic leukemia, therapeutic remission (before regeneration). Marrow devoid of hematopoietic elements. A few promyelocytes, lymphocytes and plasma cells are located close to the capillaries. ($\times$375)

which is presented in Table 3.4. In this group the transport of cells from the bone marrow into the blood depends not only on the maturity of the cells but also on the state of the interstitial tissue and the endothelial lining of the sinusoids.

Histobiopsy can contribute to:

1. The differential diagnosis of the types, groups and subgroups
2. Diagnosis of the early stages
3. Evaluation of the potential for normal hematopoiesis
4. Recognition of blastic, fibrotic, aplastic, vascular, inflammatory, necrotic and osseous complications.

The duration of the disease process alters the diagnostic parameters. Histobiopsy has documented the transitions into blastic crises, the development of terminal fibrosis as well as the transition of one type of myeloproliferative

Table 3.4 Histobiopsy classification of differentiated (chronic) leukemias[a]

Diagnosis	Histological type
Chronic myeloid leukemia = CML $n = 250$	1. Mature, predominantly neutrophilic, with increase of megakaryocytes 2. Mature, neutrophilic, megakaryocytes normal or diminished 3. Predominantly eosinophilic 4. Predominantly basophilic 5. With increase of immature megakaryocytes 6. With increase of polymorphous megakaryocytes 7. With increase of myelocytes of promyelocytes 8. With increase of blast-cells
Megakaryocytic myelosis = MM $n = 60$	1. Mature, with moderate polymorphism ⎱ = IT; idiopathic 2. Partially immature, with marked polymorphism ⎰ thrombocythemia 3. Immature—polymorphous ⎱ = 'aleukemic' megakaryoblastic myelosis 4. Immature—blastic ⎰
Mixed cellular myelosis = MCM $n = 150$	1. Promyelocytic—megakaryocytic 2. Erythroblastic—promyelocytic—megakaryocytic
Polycythemia vera = PV $n = 209$	1. Typical generalized hyperplasia 2. With prominent polymorphous megakaryocytosis
Chronic lymphatic leukemia = CLL $n = 253$	1. Follicular 2. Diffuse—mature 3. Diffuse—immature 4. Lymphocytic—immunocytic

[a] Observations from our laboratories, literature not included.

disorder into another.[37] Cooperative studies are required to evaluate the prognostic and therapeutic significance of the morphologic classifications. The histobioptic features of the main groups are considered in the following sections.

Chronic myeloid leukemia—CML

Our observations are based on biopsies from 415 cases, including 31 who underwent repeat biopsies. The mitotic activity in the bone marrow is higher than in extramedullary sites of this disease.[57-59]

   CML in the bone marrow is characterized by:

1. Increase in granulopoietic parenchyma together with an early decrease in erythropoiesis and an increase in megakaryocytopoiesis (though occasionally a decrease in megakaryocytes is seen)
2. The promyelocytic cellular proliferation originates in the peritrabecular and perivascular marrow areas with maturation of the granulocytes proceeding outwards from these regions
3. Increase in the number of arteriolar and capillary cross-sections per mm²
4. Eosinophilia and plasmacytosis
5. Osteoporosis due to diversion of the capillary supply by the leukemia
6. Tendency to myelofibrosis and osteomyelosclerosis, i.e. increase in fibrous tissue and the presence of woven bone
7. Development of AML and AMML in some of the cases.

Statistical analysis of our cases has revealed a correlation between granulopoiesis and the peripheral blood cell count,[60] though Dancey & Vadnais-Metz[61] did not find such a correlation in their study of 7 cases. In our cases there was also a correlation between the increase in number and the atypia of the megakaryocytes, marrow fibrosis and splenic enlargement. All these parameters increased during the course of the disease. However, it should be noted that Ph[1] positive cases, as well as women, have, on average, a larger number of megakaryocytes than the corresponding groups, i.e. Ph[1] negative and men.

The histological picture does not change greatly during the course of the disease, even following treatment. Watanabe[62] has reported a slight regression of the hyperplasia and thus a normalization in the proportion of immature granulopoiesis in 15 cases who went into remission after therapy. We have studied initial and follow-up biopsies in 18 cases and have not found a relationship between the duration of the disease, the therapy and the development of fibrosis. Nine cases had a consistently normal or an inconsistent fiber content, while

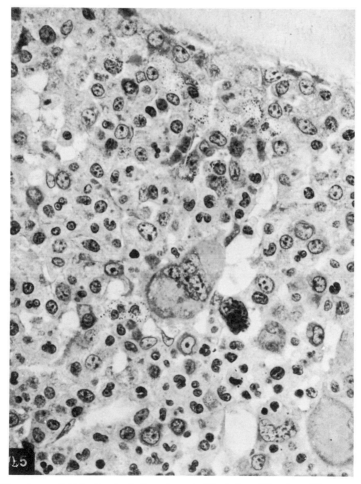

Fig. 3.20 Chronic myeloid leukemia, before therapy. Typical proliferation of immature granulocytes with many eosinophils and a few myeloblasts close to the bone. Progressive maturation of the granulocytes near the center of the marrow spaces. (Gallaminblue-Giemsa ×375)

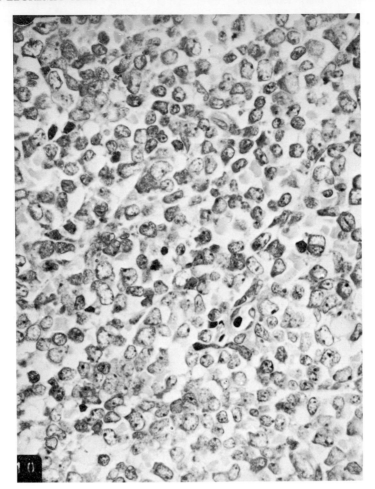

Fig. 3.21 Chronic myeloid leukemia (Ph¹ positive) in myeloblastic crisis. The typical marrow picture shows the complete replacement of the granulocytic population by myeloblasts. The aspiration biopsy of sternal marrow was a dry tap. (Gallaminblue-Giemsa × 375)

7 cases showed a steadily increasing fiber content and in 2 cases the fiber content decreased in the course of the disease, i.e. over a number of years.

The histological picture of CML is very variable, unlike that seen in smears of aspirates. The subgroups listed in the table remained constant as the disease progressed in each individual case. Devred et al[63] have concluded from 31 histologic studies that subgroups with regular development of granulocytes, with increased myelocytes, or increased myeloblasts, show no special prognostic differences. This applies also to the moderate myelofibrosis seen in 45 per cent of the cases. An unfavorable prognosis is associated with parenchymal aplasia with or without myelofibrosis, and also with extensive myeloblastic infiltration.

There is an early reduction in erythropoiesis in CML;[64] during an erythroblastic blast crisis 'streaks' are observed, which resemble those seen in Di Guglielmo's disease.[65,66] In some cases Gaucher-like histiocytes have been described which have a positive PAS reaction, contain glycolipids, siderin and cellular debris of granulo- and erythrocytes.[67,68]

Figure 3.20 shows the typical picture of CML in chronic phase and Figure 3.21 a CML in myeloblastic crisis.

We have observed a comparatively unfavourable prognosis of the subgroups 2, 3, 6, 7 and 8 (Table 3.4), though without statistical confirmation as yet. The significance of the differences between these subgroups is not clear. Possibly, ineffective granulocytopoiesis leads to intramedullary deposition of products of cellular degeneration, which evokes stromal reactions with variable features, determined by the amount of necrotic megakaryocytes, platelets, and eosinophils.

Summary

In CML histobiopsy reflects the typical blood changes found in the disease. As the disease progresses, the number of megakaryocytes and the medullary fiber content increase; concomitantly the spleen also enlarges. Conventional therapy exerts an influence on the blood picture, but hardly any in the bone marrow features. Histopathology shows a number of features whose significance is still under investigation. Biopsies are recommended prior to therapy and at regular intervals during the follow up to recognize cases likely to develop hypoplasia induced by therapy and early blast transformation.

Megakaryocytic myelosis (MM)

This condition was named by Hewer[69] in 1937, though it had been described repeatedly under various terms since the first report by Hirschfeld.[70] It is an autonomous disorder of the bone marrow[6,29,71,72] which belongs to the myeloproliferative disorders (Dameshek[73]). Moreover it may occur transiently as a transitional form during the course of other myeloproliferative disorders, e.g. PV and CML. Dameshek[73] also pointed out the tendency of the whole group to develop myelofibrotic and osteomyelosclerotic syndromes (see above).

MM is rarely listed in the modern literature.[74-76] There are several reasons for this: (1) the accompanying thrombocythemia is usually classified as the primary disorder, without consideration of the bone marrow findings; (2) the most immature megakaryoblastic forms of MM are frequently mistaken for Di Guglielmo's disease;[77] (3) other immature forms of MM are not diagnosed before the myelofibrosis has developed, at which stage the MM is listed under one of the numerous synonyms of the former disorder. Other cases are assigned to the subgroups (5) or (6) of CML. MM and CML have certain features in common as shown by Thiele et al[76] in studies with both light- and electronmicroscopy. Fickers & Speck[78] and Branehög et al[72] have found many large abnormal multinucleated megakaryocytes in MM. Fickers & Speck[78] have reported the occurrence of a blastic crisis in a case of 'primary thrombocythemia', i.e. MM, which supports the classification of MM as a differentiated myeloid hemoblastosis.

The primary diagnosis of MM is made by bone biopsy. Representative sections of the mature form of MM are shown in Figure 3.22. We have previously shown that MM may be distinguished from normal, reactive megakaryocytic

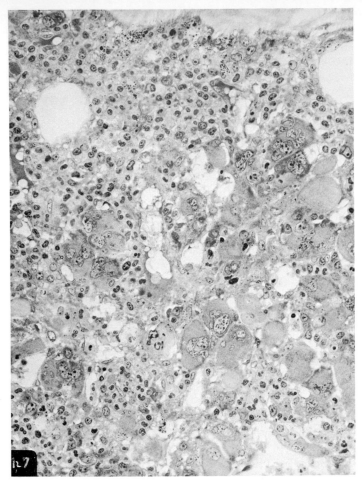

Fig. 3.22 Typical megakaryocytic myelosis, mature form. Increase of polymorphous, large megakaryocytes together with increased, predominantly mature, granulopoiesis. (Gallaminblue-Giemsa × 190)

proliferations because a six-fold increase in megakaryocytes are seen in MM as compared to normal. This increase in megakaryocytes bears no relationship to the accompanying thrombocytosis or thrombocytopenia.[29,37] The platelet count correlates with the degree of maturation of the megakaryocytes. Though some transitional forms have been described which are Ph[1] positive, MM may be distinguished from CML by bone marrow histology and the peripheral blood picture, which in MM rarely reaches leukemic levels. The initial stages of the undifferentiated forms are frequently characterized by pancytopenia. If cases of MM are treated as cases of CML, there is a high risk of a rapid development of pancytopenia. In MM there is a good correlation between the megakaryocytosis, interstitial deposition of platelets and myelofibrosis. Also in these cases it appears that the individual stromal reaction is the most important determinant of myelofibrosis (see above).

Summary

The megakaryocytic myeloses are closely related to PV and CML and may be recognized by their histological characteristics. Due to the inconsistency of the hematological picture they cannot adequately be recognized or classified without histobiopsy.

Polycythemia rubra vera (PV)

From biopsy observations on 209 patients with polycythemia, 58 of whom have been followed with a total of 169 biopsies in the course of the disease, we arrived at the following conclusions.[23,28,79] The most prominent histological findings in the bone marrow of PV are:

1. An increase in all elements of the marrow parenchyma together with a decrease in the fatty tissue
2. A striking increase, polymorphism, heterotopia and necrosis of megakaryocytes
3. An increase in the numbers of arteries, arterioles, arterial and sinusoidal capillaries
4. A mesenchymal reaction with varying amounts of lymphocytes, plasma cells and mast cells
5. A decrease in hemosiderin stores
6. A tendency, though not consistent, to develop fibrosclerosis of reticulin fibrils and of vascular stroma
7. Osteoporosis due to utilization of the capillary supply by the PV.

Of these, only the first two have been mentioned in the literature.[80] The hyperplasia of the marrow sinuses is an integral part of the polycythemic myeloproliferation.[23,81] The hyperplasia of all elements of the circulatory system was first described by our group.[23,28] We have also documented statistical correlations between the number of marrow sinusoids, the amount of erythropoiesis, the number of megakaryocytes and the increase in parenchymal mass, and between the hyperplasia of the arterial and venous capillaries. Polycythemic conditions may be regarded as autonomous and as combined parenchymatous-endothelial hyperplasias of the bone marrow. The erythropoietic cellular mass shows a positive correlation with the peripheral red cell count and an inverse proportion to the siderin content of the marrow. Relationships between the parenchymal mass in the marrow and between numbers of megakaryocytes, numbers of platelets and leukocytes in the blood, and spleen size have been observed, although not at statistically significant levels. The same is true of the increase in polymorphous megakaryocytes, necroses, inflammatory cells and fibrosis. In the course of the disease the parameters enumerated under 1, 2, 3 and 7 show an overall increase, but a clearcut tendency could not be documented; 0.4 per cent of our cases developed into undifferentiated hemoblastoses, and 28 per cent into MF and OMF. In PV, as in CML, therapy does not lead to an impressive improvement in bone marrow histology (Hauswaldt et al),[81] except for a moderate decrease in numbers of megakaryocytes and sinuses. The effect of treatment with ^{32}P on the incidence of terminal blastic crises has been under discussion since the pioneer studies of Ledlie[82] and Modan & Lilienfeld.[83] However, some investigators have shown that the higher rate of terminal leukemias is due to the therapeutic prolongation of survival.[84] It is also possible that the risk of leukemia is greater following prolonged administration of chemotherapy.[85] Hunstein et al[86] did not find a correlation between treatment with ^{32}P, duration of disease, and fibrous changes in 26 cases. Our studies of 58 cases, treated on the average for a period of 6 years with two doses of ^{32}P and monitored by biopsy 3.3 times each, demonstrate that age, therapy, and duration of the disease do not influence the fibrosis.

The development of myelofibrosis appears to be the result of individual variations, its relationship to inflammatory changes, necroses, and megakaryocytosis have been demonstrated not only in PV but also in CML and MM.[36]

The differential diagnosis of primary and secondary polycythemia is mainly supported by the difference in the histological parameters listed under 1, 2, 3 and 5 above.

Summary

In PV histobiopsy provides confirmation of the diagnosis made on clinical and hematological grounds. The marrow features show a high degree of uniformity in individual cases and change little following therapy. A terminal blastic crisis is related to the duration of the disease and, probably, to the therapy given. This does not apply to the development of myelofibrosis, a manifestation that may occur in all myeloproliferative disorders.

Chronic lymphatic leukemia (CLL)

The histobioptic bone marrow diagnosis of CLL has gained increasing recognition since the general acceptance of this procedure in every case of suspected malignant lymphoma.[87] In addition, biopsies are frequently performed in CLL because of the high rate of dry taps.

There is a broad overlap between the early aleukemic stage of CLL and various types of malignant lymphoma (well differentiated, follicular or diffuse type).[88] No criteria have yet been established which enable a distinction to be made between these two categories, or which permit a prediction in any given case, concerning the direction of its further development.[89] In addition, CLL must be distinguished from bone marrow lymphocytosis due to inflammatory or immunological stimuli: secondary bone marrow lymphocytosis is relatively frequent.[90,91]

CLL and lymphoma differ from reactive lymphocytosis in the following respects: the former shows a more uniform cell type, corresponding to its monoclonal origin, there is a tendency to spread diffusely, and the cells show a predilection for the peritrabecular areas. Biopsies from 98 cases of CLL were divided into three groups according to the peripheral blood lymphocyte counts.[92] Positive correlations were found between the lymphocyte count in the peripheral blood, the bone marrow lymphocytosis, the size of lymph nodes, spleen and liver. Similar observations have been reported by others.[93-95] There have been attempts to separate CLL into nodular or diffuse types according to the histology of the bone marrow and to attribute a different prognosis to each type.[95,96] On the other hand these two types may also be considered as the early and the late

Table 3.5 CLL—Biopsy diagnosis and leukemic picture (untreated cases)

Leukocytes in the peripheral blood	Leukocytes ($\times 10^9$/l) >100	30–100	<30	Normal blood picture
Histobiopsy characteristic of CLL $n=195$	19%	32%	36%	13%

phases of the disease process.[95,97] Hernandez-Nieto[98] has proposed a division into four types corresponding to early and late stages of the disease. It has been claimed that morphologically, the larger the lymphocytes, the more malignant the course of the disease.[95,99–101] These correlations are included among the arguments given by some authors in favor of a bone marrow origin of CLL.[100] This hypothesis is supported by the not infrequent association of CLL with myeloproliferative and immunological bone marrow manifestations.[102–104] In our

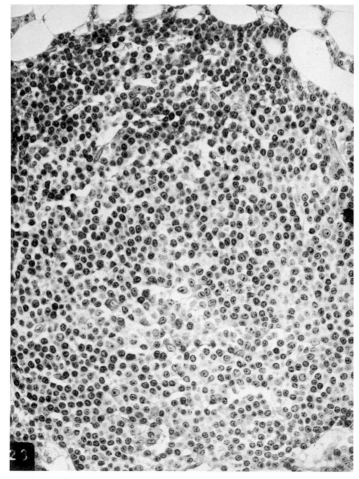

Fig. 3.23 Chronic lymphocytic leukemia; follicular type. Follicular accumulation of lymphocytes: mature cells in the margin, prolymphocytes in the center.

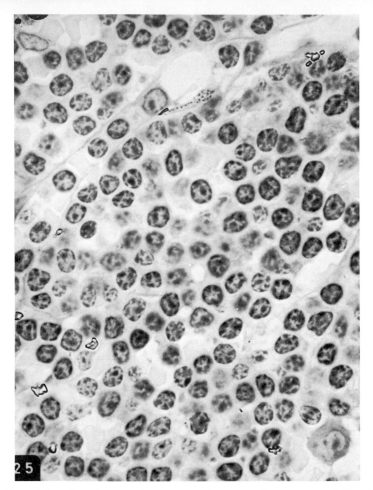

Fig. 3.24 Chronic lymphocytic leukemia; monomorphous type. Dense marrow infiltration with typical small round lymphocytes, also in the sinusoids. (Gallaminblue-Giemsa × 750)

series CLL was detected during the course of myeloproliferative disorders (PV, CML, MF) in 8 cases; 24 more cases are yet under suspicion for the same association. Multiple myeloma has been found together with CLL in five cases, three of which need further confirmation. It appears unlikely that these cases represent random occurrences. In our series of 250 patients (Table 3.5), the most important feature in the diagnosis of CLL in 49 per cent of cases with subleukemic or even normal blood counts was the bone marrow biopsy. Generally the degree of marrow infiltration reflects the progression of the disease. In some cases there is an almost homogenous distribution of the lymphocytes, in others—the minority—there are follicular structures with centers of large, 'immature' cells.

Fourteen of this 'follicular' type were compared with 35 of the diffuse type, before initiation of therapy. There was a remarkable difference in the duration of symptoms: about 20 months for the follicular, 0.9 month for the diffuse type.

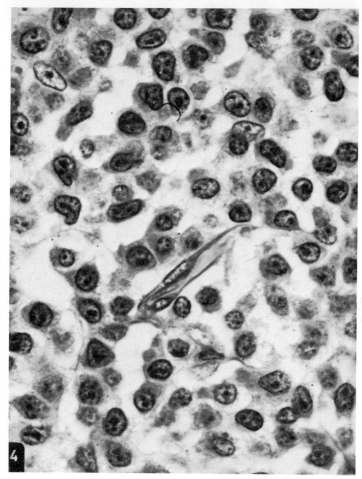

Fig. 3.25 Chronic lymphocytic leukemia; prolymphocytic type. Follicular arrangement of fairly homogeneous lymphocytic infiltration, centrally located cells with more cytoplasm and prominent nucleoli. (Gallaminblue-Giemsa × 750)

Two other variations of CLL appear of prognostic significance: the 'prolymphocytic',[105] and the mixed lymphocytic-plasmacytic with and without monoclonal dysproteinemia. Figures 3.23 to 3.25 illustrate various types of CLL in the bone marrow.

A comparison of the results of sternal punctures with those of myelotomies of the iliac crest in 58 cases of CLL has shown that: the smears of the aspirates were positive in 30 cases and suspect in 13 cases. There were dry taps in 15 cases. The biopsies showed unequivocal leukemic changes in all cases. In our series of 270 biopsies from 250 cases of CLL there was only one without lymphocytic infiltration in the bone marrow, which was later diagnosed as CLL.

Summary

The histobiopsy in CLL is diagnostic in almost 100 per cent of the cases. In the early stages, the distinction between CLL and malignant lymphoma cannot yet be made from the bone marrow biopsy; but the recognition of reactive medullary lymphocytosis is based on a number of reliable criteria. There is a close relationship between the degree of marrow infiltration and progression of the disease, as reflected in the leukocyte count and involvement of other organs. The prognostic significance of the special structural types is the subject of further investigation.

General conclusion

At the present time the following are the main indications for performing a bone marrow biopsy in leukemia. In clinical practice:

1. The early diagnosis and the differential diagnosis
2. The control of therapy, complications and accompanying disorders.

In the scientific field:

1. The understanding of the basic stromal changes of the leukemic process as a clue to a more efficient therapy.

Acknowledgments

The author is greatly indebted to Drs R. Bartl, W. Hill, K. Jäger, G. Kettner and G. Mahl for their cooperation in collecting and evaluating the material, to Dr Bertha Frisch for her help with the translation, to the technical staff of the laboratory, especially to Mrs W. Sommerfeld for the histological preparations, and to a great many colleagues for the transfer of patients.

REFERENCES

1 Mathé G, Dantchev D, Pouillart P, Florentin J 1972 De l'hématologie avec à l'hématologie sans microscope. La Nouvelle Presse Médicale 46: 3135–3139
2 Bartelheimer H, Schmidt-Rohde J M 1957 Die Biopsie des Knochens als differential-diagnostische klinische Methode. Klinische Wochenschrift 35: 429–440
3 McFarland W, Dameshek W 1958 Biopsy of bone marrow with the Vim Silverman needle. Journal of the American Medical Association 166: 1464–1466
4 Ellis L D, Jensen W N, Westerman M P 1964 Needle biopsy of bone and marrow. Archives of Internal Medicine 114: 213–221
5 Burkhardt R 1966 Technische Verbesserungen und Anwendungsbereich der Histo-Biopsie von Knochenmark und Knochen. Klinische Wochenschrift 44: 326–334
6 Burkhardt R 1970 Farbatlas der klinischen Histopathologie von Knochenmark und Knochen. Springer-Verlag, Berlin
7 Burkhardt R 1966 Präparative Voraussetzungen zur klinischen Histologie des menschlichen Knochenmarks. 1 Mitteilung: Blut XIII: 337–357. 2 Mitteilung: Blut XIV: 30–46
8 te Velde J, Burkhardt R, Kleiverda K, Leenheers-Binnendijk L, Sommerfeld W 1977 Methyl-methacrylate as an embedding medium in histopathology. Histopathology 1: 319–330
9 Bennike T, Gormsen H, Moller B 1956 Comparative studies of bone marrow punctures of the sternum, the iliac crest and the spinous process. Acta Medica Scandinavia 155: 377–396
10 Krempien B, Lemminger F M, Ritz E, Weber E 1978 The reaction of different scletal sites to metabolic bone disease—a micromorphometric study. Klinische Wochenschrift 56: 755–759
11 Capell D F, Hutchinson H E, Smith H G 1947 Marrow biopsy, preparation and use of paraffine sections from sternal puncture material. British Medical Journal 1: 403–404
12 Lukes R J, Tindle B T 1972 An approach to bone marrow evaluation by pathologists. Proceedings of the VIII World Congress of Anatomie and Clinical Pathology, Munich 12–16 September 1972, Amsterdam, Excerpta Medica, 86–92

13 Rywlin A M 1976 Bone marrow histology, aspiration versus biopsy. American Journal of Clinical Pathology 66: 617–618
14 Jamshidi K, Swaim R W 1971 Bone marrow biopsy with unaltered architecture: A new biopsy device. Journal of Laboratory and Clinical Medicine 77: 335
15 Bordier Ph, Matrajt H, Miravet L, Hioco D 1964 Mesure histologique de la masse et de la resorption des travées osseuses. Pathologie Biologie 12: 1238–1243
16 Block M H 1976 Text-Atlas of Hematology. Lea and Febiger, Philadelphia
17 Bartl R, Burkhardt R, Vondracek H, Sommerfeld W, Hagemeister E 1978 Rationelle Beckenkamm-Biopsie. Längsteilung der Proben zur Anwendung von mehreren Präparationsverfahren ohne Materialverlust. Klinische Wochenschrift 56: 545–550
18 Boellaard J W, Hirsch Thv 1959 Die Herstellung histologischer Schnitte von nicht entkalkten Knochen mittels Einbettung in Methacrylsäure-ester. Mikroskopie 13: 386–391
19 Bayerlein F 1978 Uber den Einfluß von Temperatur-, Druck- und Zeitkonstanten auf eine Methode der Methacrylateinbettung organischer Gewebe. Inauguraldissertation. University Munich
20 Staples W G, Gétaz E P 1977 Bone marrow involvement in malignant lymphoma without peripheral lymphadenopathy. South African Medical Journal 52: 60–63
21 Burkhardt R, Bartl R, Zettl R, Hill W, Jäger K, Frisch B 1978 The significance of single large scale bone marrow biopsies in malignant lymphoma, myeloma and metastatic growth. XII International Cancer Congress, Buenos Aires (Argentina) 5–11.10
22 Burkhardt R 1964 Die klinische Histologie der normalen und pathologischen Erythropoese im menschlichen Knockenmark. Folia haematologica, Neue Folge 9: 353–365
23 Burkhardt R, Pabst W, Kleber A 1969 Knochenmark-Histologie und Klinik der Polycythaemia vera. Archiv für Klinische Medizin 216: 64–104
24 Wienbeck J 1937 Das Zellbild des kindlichen Knochenmarkes bei Infektionskrankheiten. Verhandlungen der Deutschen Gesellschaft für Pathologie 37: 127–130
25 Burkhardt R 1974 Wechselwirkungen zwischen Knochenmark und Knochen. Verhandlungen der Deutschen Gesellschaft für Pathologie 58: 205–218
26 Demmler K, Burkhardt R 1974 Gefäßveränderungen im Knochenmark bei granulozytären Myelosen. Blut XXVIII: 178–186
27 Demmler K 1976 Das Gefäßsystem des Knochenmarkes. Ferdinand Enke-Verlag, Stuttgart
28 Burkhardt R, Bartl R, Frisch B, Hill W, Jäger K, Mahl G, Zettl R 1978 The role of the vascular system in proliferative and aplastic bone marrow disorders. XVII Congress of the International Society of Haematology. Paris (France) 23–29.7
29 Burkhardt R, Kronseder A 1977 Megakaryozytäre Myelose—Ursache der 'idiopathischen' Thrombozythämie. Fortschritte der Medizin 95: 1261–1266
30 Trentin J J 1971 Determination of bone marrow stem cell differentiation by stromal hemopoietic inductive microenvironments (HIM). American Journal of Pathology 65: 621
31 Tavassoli M 1975 Studies on hemopoietic microenvironments. Experimental Hematology 3: 213–226
32 Dreyfus B 1973 Editorial: preleukaemia, Lancet 1: 1426
33 Dreyfus B 1976 Preleukemic states: definition and classification. Refractory anemia with excess of myeloblasts in the bone marrow. Blood Cells 2: 33–55
34 Bernard J, Izrael V, Jacquillat C 1975 Les leucémies oligo-blastiques. La Nouvelle Presse médicale 4: 943–945
35 Gralnick H R, Galton D A G, Catovsky D, Sultan C, Bennett J M 1977 Classification of acute leukemia. Annals of Internal Medicine 87: 740–753
36 André J, Schwartz R, Dameshek W 1961 Tuberculosis and myelosclerosis with myeloid metaplasia. Journal of the American Medical Association 178: 1169–1174
37 Burkhardt R, Bartl R, Beil E, Demmler K, Hofmann E, Irrgang U, Kronseder A, Langegger H, Saar U, Ulrich M, Wiemann H 1975 Myelofibrosis—Osteomyelosclerosis Syndrome—Review of Literature and Histomorphology. Advances in the Biosciences 16: 9–56 (Vieweg: Pergamon Press)
38 Burkhardt R (in press) Myelogene Osteopathien. In: Bartelheimer H, Kuhlencordt R (eds) Handbuch der inneren Medizin, vol VI, 1 Klinische Osteologie. Springer-Verlag, Berlin
39 Burkhardt R (in press) Knochenveränderungen bei Erkrankungen des Knochenmarkes. Verhandlungen der Deutschen Gesellschaft für innere Medizin 85
40 Hayhoe F G J, Quaglino D, Doll R 1964 The Cytology and Cytochemistry of Acute Leukaemias. HMSO, London
41 Galton D A G, Dacie J V 1975 Classification of the acute leukaemias. In: Bessis M, Brecher E (eds) Unclassifiable Leukemias. Springer-Verlag, Berlin. p. 17–24

42 Beard M E J 1973 Classification of acute leukaemias using Romanowsky, Sudan black and periodic acid Schiff stains. In: Mathé G, Pouillart P, Schwarzenberg L (eds) Recent results in cancer research, vol 43, Nomenclature, methodology and results of clinical trials in acute leukemias. Springer-Verlag, Berlin. p 21–22

43 Brincker H 1973 Clinical classification and evaluation of treatment response in acute myeloid leukaemia on the basis of differences of leukaemic cell differentiation. Scandinavian Journal of Haematology 11: 383–390

44 Bennett J M, Catovsky D, Daniel MTh, Flandrin G, Galton D A G, Gralnick H R, Sultan C 1976 Proposals for the classification of the acute leukaemias. French-American-British (FAB) Co-operative Group. British Journal of Haematology 33: 451

45 Löffler H 1978 Die akuten (unreifzelligen) Leukämien. In: Queisser W (ed) Das Knochenmark Morphologie—Funktion—Diagnostik. Georg Thieme Verlag, Stuttgart. p 273–294

46 Mathé G, Belpomme D, Dantchev D, Pouillart P, Schlumberger J R, Lafleur M 1975 Leukaemic lymphosarcomas. Respective prognosis of the three types: prolymphocytic, lymphoblastic (or lymphoblastoid) and immunoblastic. In: Bessis M, Brecher G (eds) Unclassifiable leukemias. Springer-Verlag, Berlin. p 25–36

47 Mathé G, Belpomme D, Dantchev D, Pouillart P, Navares L, Hauss G, Schlumberger J R, Lafleur M 1975 Search for correlations between cytogical types and therapeutic sensitivity of acute leukaemias. In: Bessis M, Brecher B (eds) Unclassifiable leukemias. Springer-Verlag, Berlin. p 37–52

48 Rappaport H 1973 Histologic criteria for diagnosis and classification of acute leukemias. In: Mathé G, Pouillart P, Schwarzenberg L (eds) Recent results in cancer research, vol 43, Nomenclature, methodology and results of clinical trials in acute leukemias. Springer-Verlag, Berlin. p 35–42

49 Skeel R T, Bennett J M, Henderson E S 1970 Bone marrow lymphocytosis in acute leukemia. Blood 35: 356–360

50 Pushpa V, Till M M, Raynsford G, Hardistry R M 1973 Bone-marrow lymphocytes in acute leukaemia: Effect of therapeutic regimes. Biomedicine 19: 11–15

51 Green A A 1974 The prognostic value of bone marrow lymphocytes in acute lymphocytic leukemia of childhood. Cancer 34: 2009–2013

52 Oshima T 1975 Treatment of acute leukemia by quantitative observation of leukemic cells and normal hematopoietic cells in the bone marrow. Acta Haematologica Japonica 37: 773–774

53 Reddemann H 1978 Quantitative behavior of eosinophilic granulocytes in the bone marrow of children with acute lymphoblastic leukoses. Folia hematologica (Leipzig) 105: 43–51

54 Hann I M, Evans D I, Marsden H B, Morris Jones P, Palmer M K 1978 Bone marrow fibrosis in acute lymphoblastic leukaemia in childhood. Journal of Clinical Pathology 31: 313–315

55 Bloomfield C D, Theologides A 1973 Acute granulocytic leukemia in elderly patients. Journal of the American Medical Association 226: 1190–1193

56 Kawada S 1967 Histopathological Study of the bone marrow by needle biopsy. Nihon University Journal of Medicine 26: 798–808

57 Baccarini M, Zaccaria A, Santucci A M, Bagnara G P, Ricci P, Gobbi M, Ruggero D, Brunelli M A, Tura S 1975 A simultaneous study of bone marrow spleen and liver in chronic myeloid leukemia: Evidence for differences in cell composition and karyotypes. Series Haematologica 8: 81–112

58 Pareishvili E A, Akopova M A, Kalantar N R, Murdyan L B, Pogsyan A S, Eliyan L N 1977 Mitotic activity of bone marrow cells in patients with myeloid leukemia. Problemy Gematologii Perelivaniya Krovi 22: 19–21

59 Brandt L, Mitelmann F, Beckmann G, Laurell H, Nordenson I 1977 Different composition of the eosinophilic bone marrow pool in reactive eosinophilia and eosinophilic leukaemia. Acta Medica Scandinavia 201: 177–180

60 Arzberger A (in preparation) Knochenmarkhistologie und Klinik der CGL. Inaugural dissertation. University Munich

61 Dancey I T, Vadnais-Metz L H 1978 A quantitative assessment of neutrophil marrow in seven patients with chronic granulocytic leukaemia. British Journal of Haematology 39: 325–338

62 Watanabe K 1967 Histopathological study of the bone marrow by needle biopsy. Nihon University Journal of Medicine 26: 784–797

63 Devred C, Bentata J, Diebold J, Bernadou A, Bilski-Pasquier G 1977 Bone marrow biopsy in chronic myeloid leukemia. I Value of initial examination. Semaines Hôpitaux Paris 53:

119–124, II Its value during the course of the disease. Semaines Hôpitaux Paris 53: 125–131

64 Buyssens N, Bourgeois N H 1977 Chronic myelocytic leukemia versus idiopathic myelofibrosis. A diagnostic problem in bone marrow biopsies. Cancer 40: 1548–1561

65 Srodes C H, Hyde E H, Boggs D R 1973 Autonomous erythropoiesis during erythroblastic crisis of chronic myelocytic leukemia. Journal of Clinical Investigation 52: 512–515

66 Rosenthal S, Canellos G P, Gralnick H R 1977 Erythroblastic transformation of chronic granulocytic leukemia. American Journal of Medicine 63: 116–124

67 Keyserlingk D Graf, Boll I, Albrecht M 1972 Elektronenmikroskopie und Cytochemie der 'Gaucher-Zellen' bei chronischer Myelose. Klinische Wochenschrift 50: 510–516

68 Kirchen M E, Marshall G J 1976 Marrow storage cells: An ultrastructural study. Journal of the Reticuloendothelial Society 19: 109–119

69 Hewer T F 1937 Megakaryocytic myelosis with osteosclerosis. Journal of Pathology and Bacteriology 45: 383–390

70 Hirschfeld H 1914 Die generalisierte aleukämische Myelose und ihre Stellung im System der leukämischen Erkrankungen. Zeitschrift für klinische Medizin 80: 126–173

71 Georgii A, Vykoupil K F 1973 Histologisch-bioptische Klassifizierung myeloproliferativer Erkrankungen. In: Stacher A, Höcker P (eds) Erkrankungen der Myelopoese 'Leukämien, Myeloproliferative Syndrome, Polycythaemia'. Urban und Schwarzenberg, Munchen. p. 47

72 Branehög I, Ridell B, Swolin B, Weinfeld A 1975 Megakaryocyte quantifications in relation to thrombokinetics in primary thrombocythaemia and allied diseases. Scandinavian Journal of Haematology 15: 321–332

73 Dameshek W 1951 Some speculations on the myeloproliferative syndromes. Blood 6: 372–375

74 Zucker J M, Lesage B, de Montis G, Rossier A 1972 Thrombocytémie de l'enfant. (A propos d'une observation. Revue de la littérature) Annales de Pédiatrie 19: 393–400

75 Iizumi T, Ohnishi Y, Higuchi M 1973 An autopsy case of megakaryocytic myelosis. Acta Pathologica Japonica 23: 367–383

76 Thiele J, Georgii A, Vykoupil K F 1976 Ultrastructure of chronic megakaryocytic-granulocytic myelosis. Blut 32: 433–438

77 Demmler K, Burkhardt R, Prechtel K 1970 Megakaryoblastische Myelose. Klinische Wochenschrift 48: 1168–1173

78 Fickers M, Speck B 1974 Thrombocythaemia. Familial occurrence and transition into blastic crisis. Acta Haematologica 51: 257–265

79 Cirl C (in preparation) Knochenmarkshistologie und Klinik der Polycythaemie. Inaugural dissertation. University Munich

80 Lagerlöf B, Franzén S 1972 The ultrastructure of megakaryocytes in polycythaemia vera and chronic granulocytic leukaemia. Acta pathologica et microbiologica scandinavica Section A 80: 71–83

81 Hauswaldt C, Hunstein W, Uhl N, Doering P 1967 Histological bone marrow findings in polycythemia vera before and after ^{32}P therapy. Archiv für klinische Medizin 213: 219–236

82 Ledlie E M 1960 The incidence of leukaemia in patients with polycythaemia vera treated by ^{32}P, Clinical Radiology 130–133

83 Modan B, Lilienfeld A M 1965 Polycythemia vera and leukemia—the role of radiation treatment A study of 1222 patients. Medicine 44: 305–344

84 Szur L, Lewis S M 1966 The haematological complications of polycythaemia vera and treatment with radioactive phosphorus. British Journal of Radiology 39: 122–130

85 Weinfeld A, Westin J, Ridell B, Swolin B 1977 Polycythaemia vera terminating in acute leukaemia A clinical, cytogenetic and morphologic study in 8 patients treated with alkylating agents. Scandinavian Journal of Haematology 19: 255–272

86 Hunstein W, Hauswaldt C, Pixberg H U, Uhl N 1967 Biopsy investigations of fiber increase in the bone marrow in polycythemia treated with ^{32}P. Verhandlungen der Deutschen Gesellschaft für innere Medizin 72: 280–283

87 Rosenberg S A 1975 Bone marrow involvement in the non-Hodgkin's lymphomata. British Journal of Cancer 31 (suppl II): 261–264

88 Brunning R D 1975 Bone marrow and peripheral blood involvement in non-Hodgkin's lymphomas. Geriatrics Oct: 75–80

89 Pangalis G A, Nathwani B N, Rappaport H 1977 Malignant lymphoma, well differentiated lymphocytic. Its relationship with chronic lymphocytic leukemia and macroglobulinemia of Waldenström. Cancer 39: 999–1010

90 Dick F, Bloomfield C D, Brunning R 1974 Incidence, cytology, and histopathology of non-Hodgkin's lymphomas in the bone marrow. Cancer 33: 1382–1398

91 Burkhardt R 1976 Knochenmarkveränderungen bei malignen Lymphomen. In Hämatologie und Bluttransfusion, vol 18. J F Lehmanns Verlag, München. p 281–301

92 Hahner U, Burkhardt R 1977 Knochenmarksdiagnostik bei Haarzell-Leukämie. Klinische Wochenschrift 55: 933–944

93 Demmler K, Vykoupil K F, Georgii A 1969 Über die Beziehungen von leukämischem Blut und leukotischer Organinfiltration bei lymphatischen Leukämien. Hämatologie und Bluttransfusion, vol 8. J F Lehmanns Verlag, München. p 159–161

94 Bernadou A, Bernard J, Bilski-Pasquier G, Bousser J 1973 A propos du pronostic des leucémies lymphoides chroniques. Annales de Médicine interne 124: 549–560

95 Gray J L, Jacobs A, Block M 1974 Bone marrow and peripheral blood lymphocytosis in the prognosis of chronic lymphocytic leukemia. Cancer 33: 1169–1178

96 Carbone A, Santoro A, Pilotti S, Rilke F 1978 Bone-marrow patterns and clinical staging in chronic lymphocytic leukaemia (letter to editor). Lancet i: 606

97 Charron D, Dighiero G, Raphael M, Binet J L 1977 Bone-marrow patterns and clinical staging in chronic lymphocyte leukaemia (letter to editor). Lancet 2: 819

98 Hernandez-Nieto L, Montserrat-Costa E, Muncunill-Ribas J, Brugues M R, Granena A, Nomdedeu B, Feliu-Frasnedo E, Rozman C 1977 Chronic lymphocytic leukemia. Patterns of bone marrow involvement and their relationship with the clinical stages. Sangre (Barcelona) 22: 882–889

99 Basu A K, Repka E, Raik E, Gordon S, Vincent P C, Gunz F W 1976 Changing clinical, morphological and immunological patterns in chronic lymphocytic leukaemia. Pathology 8: 211–219

100 Sanchez-Fayos J, Outerinio J, Escudero A, Calabuig T, Perez-Pino T, Perec S C, Paniagua G 1978 Cytoproliferative activity of bone-marrow and peripheral blood compartments in chronic lymphocytic leukemia. Preliminary report on the analysis of fifteen cases. Sangre (Barcelona) 23: 411–417

101 Dubner H N, Crowley J J, Schilling R F 1978 Prognostic value of nucleoli and cell size in chronic lymphocytic leukemia. American Journal of Hematology 4: 337–341

102 Catovsky D, Galton D A G 1971 Myelomonocytic leukaemia supervening on chronic lymphocytic leukaemia. Lancet i: 478

103 Roberts P D, Forster P M 1973 Chronic lymphocytic leukaemia associated with acute myelomonocytic leukaemia. British Journal of Haematology 25: 203–206

104 Abelott M D, Waterbury L 1974 Pure red blood cell aplasia and chronic lymphocytic leukemia. Archives of Internal Medicine 134: 721–724

105 Galton D A G, Goldman J M, Wiltshaw I, Catovsky D, Henry K, Goldenberg G J 1974 Prolymphocytic leukaemia. British Journal of Haematology 27: 7–23

4

Ultrastructure of the Leukemic Cell

J. Breton-Gorius   M. F. Gourdin   F. Reyes

INTRODUCTION

For one century, histochemical reactions have been widely used in association with the Giemsa stain for the recognition of normal and leukemic hematopoietic cells. However, the study by light microscopic examination of films has some limitations.

As a consequence, hematologists have turned increasingly to electronmicroscopy for the analysis of the fine structure of cells and for determining the nature of some poorly differentiated cells. During 20 years, many papers have appeared on the ultrastructural aspect of leukemic cells and on the search for possible virus particles. The latter has been disappointing in the case of human leukemia. With the development of ultrastructural cytochemical methods, a new field of investigation was opened. More recently, the synthesis and the localization of immunoglobulins were assessed by the application of immunocytochemical methods at electronmicroscopy.

It is our intention to review the contribution of conventional transmission electronmicroscopy, cytochemical and immunoperoxidase methods to the knowledge of normal and leukemic cell differentiation.

CONTRIBUTION OF CONVENTIONAL ELECTRONMICROSCOPY TO THE KNOWLEDGE OF LEUKEMIC CELLS

METHODS

The preparation of bone marrow cells

Bone marrow specimens are usually obtained by sternal aspiration as a suspension of marrow particles, contaminated by some blood, which are immediately immersed into a fixative solution. The sample is put into a petri dish; then the marrow particles can be collected with a Pasteur pipette and resuspended into a fresh fixative solution. Since no anticoagulant is added, coagulation may occur in some cases. Marrow fragments can be distinguished easily from clots which appear stained as red cells.

In advanced myelofibrosis or in aplasia in which the aspiration is unsuccessful, marrow biopsy can be performed; after prefixation, marrow particles may be separated from the bone marrow spicules under microscopic examination.

Collection of peripheral blood leukocytes

Twenty ml of venous blood is obtained in polyethylene syringes wet with aqueous heparin. The buffy coat may be separated by several procedures.

When a normal or increased number of leukocytes is present the usual procedure to concentrate the nucleated cells consists of sedimentation at room temperature in a tube slanted at 45° for 1 h. The buffy coat is then removed with a thin Pasteur pipette and fixed.

A good concentration of cells is also obtained by centrifugating in narrow Kaplow tubes[1] at 2000 r/min for 10 min which increases the thickness of the buffy coat.

Separation of leukocytes from erythrocytes can also be enhanced by increasing the sedimentation in the presence of macromolecules. The heparinized blood is mixed with an equal volume of 2 per cent dextran (Abbott Laboratories, North Chicago, Ill.) in heparinized physiologic saline. After sedimentation the white layer and supernatant platelet-rich plasma are collected and centrifugated for 5 min at 200 g to concentrate the leukocytes while platelets remain in suspension.[2]

Anderson's[3] method is a very good one when the leukocyte count is low or when the cells under study are rare. It is based on the fact that glutaraldehyde added to the buffy coat causes the solidification of the plasma; subsequently, this zone may be cut into small blocks which will be oriented in the embedding material. In this procedure, the specimen is centrifuged to cause layering of erythrocytes, leukocytes, platelets and plasma. The plasma is then removed and replaced with glutaraldehyde fixative. The buffy coat can be removed as a solid disk and cut into slices.

Fixation, dehydration and embedding

The marrow particles and the leukocyte suspension are prefixed by aldehyde solutions. The most commonly used is glutaraldehyde 1.25 per cent freshly prepared from the distilled glutaraldehyde (TAAB Laboratories) in 0.1 mol/l phosphate buffer (pH 7.2) or in 0.1 mol/l cacodylate-HCl buffer (pH 7.4) with 1 per cent sucrose.[4] Good results may also be obtained in a mixture of 1 per cent freshly prepared paraformaldehyde and 3 per cent glutaraldehyde in 0.1 mol/l sodium cacodylate buffer, pH 7.4 with 0.05 per cent $CaCl_2$.[5]

In order to preserve the integrity of microtubules, the fixation in aldehydes is made at the room temperature for 30 min. Subsequently, marrow particles or leukocytes are washed three times in the same buffer. Washing a cell suspension requires centrifugation and resuspending the cell pellet in buffer.

Subsequently, cells are postfixed in 1 per cent OsO_4 in phosphate or cacodylate buffer for 30 min at 4°C, and are then rinsed in distilled water. The treatment with buffered 0.5 per cent uranyl acetate for 30 min increases the density of DNA, ribosomes and all membranes; however, this procedure is not recommended for studying neutrophil leukocytes since the azurophilic granules appear extracted. Dehydration is accomplished at room temperature in graded ethanols (70°, 90° and absolute ethanol, two baths of 20 min for each). Most plastic embedding mixtures are not miscible with ethanol; therefore propylene oxide is used as intermediate solvent; after two short passages, equal volumes of epon and propylene oxide for 1 h facilitate the infiltration of the resin. The hardness of the final block can be adjusted by the ratio of two mixtures.

$$
\text{Solution A} \begin{cases} \text{Epikote (epon) 812} & \text{31 ml} \\ \text{DDSA (Ciba Labs. or} & \text{50 ml} \\ \text{Ladd Res. Indust.)} \end{cases}
$$

$$
\text{Solution B} \begin{cases} \text{Epikote 812} & \text{100 ml} \\ \text{Methyl nadic anhydride} & \text{89 ml} \end{cases}
$$

Usually 7 ml of B and 3 ml of A are mixed with a final addition of 6 big drops of the activator DMP-30 (Ciba Labs. or Ladd Res. Indust.) Each marrow particle is put at the bottom of gelatin capsules which are filled with the final mixture of A, B and DMP. In order to pack cells, one drop of cell suspension is disposed in the capsule and centrifugated for 15 min at 10 000 g, before filling with epon. The polymerization is made at 60°C for 20 h. Thin sections cut on an ultramicrotome are counterstained with alkaline lead citrate for 5 s preceded by uranyl acetate for 10 min (except when samples have been previously treated by uranyl acetate after the postfixation step).

For this purpose, the grids containing the sections are set on drops of solution in a plastic film. The counterstaining solutions are the following:

Uranyl acetate: saturated aqueous uranyl acetate diluted in half with distilled water is filtered.
Alkaline lead citrate (modified Reynolds[6] method).

$$
\begin{aligned}
&33.1 \text{ g of lead nitrate mol/l} \\
&29.4 \text{ g of sodium citrate mol/l} \\
&4 \text{ g of sodium hydroxide mol/l}
\end{aligned}
$$

Mix 16 ml of water, 3 ml of sodium citrate and 2 ml of lead nitrate. A precipitate is formed. The solution is shaken and after addition of 4 ml of sodium hydroxide, the solution becomes clear. This solution is kept at 4°C under Vaseline oil. Before use, the solution is centrifugated 5 min.

After staining, the grids are washed with distilled water and dried on filter paper.

MAIN RESULTS

Morphologic examination of leukemic cells has permitted the assembly of an inventory of quantitative and qualitative alterations of the cell organelles. Numerous lesions or inclusions have been demonstrated which are otherwise undetectable by light microscopy. Abundant examples of the ultrastructural contributions to the knowledge of various leukemic cells can be found in several atlases.[7-9] It is not our intention to review all the abnormalities described in leukemic cells. However, Table 4.1 indicates the most frequent and striking features.

Table 4.1 Some contributions of conventional electronmicroscopy to the study of leukemic cells.

Types of leukemia	Abnormalities which may be present
Chronic lymphocytic leukemia	Crystalline inclusions in ER with IgM content[7, 8, 10]
Myeloma and Waldenström's disease	Nuclear inclusions[7-9, 11]
Hairy cell leukemia	Ribosome-lamellar complexes[12, 13]
Acute myeloblastic leukemia	Fibrillar bodies[3, 7] Abnormal granules[14] Asynchrony and anarchy of development of organelles[14] Periodicity array of dense lines in Auer bodies[8, 14, 15] Nuclear pockets[7]

CONTRIBUTION OF CYTOCHEMICAL TECHNICS TO THE KNOWLEDGE OF NORMAL CELLS

METHODS

Peroxidases

Graham & Karnovsky[16] have introduced in 1966 a new substrate, the 3-3' diaminobenzidine (DAB). This substance, derived from benzidine, is oxidized by heme enzymes in the presence of H_2O_2. Oxidized DAB is an electron dense insoluble polymer, the density of which increases after osmium tetroxide post-fixation. Myeloperoxidase (MPO) present in the monocyte and neutrophil series and peroxidases from eosinophil and basophil series can be easily detected by the Graham-Karnovsky method after the usual prefixation by glutaraldehyde. However, some other peroxidase or peroxidase-like enzymes can be inhibited by glutaraldehyde and their demonstration requires special methods. Thus, the platelet peroxidase (PPO) present in endoplasmic reticulum of megakaryocytes and platelets[17, 18] and the peroxidase-like enzyme of hairy cells[19] are only revealed with good reproducibility by the method introduced by Roels[20] in which unfixed cells are directly incubated in buffered DAB medium. The cell morphology is not always well preserved but all heme enzymes are revealed. PPO is also regularly demonstrated by Anderson's method[21] in which low concentration of aldehydes are mixed with tannic acid. We will describe these three methods.

Graham & Karnovsky technic[16]
Bone marrow particles or buffy coat cells are fixed for 30 min at 4°C with 1.25 per cent distilled glutaraldehyde in 0.1 mol/l phosphate buffer. The marrow blocks and blood leukocytes are subsequently washed three times in 0.1 mol/l phosphate buffer. As DAB penetrates slowly into the bone marrow particles, 40 μm thick sections of bone marrow cut on a Smith-Farquhar TC-2 tissue sectioner, are incubated in the DAB medium (see below). One can also pre-incubate marrow particles for a long period (24 h) in DAB alone at 4°C in order to facilitate the penetration, before final incubation in fresh DAB medium. Samples

are incubated for 30 min at room temperature, in the dark, in the DAB medium prepared as follows:

0.05 mol/l, Tris-HCl buffer, pH 7.6 containing DAB, and 0.1 ml 1 per cent H_2O_2 (freshly diluted from a 30 per cent solution).

If free base DAB (K and K Laboratories, Plainview, New York) is used, a saturated solution is prepared by shaking 2 to 3 mg of DAB with 10 ml of buffer. This solution is filtered before use.

DAB-tetra-HCl (Sigma Chemical Company, St Louis, Missouri) is more soluble; 5 mg are dissolved in 10 ml of buffer. The pH is adjusted to pH 7.6 with 1 mol/l solution of sodium hydroxide.

The specificity of the reaction is determined from control incubations, in which either DAB or H_2O_2 have been omitted. All incubations are followed by two washes of the tissue or cells in 0.1 mol/l phosphate buffer and then by postfixation for 30 min in 1 per cent osmium tetroxide solution. The cells are then processed as indicated previously. In order to evaluate the dense reaction product of oxidized DAB, sections are examined first without lead citrate counterstaining.

Roels technic[20]

Unfixed cells are incubated for 1 h in a medium containing 20 mg DAB, 0.01 ml 3 per cent H_2O_2 in 10 ml Ringer-Tris buffer 0.05 mol/l, pH 7.3. After washing in Ringer-Tris buffer, cells are fixed by glutaraldehyde followed by osmium tetroxide.

Anderson technic[21]

Prior to fixation, the buffy coat must be centrifuged at low speed for 10 min and then washed twice in Hanks' balanced salt solution in order to eliminate plasma proteins that would precipitate with the fixative. The bone marrow fragments obtained by aspiration in a heparinized syringe are washed several times in Hanks' solution. The fixative consists of 1 per cent tannic acid (E. Merck, Darmstadt), 2 per cent paraformaldehyde, and 0.5 per cent distilled glutaraldehyde (25 per cent biologic grade, TAAB, England) in 0.1 mol/l phosphate buffer at pH 7.2. The fixative is prepared just prior to use, filtered and chilled at 4°C. Cells are fixed for 1 h at 4°C, washed in phosphate buffer and are incubated in DAB medium or can be stored at 4°C for prolonged periods before incubation in DAB medium; this medium contains 20 mg of DAB and 0.1 ml H_2O_2 at 1 per cent in 10 ml 0.05 mol/l Tris-HCL buffer. The pH is readjusted to 7.6 with a 1 mol/l solution of sodium hydroxide. Incubation is carried out in a dark room at room temperature for 1 h. The cells are then rinsed in several changes of phosphate buffer (0.1 mol/l, pH 7.2) and postfixed for 30 min in 1 per cent osmium tetroxide in phosphate buffer.

Catalase

The cytochemical methods using DAB media are not specific for peroxidases; several heme-containing molecules including catalase can oxidize DAB in the presence of H_2O_2. In a number of cell types, catalase and hydrogen peroxide generating oxidase have been found associated with sedimentable particles termed peroxisomes. The peroxisomal catalase has been visualized cytochemically[22,23] in organelles with a nucleoid by modifications of the DAB technics. Incubation of fixed cells in DAB medium at a pH higher than that used for staining peroxisomes facilitates identification of other smaller peroxisome-like particles which stain positively for catalase.[24] Their small size and close association with smooth endoplasmic reticulum have led Novikoff et al[25] to introduce the term 'microperoxisome'. Microperoxisomes have been described in normal bone marrow cells; erythroblasts,[26] macrophages,[26] megakaryocytes and platelets[27] and granulocytes.[28,29] The method is the following:

Bone marrow particles and cells from the buffy coat are fixed for 30 min or longer at 4°C with 1.25 per cent distilled glutaraldehyde in 0.1 mol/l phosphate buffer. The marrow blocks and blood leukocytes are subsequently washed three times in 0.1 mol/l phosphate buffer. Incubation is carried out in alkaline DAB.[24] The medium contains: 20 mg of DAB and 0.2 ml of 2.5 per cent H_2O_2 (freshly diluted from a 30 per cent solution) in 10 ml of 0.05 mol/l propanediol buffer pH 9.7. Incubation is carried out at 37°C for 3 h in a dark room. Following the incubation, the bone marrow fragments are rinsed in the buffer and postfixed in 1 per cent osmium tetroxide at 4°C for 30 min. As controls, cells are incubated in the medium lacking either DAB or H_2O_2. In order to test the inhibitory effect of 3-amino 1,2,4-triazole (AMT) on catalase, the specimens are maintained in buffer containing 2×10^{-2} mol/l AMT for 30 min at 4°C prior to incubation and are subsequently incubated in the appropriate medium to each of which 2×10^{-2} mol/l AMT has been added. In contrast, potassium cyanide at a concentration of 1×10^{-2} mol/l has no effect on microperoxisome staining.

Glycogen

Polysaccharides can be specifically stained by a reaction derived from that used for PAS. For electronmicroscopy, the Schiff is replaced by the thiosemicarbazide or the thiocarbohydrazide revealed by the silver proteinate.[30]

The sections of embedded material are treated by laying them on the surface of different reagents and transfering them from one to another by a platinium loop as follows:

1. Treatment of sections by periodic acid at 1 per cent in distilled water for 20 min at room temperature
2. Washing twice rapidly, then three times for 10 min each in distilled water
3. Treatment by the thiocarbohydrazide at 1 per cent in 10 per cent of acetic acid for 30 min
4. Washing with acetic acid at 10 per cent; two washes rapidly then two others of 15 min each followed by three washes with distilled water
5. Silver proteinate at 1 per cent in distilled water for 30 min in a dark room.

RESULTS

1. Localization of myeloperoxidase (MPO) in the monocyte and neutrophil series

As suggested by the peroxidase reaction seen by light microscopic examination, electronmicroscopic studies after incubation in Graham-Karnovsky medium

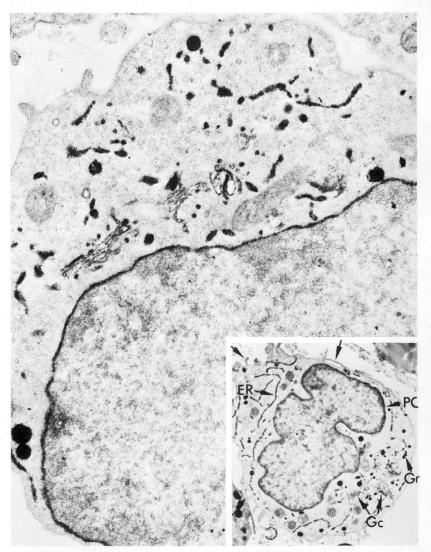

Fig. 4.1 Normal promonocyte incubated for peroxidase (Graham and Karnovsky method). **Inset:** as in the promyelocyte, peroxidase reaction product is distributed in the perinuclear cisterna (PC), all segments of the endoplasmic reticulum (ER), the Golgi cisternae (Gc) and all cytoplasmic granules (Gr). Hence the promonocyte is sometimes difficult to distinguish from early neutrophil precursors. However, in promonocytes some characteristics are typical: granules are smaller, the nucleus is deeply indented and numerous microvillous extensions of the plasma membrane (arrows) can be seen related to the endocytosis capacity. ($\times$5200) **Enlargement of the Golgi zone:** all the cisternae and vesicles contain the dense reaction product. ($\times$17 600)

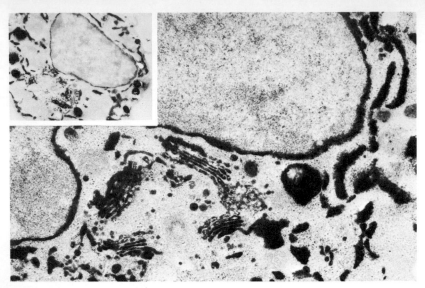

Fig. 4.2 Normal promyelocyte incubated for the demonstration of peroxidase. **Inset:** at low magnification, a strong reaction is seen in the nuclear envelope, endoplasmic reticulum, Golgi apparatus and azurophil granules. (× 4900) **Enlargement of the Golgi zone:** all the cisternae, vesicles and granules are filled with the dense reaction product. (× 18 300)

have confirmed that MPO is contained in granules. In addition, in promonocytes and neutrophil promyelocytes, the enzyme can be detected during its synthesis in the entire secretory apparatus: rough endoplasmic reticulum (RER), Golgi apparatus and its associated vesicles. This indicates that MPO is synthesized and packaged into granules by the same pathway which has been defined for other secretory proteins (Ref. 31 gives a general review). The promonocyte resembles the promyelocyte in that they are both defined by the presence of MPO in RER, Golgi apparatus and all granules (Figs 4.1 and 4.2). Distinguishing features of the promonocyte are the irregular shape of the nucleus, membrane ruffling related to their capacity of ingestion, and the small size of their reactive granules.

After the arrest of MPO synthesis the RER and Golgi apparatus become unreactive while the enzyme is detected only in azurophil granules. A new category of granules is produced which has a different content.

Eosinophils contain a peroxidase genetically and biochemically distinct from MPO. The Graham-Karnovsky technic reveals its presence in the RER and Golgi apparatus of developing eosinophils; the enzyme is seen in the matrix of granules, the crystal being devoid of reaction.

Basophil promyelocytes exhibit peroxidase activity in their granules and cisternal compartments. The granules can be recognized by their typical stippled appearance. Imperfect fixation of basophil granules with extraction makes detailed conclusions about granulogenesis difficult.

2. Localization of platelet peroxidase (PPO) in the megakaryocyte lineage

Using the Roels and Anderson technic, PPO has been detected in the RER and smooth endoplasmic reticulum (SER) of megakaryocytes and platelets (Fig.

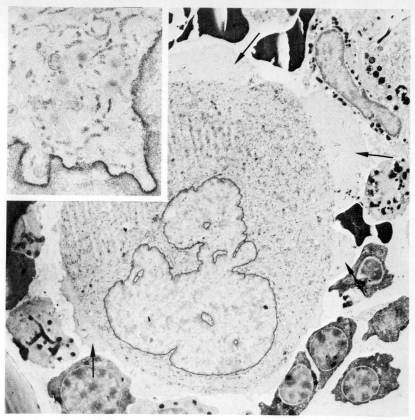

Fig. 4.3 Normal megakaryocyte reacted for platelet peroxidase (prefixation by the tannic acid-aldehyde mixture). The enzyme activity is seen in the nuclear envelope and small saccules of endoplasmic reticulum. The peripheral blebs (arrows) appear without organelle content. ($\times 2300$)
Inset: Golgi cisternae and granules are unreactive, a positive reaction being present in the perinuclear space and in the endoplasmic reticulum cisternae. ($\times 13\,550$)

4.3). This technic also reveals granulocytic peroxidases (MPO). However, some distinctions can be made between these two enzymes having the same reactivity. The most important difference is that MPO is always located in the Golgi cisternae and granules of promonocytes and promyelocytes (Fig. 4.2) while PPO is only detected in RER and SER. The genes coding for MPO and PPO biosythesis are different since PPO has been detected in platelets and megakaryocytes from patients with MPO deficiency.[28] The functions of MPO and PPO are also different; PPO is implicated in platelet prostaglandin biosynthesis, while the MPO-H_2O_2 system plays a role in bactericidal function. Finally PPO is very sensitive to fixation with glutaraldehyde and its detection requires the use of peculiar methods.[18] In contrast, MPO is very resistant. Thus, PPO appears to be characteristic of the megakaryocyte line. It can be detected in RER of bone marrow cells with a blastic or lymphoid appearance.[31] These very infrequent cells have a size similar to that of proerythroblasts and they should be considered as small precursors (2N or 4N) of megakaryocytes, unrecognized by conventional methods (Figs 4.4 and 4.5). Their number is increased in the bone marrow of patients with thrombocytopenia. Since the term megakaryoblast has

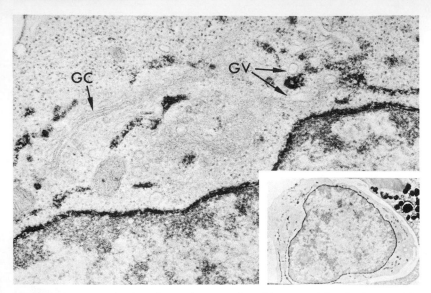

Fig. 4.4 Inset: low magnification of normal promegakaryoblast, tested for platelet peroxidase. A positive reaction is seen in the perinuclear space and endoplasmic reticulum. (×3850) A higher magnification shows that the Golgi cisternae (GC) and Golgi vesicles (GV) are unreactive as it is the case in more mature megakaryocytes. (×25 300)

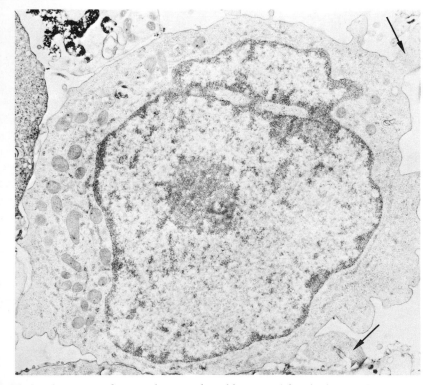

Fig. 4.5 Another aspect of a normal promegakaryoblast, tested for platelet peroxidase. The enzyme is localized in the perinuclear envelope and in all short segments of endoplasmic reticulum. Note the indented nucleus and cytoplasmic blebs (arrows). (×9300)

been used to define the earliest precursor of megakaryocyte which can be identified by its large size, we propose to term the small precursors recognized by the PPO reaction as promegakaryoblast (Pro MKB).

3. Localization of catalase and glycogen

Catalase containing particles have been identified early in the maturation of granulocytes, erythroblasts and megakaryocytes. In promegakaryoblasts, they are produced before the occurrence of α-granules.

Glycogen molecules can be revealed in cells treated for the morphologic examination and also in cells incubated in the DAB media. In such cases, neutrophil promyelocytes synthesizing MPO are seen to contain free glycogen molecules. During maturation their production increases and in the neutrophil polymorphonuclear leukocytes they are grouped in clusters. Glycogen molecules are also detected in erythroblasts. They disappear in red cells. In megakaryocytes, their number increases with maturation, and in platelets they are present in aggregates.

CONTRIBUTION OF THE CYTOCHEMICAL DEMONSTRATION OF PEROXIDASES TO THE KNOWLEDGE OF LEUKEMIC CELLS

Megakaryoblastic leukemia

The presence of a peroxidase activity similar in all its characteristics to PPO was recently detected in 80 per cent of blasts from a case of acute leukemia.[32] The small blasts possessing PPO exhibited undifferentiated or lymphoid appearance on light and electronmicroscopy and no granules or demarcation membranes could be detected by conventional electronmicroscopy (Figs 4.6–4.8). The presence of PPO has allowed the classification of this acute leukemia as pure megakaryoblastic leukemia. Normal or malignant B- and T-lymphocytes, including lymphoblasts, at various maturation stages do not exhibit PPO activity.[19]

Some PPO positive blast cells exhibited cytoplasmic blebs. These pseudopodial protuberances are frequently observed in the megakaryocyte line; however, they may also be encountered in cells of other series, and thus do not constitute a specific morphologic marker. Such observations emphasize the difficulty in distinguishing the Pro MKB from a lymphoblast by conventional methods. However, other features detected by light microscopy may be useful to suspect acute megakaryoblastic leukemia. (1) The marrow biopsy discloses a low cellular density and a dense reticulum network; the sclerosis of the bone explains the difficulty in aspirating bone marrow (see Ch. 3). (2) The small blasts which are peroxidase-negative at light microscopy constitute the majority of the cells. However, numerous large typical megakaryocytes with one or several round and independent nuclei are present. The observation of cells whose size is intermediate between large megakaryocytes and small blasts suggests an increased number of megakaryoblasts. (3) The blood picture shows pancytopenia with a majority of blasts cells and a very low count of large abnormal platelets.

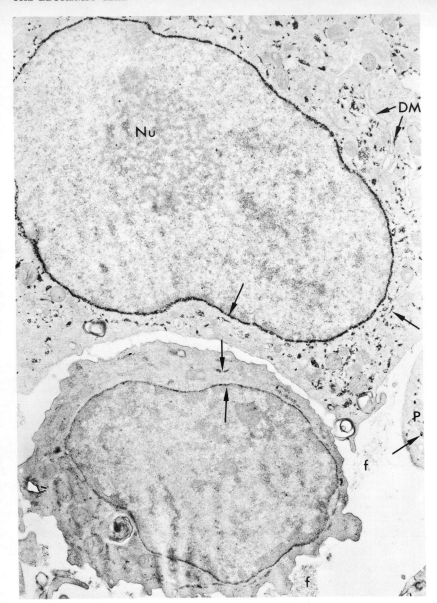

Fig. 4.6 Bone marrow from a patient with megakaryoblastic leukemia treated with the PPO reaction (prefixation by the tannic acid-aldehydes mixture). A large megakaryocyte possesses a round nucleus with a nucleolus (Nu). The dense reaction of DAB oxidized by platelet peroxidase is localized in the nuclear envelope, and short segments of endoplasmic reticulum (arrows). Some demarcating membranes (DM) are present while α-granules are not produced. At the bottom, a promegakaryoblast with a lymphoid morphology can be identified only by the presence of a weak platelet peroxidase reaction (arrows). Part of a platelet (P) shows a positive reaction in the dense tubular system (arrow). Note the presence of numerous extracellular fibrils (f). (× 10 300)

Fig. 4.8 (*opposite*) Promegakaryoblast from the same patient (incubation in DAB medium after fixation by tannic acid-aldehydes mixture). The morphology is better than in Figure 4.7 but the peroxidase reaction is weaker. The Golgi cisternae (Go) are unreactive, except in one peripheral cisterna (arrow). (× 11 600) **Inset:** a thick section of the same material. A brown ring surrounds the nucleus of one cell indicating that the peroxidase in the nuclear cisterna could be visualized by lightmicroscopic examination.

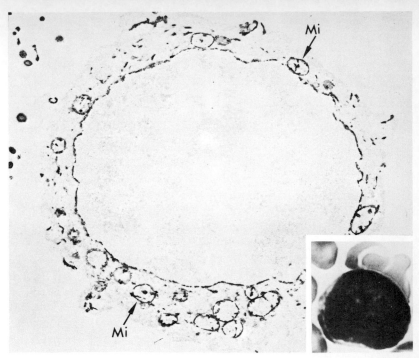

Fig. 4.7 Promegakaryoblast from a patient with acute megakaryoblastic leukemia (incubation in DAB medium without prefixation). A strong reactivity is present in the nuclear envelope and in all segments of endoplasmic reticulum. As in every cell type mitochondria (Mi) exhibit a reaction due to their cytochrome content ($\times$ 11 600). **Inset:** similar cell observed on Romanovsky stained smears. Note the undifferentiated aspect and the high nucleocytoplasmic ratio.

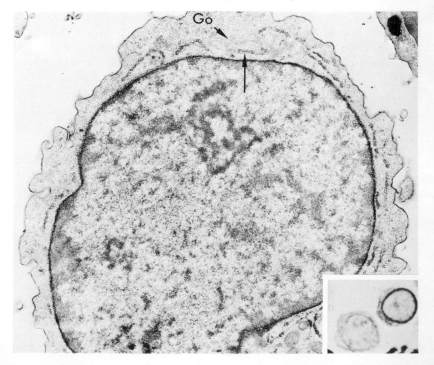

In the majority of previous reports of acute megakaryoblastic leukemia the peripheral blood cells were megakaryocyte precursors identified by their large size, mononuclear blast cells and cells which were considered as lymphocytes.[33] In contrast with our patient, the platelet count was often in the range of $1000 \times 10^9/l$. Our case seems similar to those described by Fabich et al[34] as acute myelofibrosis.

Eleven cases of acute leukemia, highly suggestive of megakaryoblastic leukemia have been recently reported.[35] This diagnosis was suspected by light-microscopy; only in two cases in which the PPO content was determined, the Pro MKB nature of the blasts could be confirmed. Bone marrow fibrosis was a constant finding in these 11 patients, including 3 children in whom major radiologic bone lesions were present. The morphologic aspect of blasts could have led to a confusion with acute lymphoblastic leukemia. The rapid clinical course and the poor response to chemotherapy were a constant feature.

Recently, three new cases were reported.[36] However, since the detection of PPO was not performed, only MKB, having started their cytoplasmic maturation, were identified.

Acute myelomegakaryoblastic leukemia

In some cases of acute leukemia described as acute myeloblastic leukemia (M_1 in the FAB classification).[37] Pro MKB could also be mixed with a small percentage of myeloblasts (Figs 4.9 and 4.10). We feel that such acute leukemias could be better classified as acute myelomegakaryoblastic leukemias.

The megakaryoblastic nature of cells in the blast crisis of chronic myeloid leukemia (CML)

The origin of cells in the blast crisis of CML remains controversial. Difficulties arise from the lack of cytochemical characteristics of differentiation. In one case in which blast cells exhibited an undifferentiated or lymphoid appearance by light and electronmicroscopy, 90 per cent of blast contained PPO.[38] In addition to Pro MKB, some micromegakaryocytes could be recognized among the reactive cells, by the presence of typical α-granules and demarcation membranes (Fig. 4.11). A circulating naked nucleus of a micromegakaryocyte after platelet shedding could be recognized by the PPO present in the nuclear envelope (Fig. 4.12).

The occurrence of Pro MKB has been documented in another study in which Pro MKB and micromegakaryocytes were found in the blast population of 7 patients out of 12 in apparent 'lymphoid' blast crisis of CML.[39] The blasts had a lymphoid appearance and were peroxidase negative by lightmicroscopy. Pro MKB were predominant in 2 cases and present in 5 other cases, mixed with other early myeloid blasts. In such patients, our findings suggest that in spite of the lymphoid appearance of the blasts, they were derived from pluripotent myeloid stem cells.

In several other studies, the presence of small megakaryoblasts, i.e. Pro MKB in the blast crisis of CML, has been suggested without cytochemical identification. This megakaryoblastic transformation was suggested by the abundance of blasts with undifferentiated morphology and micromegakaryocytes which

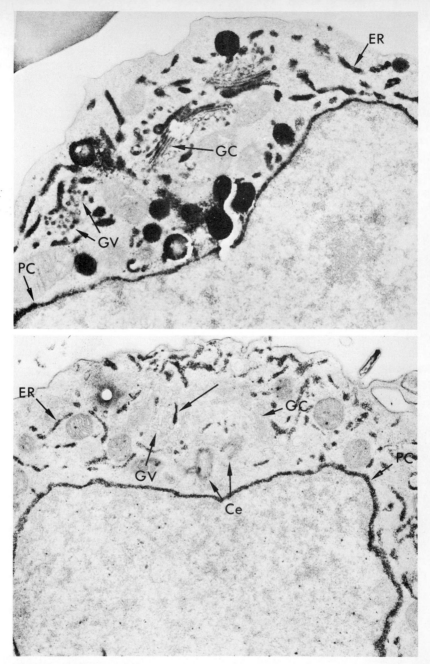

Figs 4.9 (*above*) **and 4.10** (*below*) Blood blasts in a case of acute myelomegakaryoblastic leukemia reacted for platelet peroxidase (prefixation by the tannic acid-aldehydes mixture). **Fig 4.9:** Golgi zone of a promyelocyte. Myeloperoxidase reaction fills the whole secretory apparatus, i.e. perinuclear cisterna (PC), endoplasmic reticulum (ER), Golgi cisternae (GC) and vesicles (GV) and azurophil granules. (×16 250) **Fig. 4.10:** Golgi zone of promegakaryoblast. The enzyme activity is seen in the perinuclear space (PC) and endoplasmic reticulum (ER). Note that the intensity of the reaction is weaker than in promyelocyte. Another distinction is the total lack of reaction product in Golgi cisternae (GC) and vesicles (GV), except for one cisterna (arrow). Two centrioles (Ce) are located in the Golgi zone. (×16 250)

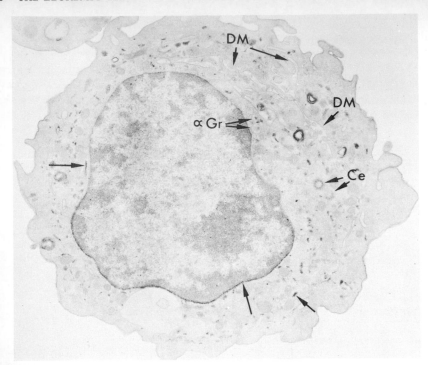

Fig. 4.11 Circulating micromegakaryocyte treated for the detection of platelet peroxidase (patient with blast crisis of CML). In addition to the presence of PPO (arrows) the cytoplasmic maturation has started by the production of α-granules (α-Gr) and demarcation membranes (DM). Two centrioles (Ce) suggest the diploid pattern of this small cell. (×9400)

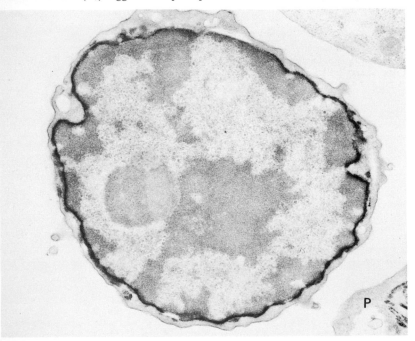

Fig. 4.12 Circulating naked nucleus originating from a micromegakaryocyte after platelet shedding (patient with blast crisis of CML). A thin rim of cytoplasm surrounds the nucleus. The PPO reaction fills the perinuclear cisterna. Portion of a platelet (P) contains reactive dense tubules. (×15 300)

exhibited by electronmicroscopic examination, characteristic demarcation membranes and abundant α-granules. The critical role of conventional electron-microscopy was to demonstrate transitional forms between these blasts and micromegakaryocytes.[40] Thus, on this basis, the megakaryoblastic nature of the cells was recognized in 15 per cent of blast crisis in a recent study of 19 patients.[41]

In conclusion, PPO, a marker for the normal Pro MKB, has been most useful

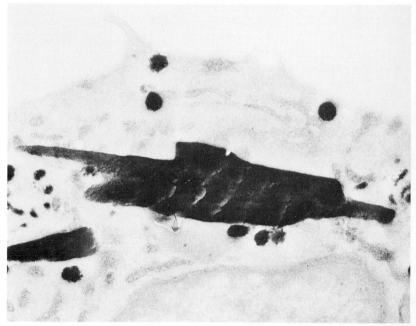

Fig. 4.13 Auer bodies in a blast from AML (MPO reaction). Two Auer bodies and granules are strongly reactive as indicated by the black deposit of oxidized DAB. (× 22 150)

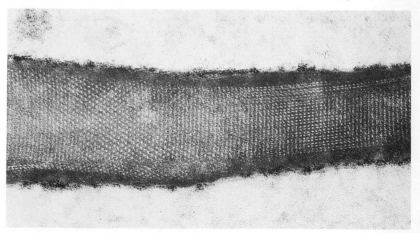

Fig. 4.14 Higher magnification of Auer body. Unreactive proteins regularly arranged with a well-defined periodicy are seen. This pattern differs totally from that observed in Auer bodies from acute promyelocytic leukemia. (See Fig. 4.16.) (× 11 000)

for the recognition of leukemic Pro MKB which could be confused with un-differentiated or lymphoid blasts by conventional methods.

Acute myeloblastic leukemia (AML)

Granule formation is often abnormal in AML.[42] Firstly, an abnormal concentration and packaging of azurophil granules may occur resulting in the formation of Auer rods. The existence of a periodicity in Auer rods was proven some 20 years ago. The arrangement of molecules constituting the crystalline material has been demonstrated with greater precision by means of the MPO reaction.[43] The dense reaction product has been used as a dark field to visualize the un-reactive protein of Auer bodies which may then be easily identified by its nega-tive contrast. In four cases of AML, an identical pattern of protein associated in a regular linear arrangement with well-defined periodicity was identified (Figs 4.13 and 4.14). Secondly, numerous giant granules resembling those of the Chediak-Higashi syndrome may be present.[44,45] These giant granules are also formed by fusion of azurophil granules, as in Chediak-Higashi; however, they appear different in that they contain numerous microcrystalline structures like those of Auer bodies.[45] However, the configuration, size and organization of the protein in the microcrystal are distinct from that seen in Auer bodies in AML.[43] These features suggest that the nature of the protein which crystallizes in Auer bodies may be heterogeneous.

Another anomaly concerns the granule production which may be absent[14] or a selective absence of MPO within the azurophil granule. [46,47]

Acute promyelocytic leukemia (APL)

In the hypergranulated cells of APL, "bundles of firewood" of Auer bodies are seen (Fig. 4.15). In all cases, Auer bodies reveal an identical substructure which consists of a hexagonal arrangement of tubes with a periodicity of 250 Å.[15] This has also been confirmed by examination after the cytochemical detection of MPO[43] (Fig. 4.16).

The presence of disseminated intravascular coagulation is always associated with this organization of Auer rods suggesting that some crystallized proteins of these bodies may trigger the coagulation process.

Acute leukemia with proliferation of eosinophil and basophil precursors

The diagnosis of eosinophil leukemia is based on the presence of immature eosinophil precursors in the blood with proliferation of these cells in different tissues.

Examination by electronmicroscopy reveals large granules typical of immature eosinophils.[48]

During the chronic phase of CML an increased number of basophils can be seen. When the percentage reaches 50 per cent, many authors use the term of basophil leukemia.[7] The ultrastructural study reveals granules with variable structure, show in their immaturity. These granules exhibit the characteristic metachromasia with the toluidine blue stain.

During the blast crisis of CML, among vacuolated blasts negative with the toluidine blue reaction, the MPO reaction can reveal cells actively synthesizing

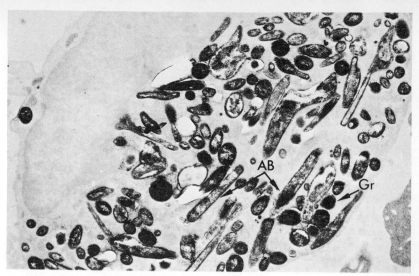

Fig. 4.15 Neutrophil promyelocyte from a patient with APL reacted for peroxidase. Both granules (Gr) and Auer bodies (AB) are positive. (×9000)

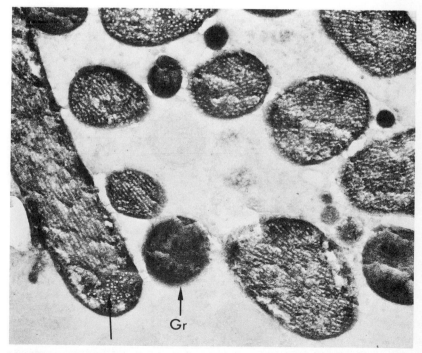

Fig. 4.16 Higher magnification of Auer bodies (same sample). While the matrix appears homogeneously dense in the granules (Gr), the crystallized proteins appear in negative contrast against the dark reaction product in the numerous Auer bodies. Thus, proteins without peroxidase activity are well defined. In longitudinal section, the crystal is constituted by a parallel arrangement of tubes which appear hollow on tranverse section (arrows). (×33000)

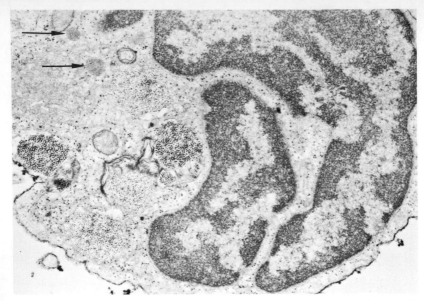

Fig. 4.17 Normal basophil granulocyte prefixed with the tannic acid-aldehyde mixture and incubated in DAB medium. Large granules exhibit a positive reaction with a characteristic stippled appearance. Two smaller granules (arrows) are peroxidase negative. ($\times$ 18 340)

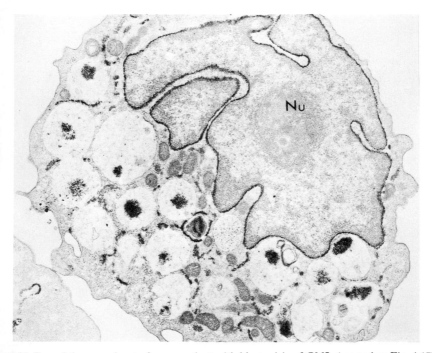

Fig. 4.18 Basophil promyelocyte from a patient with blast crisis of CML (reacted as Fig. 4.17). The very indented nucleus contains a large nucleolus (Nu). The endoplasmic reticulum including the perinuclear cisterna is reactive. The majority of granules are extracted; only in the center persists a dense reaction product with a stippled pattern. ($\times$ 10 600)

peroxidase in the perinuclear envelope and RER. Using the Anderson method, the vacuoles contain reactive punctate material in the center which resembles basophil granules (Figs. 4.17 and 4.18). In the absence of fixation, the granular reaction is clear and no vacuoles are seen. The stippled appearance of the granules is identical to normal basophil granules. A possible explanation is that early basophil precursors do not acquire the characteristic metachromasia of more mature basophils and the soluble material of the granules is extracted during the fixation; in contrast, this solubility is circumvented by reacting the cells with DAB medium before the fixation, thus preventing the dissolution of the granular content.[39] Out of 12 cases of blast crisis of CML with peroxidase negative blasts at lightmicroscopy, 9 contained a variable percentage of such early basophil promyelocytes (from 5 to 75 per cent) unidentified by usual methods, and detected by ultrastructural cytochemistry.[39] These precursors could also be detected by cultures in diffusion chambers. On day 30, 87 per cent of the cells were mature basophils and all the metaphases contained the Philadelphia chromosome. This demonstrates that in the acute phase of CML, leukemic basophil precursors may grow and mature *in vitro*.[49]

Acute monoblastic leukemia

As in AML, leukemic monocytic precursors may exhibit a complete absence of peroxidase in the cytoplasmic granules.[50] In other cases there is a discrepancy between positivity by electronmicroscopy and negativity at the lightmicroscope; this could, however, be due to the small size and low number of cytoplasmic granules.[51]

In some cases, the majority of blasts are seen synthesizing MPO (Fig. 4.19). Among these cells, few are starting the MPO synthesis; their secretory apparatus is filled with reaction product but they do not yet produce granules (Fig. 4.20).

In some cases of blast crisis of CML and of acute leukemia with blasts appearing as undifferentiated on the basis of standard cytochemistry, ultrastructural peroxidase cytochemistry has revealed blasts with very small granules containing MPO.[39] It was not possible to ascertain whether they were granulocyte or monocyte precursors. Both the small size of these granules (0.1 to 0.3 μm) and their infrequent occurrence explain why these cells may not be recognizable by standard lightmicroscopic cytochemistry.

Hairy-cell leukemia (HCL)

This chronic lymphoproliferative disorder, a well-defined clinical and cytological entity[52-54] will be considered now in view of the ongoing debate about the origin of the proliferative cells. Despite abundant morphologic cytological, functional and immunological data (reviewed in Ref. 19) difficulties still exist in the characterization of hairy cells (HC) as derived exclusively from one known normal series, i.e. lymphocytes or monocytes.

As mentioned above (Table 4.1) conventional electronmicroscopy has provided some information about the nature of hairy cells. The finding of ribosome-lamellar complexes[12, 13] pointed to an abnormal ribosomal distribution. This feature was initially thought to be specific for HCL but has now been described

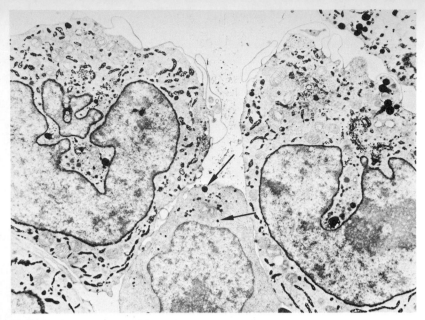

Fig. 4.19 Blasts from acute monoblastic leukemia tested for peroxidase. Two cells with very indented nuclei are seen actively synthesizing MPO. Their whole secretory apparatus and granules are strongly stained by the reaction product. Note the microvillous extensions of the plasma membrane. A third blast has completed the synthesis and only the granules (arrows) are reactive. (× 5400)

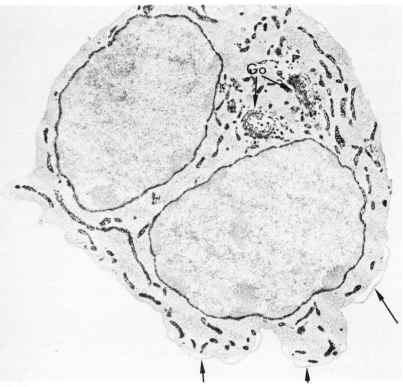

Fig. 4.20 Blast starting the MPO synthesis (same sample). This cell, without any granule can be considered as belonging to the monocytic series by the presence of MPO in the endoplasmic reticulum and the Golgi apparatus (Go). As in the more mature promonocytes, numerous invaginations of the plasma membrane are observed at the periphery (arrows). (× 7750)

in a few cases of B-lymphocytic proliferations[55] and its significance remains unknown. More closely related to the functional characterisation of HC was the finding of endocytosis properties although less marked than in normal macrophages. Evidence for this was given by ultrastructural studies of HC showing bacteria and latex particles enclosed in cytoplasmic vacuoles.[13] The significance of this finding has recently been questioned because pictures of material within a vacuole—as it appears on ultrathin sections—may just result from the adherence of material to the deeply invaginated surface membrane rather than from true endocytosis.[56] Attention has also been drawn to the fact that some leukemic B-lymphocytes can exhibit similar features on conventional electron-microscopy, i.e. particles apparently enclosed within vacuoles. This suggests that 'endocytosis' could as well occur to some extent in lymphocytes.[57]

At the present time, available data lead to the conclusion that HC may be endowed with both monocytic and lymphocytic characteristics. As to lymphocytic characteristics the demonstration of surface immunoglobulins (SmIg) has been an important finding.[58] Some difficulties arose when it became clear that the SmIg in HC could result from cytophilic binding[59] (see Ch. 5). Recent data support the view that at least some SmIg are a genuine product of HC.[60] These B-lymphocyte features do not preclude HC from expressing other non-lymphocytic features, such as the peroxidase activity recently demonstrated in this laboratory by means of ultrastructural cytochemistry.[19]

When glutaraldehyde-fixed HC are reacted with the Graham and Karnovsky medium,[16] i.e. in conditions that reveal MPO in the granulocyte and monocyte series,[31] no reactive organelles are found. However, peroxidase reactivity is detectable in HC when investigated by the more sensitive methods described above. Using the tannic acid-aldehyde mixture[21] peroxidase is demonstrated in some, but not all, HCL samples being localised in ER strands (Figs 4.21 and 4.22). This activity is best demonstrated when HC are incubated in DAB as unfixed cells;[20] with this method peroxidase is detectable in most HCL samples, and in all after a few hours in vitro culture.[19] The reactivity is retained in cultures up to 4 weeks. It is located in perinuclear and ER strands, but never in Golgi saccules or any granule; mitochondria are also reactive as a result of the cytochrome reactivity, the latter being clearly distinguished from ER reactivity by suitable inhibitors.[19]

These results establish that HC exhibit a peroxidase activity when studied by sensitive methods. The exclusive distribution of HC peroxidase in ER constitutes another main difference with the MPO of maturing bone marrow and blood monocytes. On the basis of its subcellular distribution, sensitivity to fixatives and to inhibitors, HC peroxidase appears to be similar to peroxidases of various tissues,[20,21] megakaryocyte series,[32] and various animal and human tissue macrophages (reviewed in Ref. 19). Furthermore it was recently shown that human blood monocytes (already equipped with MPO-positive granules) developed after a short in vitro adherence (as it was the case for some HCL samples), an additional peroxidase activity with an identical distribution and similar cytochemical features to that of HC.[61,62] Such 'activated' monocytes retain their phagocytosis ability and, interestingly, the newly acquired peroxidase activity does not enter into ingestion vacuoles, this being another distinctive

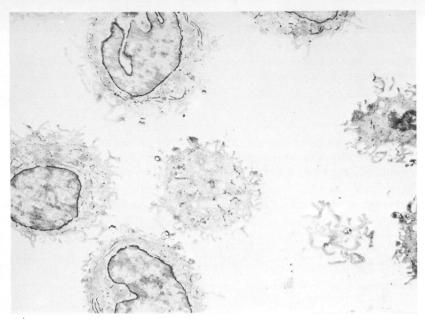

Fig. 4.21 HCL blood sample treated by the tannic acid-aldehyde fixative and incubated in DAB. HC peroxidase is seen as a black reaction product in the perinuclear space and narrow cytoplasmic endoplasmic reticulum strands, seen as elongated profiles or as dots when cross-sectioned. (× 4650)

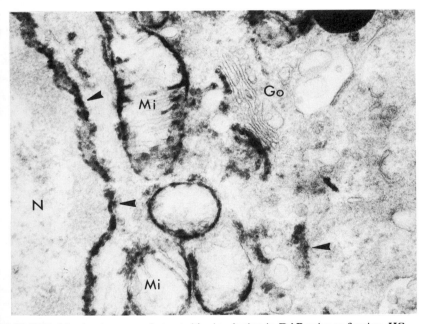

Fig. 4.22 HCL blood culture sample treated by incubating in DAB prior to fixation. HC peroxidase is visible in the perinuclear space and endoplasmic reticulum (arrows) but not in the Golgi lamellae (Go). Cytochrome activity is obvious in mitochondria (Mi); N, nucleus. (× 41 000)

feature with MPO.[62] An identical fate of peroxidase was found in HC induced to ingest latex particles, emphasizing that ER-bound peroxidase has a pathway distinct from the usual lysosomal enzymes.[63]

Our study has failed to detect any peroxidase activity in a large variety of T- and B-lymphocyte samples (including cultured samples so that a delayed *in vitro*-induced reactivity can be excluded) from human normal individuals and patients with immunoproliferative states. The same occurs in normal mitogen-induced immunoblasts and in Burkitt-derived cell lines.[19]

In conclusion a new enzymatic marker has been demonstrated in HCL by means of ultrastructural cytochemistry. This marker appears to be related to differentiation characteristics of the macrophage cells. It is to be added to the already demonstrated B- (and occasionally T-)[64] lymphocyte features of HC which therefore constitute a puzzling example of cells with a hybrid phenotype.

CONTRIBUTION OF IMMUNOELECTRONMICROSCOPY

INTRODUCTION

After Coons[65] had introduced the immunofluorescence technic which allowed the detection of cell components by means of appropriate antibody, the search for a similar methodology was to be anticipated at the ultrastructural level. As a matter of fact immunofluorescence does not allow a morphologic analysis of cells or a precise localization of antigen at the subcellular level. The development of immunoelectronmicroscopy (IEM) was linked to the finding of suitable markers,[66] i.e. electron-dense substances conjugated to functional antibody. Ferritin was first introduced by Singer[67] after conjugation to antibody by means of covalent bonds.

Although ferritin-conjugated antibody was used to trace cytoplasmic immunoglobulins in plasma cells,[68] few IEM studies have been performed by using this marker for the detection of cytoplasmic antigens,[69] presumably because of a limited penetration of the conjugate within the cells. Ferritin-coupled antibodies were rather used in IEM detection of cell surface antigens.[70–72]

Immunoperoxidase technics were developed more than 10 years ago independently by Avrameas[73] and Nakane.[74] It has become widely accepted since that horseradish peroxidase (HRP), which is the enzymatic marker coupled to antibody in these technics, was even more suitable for IEM studies than ferritin.[75] As an example, IEM studies of immunoglobulin-producing cells in HRP-immunized animals showed that HRP (in this system acting as antigen) allowed an excellent visualization of immunoglobulins (antibodies to HRP) within the secretory organelles of plasma cells.[76] Because of this excellent visualization HRP-coupled antibodies or lectins have been largely used in IEM studies, most of them being, however, devoted to surface antigen staining.[77,78] As for ferritin conjugates, some difficulties were indeed encountered in the staining of cytoplasmic antigens, that were also believed to result from a limited penetration of conjugates. It became accepted that correct fixation (in order to get satisfactory ultrastructural preservation) and conjugate penetration were to some extent contradictory goals.[79] Therefore various attempts were made in order to enhance intracellular staining by (1) modifying tissue sampling in 'pre-embedding' technics (use of fixed or frozen tissue sections) and (2) reducing the size of conjugates by using monovalent Fab fragments of antibody or, conversely, tracers with smaller molecular weight.[80,81] It should be outlined that such attempts were done by workers involved in IEM studies of tissue sections.

In this laboratory, IEM studies started some years ago by studying the appearance of blood group antigens on the surface of human maturing normoblasts. This study was undertaken to analyze the mechanism of antigenic loss in leukemia and pre-leukemic states and included a parallel study of normal erythroid series. For that purpose, cell suspensions have been used. Subsequently we have used a similar methodology on lymphocyte cell suspensions and this simple technic, initially devised for studying SmIg, has been shown to detect simultaneously both surface and cytoplasmic immunoglobulin of maturing B-lymphocytes. In the following sections we will describe our experience in IEM studies of (1) blood group antigens using a two step-indirect method and (2) B-cell immunoglobulins (Ig) using a one-step direct method.

MATERIAL

Cell suspensions
They are obtained from various sources. All centrifugations are performed at 200 g at room temperature. Erythrocyte suspensions are prepared by allowing fresh heparinized blood to sediment 1 h at room temperature. After discarding buffy coat cells, the erythrocyte pellet is washed three times in large volumes of phosphate buffered saline (PBS) pH 7.4, 0.1 mol/l, and processed to fixation. Leukocyte suspensions are prepared by aspirating the buffy coat cells in plasma, centrifuging and resuspending in a large volume of Hank's balanced salt solution (HBSS), 1 h at room temperature, before being washed twice further in HBSS. This procedure is known to enhance the elution of cytophilic Ig from the cell surface which may interfere with the demonstration of SmIg on B-lymphocytes[82] (see also Ch. 5). No attempt is made to purify lymphocytes from other leukocytes since the cells will be identified under EM. Bone marrow cell suspensions are obtained by aspiration; marrow particles are separated from contaminating blood and dissociated by repipetting in HBSS; they are then washed three times in large volumes of HBSS before fixation. Thymus and spleen cell suspensions are obtained by teasing the tissue with fine forceps in HBSS and concentrating the cells by repeated centrifugations and washes. According to the experimental procedure (see below) washed lymphocyte cell suspensions can be fixed or prior reacted with conjugates as live cells.

Cell fixation
Washed suspensions are fixed by resuspending the cell pellet in glutaraldehyde (TAAB Lab.) 1.25 per cent in PBS for 30 min at room temperature and washed twice in PBS. Such fixed cells can be stored in cold PBS for long periods of

time before being reacted with conjugates, this being of valuable help for laboratories involved in the study of rare leukemic samples.

Conjugates

Coupling of HRP (Sigma Lab.) to antibodies is carried out by the two-step procedure of Avrameas and Ternynck using glutaraldehyde as a cross-linking agent.[81] In this procedure the ratio of HRP to antibody is 3 : 1, 5 mg of antibody being usually conjugated. In the first step, HRP is reacted with an excess of glutaraldehyde by dissolving 15 mg of peroxidase in 0.2 ml of a 1 per cent glutaraldehyde solution in 0.1 mol/l phosphate buffer, pH 6.8. After the preparation has been left for 18 h at room temperature, it is filtered through a small (0.9 × 60 cm) G-25 Sephadex column equilibrated with 0.15 mol/l saline in order to eliminate unreacted glutaraldehyde. Fractions containing HRP (brown colored) are collected and pooled up to about 1 ml. One ml of solution containing 5 mg of antibody previously dialyzed against 0.15 mol/l saline is added to the pooled glutaraldehyde-treated HRP and to 0.2 ml of 0.5 mol/l carbonate bicarbonate buffer, pH 9.5; the mixture is kept in the cold for 24 h and dialyzed against PBS.

As a rule the solution of HRP-coupled antibody is further fractionated before use in order to eliminate the excess of free (non-coupled) HRP. This is performed by 50 per cent ammonium sulfate precipitation as follows: reacting the conjugate with an equal volume of saturated ammonium sulfate for 24 h in the cold, three washes in 50 per cent ammonium sulfate diluting down proteins to 5 mg/ml, and dialysis against distilled water for 1 h and for one night against PBS; fractionated conjugates are stored in the cold before use. This fractionation procedure has been devised in order to prevent the reaction of free HRP with glutaraldehyde-fixed cells responsible for non-specific staining either at the surface[83] or in the cytoplasm (unpublished observations).

Anti-human Ig antibodies

It has been shown that the results of IEM studies are more reproducible and non-specific staining less pronounced with pure labelled antibodies than with the labelled IgG fraction of antisera.[84] Therefore in this laboratory anti-Ig antibodies have been purified from rabbit or sheep hyperimmune antisera by an immunoadsorption procedure.[85] Immunoadsorbents are prepared by crosslinking 400 mg bovine serum albumin of (BSA) and 100 mg of the appropriate purified human Ig, following the technic described by Avrameas and Ternynck;[86] this technic leads to the insolubilization of Ig which is obtained as small particles resuspended and stored in cold buffer. An immunoadsorption procedure consists in resuspending the washed immunoadsorbent particles in 20 ml of antiserum by stirring for 1 h at room temperature; all subsequent steps are then performed at +4°C. The batch containing antiserum and immunoadsorbent is centrifuged for 15 min, the antiserum pipetted off and particles resuspended in 100 ml cold PBS and washed. This is repeated until the optical density of the supernatant becomes lower than 0.05, indicating that the antiserum proteins have been washed off. The following step consists of eluting by acidification the anti-Ig antibodies that are specifically fixed on the immunoadsorbent particles. This is performed by resuspending particles in 50 ml of

HCl-glycine buffer 0.2 mol/l, pH 2.8 for 15 min; after pipetting off the supernatant containing eluted antibody, the optical density is determined and the eluate neutralized by adding 10 ml of K_2HPO_4, 1 mol/l. The procedure is repeated once or twice at pH 2.8 until the optical density of the eluate becomes lower than 0.050 and then further at pH 2.2, once or twice according the optical density of the eluates. At the end of the procedure, immunoadsorbent particles are neutralized by resuspending in 10 ml K_2HPO_4, 1 mol/l, 40 ml distilled water and after centrifugation stored in cold PBS. Eluates with protein content (i.e. pure antibody) are dialyzed against PBS for 24 h, twice pooled and concentrated to 5 mg/ml with an ultrafiltration cell equipped with a Diaflo UM-10 membrane (Amicon, Lexington, Mass., USA). Pure antibodies are frozen at $-20°C$ until conjugation. By these procedures anti-Ig antibodies are obtained, either polyspecific to several Ig isotypes (for example reacting with both κ and λ light chains) or monospecific for heavy or light chains, depending upon the appropriate immunoadsorbent. (For details of preparation of antibodies see also Ch. 5.)

As an example anti-μ antibody is prepared as follows: rabbits are immunized with an IgMκ serum (from a patient with Waldenström disease) and the resulting hyperimmune serum (thus containing among others anti-μ+anti-κ antibodies) is passed on a IgMκ immunoadsorbent (prepared by insolubilization of pure IgMκ); eluted pure anti-μ+anti-κ antibodies are then adsorbed on a IgGκ immunoadsorbent (IgGκ being purified from a myeloma serum) thus leaving pure monospecific anti-μ antibody in the supernatant. A slightly different procedure used for preparing anti-δ antibody, will also be detailed here as another example of antibody purification: monospecific whole anti-IgD antiserum is obtained commercially (CDTS, Bois-Guillaume, Rouen, France). The antiserum is first adsorbed on a normal human serum immunoadsorbent (prepared by cross-linking with BSA as indicated above for any purified Ig) then on an IgM immunoadsorbent; the resulting supernatant, i.e. the extensively adsorbed anti-IgD serum is then passed on a IgD immunoadsorbent (prepared by copolymerizing an IgD myeloma serum with BSA) and pure anti-δ antibody eluted following the acidification procedure detailed above. Normal rabbit IgG is prepared by ammonium sulfate precipitation of pooled serum; this crude IgG fraction is conjugated to HRP as described above and can be used in control experiments.

METHODS

For the immunocytochemical demonstration of cell antigens, a 3 per cent cell suspension is prepared by resuspending three volumes of cell pellet of either fixed or live cells (according to the experimental procedure) in 100 vol of PBS; 1 ml of this 3 per cent cell suspension is used in the following steps listed in Table 4.2. Reacting with specific reagents consists of centrifuging the 3 per cent suspension and resuspending the cell pellet in 1 ml of the appropriate reagent. Before use, conjugates have been centrifuged at 150 000 g for 20 min in order to remove precipitates occurring during storage. It should be noted that steps of brief glutaraldehyde post-fixation lead to the immobilization of

Table 4.2 Immunoelectronmicroscopy procedures

Indirect	Direct	
	Fixed cell suspension in PBS[a]	Unfixed cell suspension in HBSS
Fixed cell suspension in PBS[a]		
↓		
Cell pellet resuspended in primary layer, 1 h, room temp.		
↓		
3 washes in cold PBS		
↓		
Brief glutaraldehyde (1.25%) postfixation, 10 min, room temp.		
↓		
2 washes in cold PBS[a]	→	→
↓		
Cell pellet resuspended in HRP conjugated anti-Ig (0.5–1 mg/ml) 1 h, room temp.	Cell pellet resuspended in HRP conjugated anti-Ig (0.5–1 mg/ml), room temp.	Cell pellet resuspended in HRP conjugated anti-Ig varying time and temp. of incubation; with or without Na azide
↓	↓	↓
3 washes in cold PBS	3 washes in cold PPS	3 washes in cold PBS
↓	↓	↓
Brief glutaraldehyde postfixation	Brief glutaraldehyde postfixation	Glutaraldehyde postfixation, 30 min in the cold.
↓	↓	↓
2 washes in cold PBS[a]	2 washes in cold PBS	2 washes in cold PBS[a]
↓	↓	↓
Cytochemical detection of HRP, 30 min, room temp., in the dark	Cytochemical detection of HRP, 30 min, room temp. in the dark	Cytochemical detection of MRP, 30 min, room temp. in the dark
↓	↓	↓
1 wash in distilled water	1 wash in distilled water	1 wash in distilled water
↓	↓	↓
1% OsO$_4$ postfixation, 30 min	1% OsO$_4$ postfixation, 30 min	1% OsO$_4$ postfixation, 30 min
↓	↓	↓
Graduate alcohols and embedding	Graduate alcohols and embedding	Graduate alcohols and embedding

[a] May be stored until further processing

antibody specifically attached to the cells and allow storage of cell suspensions for periods of time before further processing. The cytochemical reaction detecting HRP is developed by resuspending the cell pellet in the dark for 30 min in a few ml of the Graham and Karnovsky medium[16] containing 10 mg diaminobenzidine, 10 ml Tris-HCl buffer 0.05 mol/l pH 7.6, and 1 ml 0.1 per cent H_2O_2; when preparing the medium, the pH has to be adjusted to 7.6 by adding 1 mol/l NaOH. Osmium post-fixation as indicated in Table 4.2 is not an obligatory step. As a rule ultrathin sections are not counterstained, in order to avoid a possible underestimation of some weak surface stainings.

A and A_1 blood group antigens

These are detected by a two-layer indirect method. The primary layer consists of IgM human allo-antibodies from various sources;[87] the second layer consists accordingly of rabbit anti-human IgM conjugate. In this system of erythrocyte staining, the prior fixation of cells has several specific advantages. First, glutaraldehyde-fixed erythrocytes retain their ability to bind specific antibody but become non-agglutinable, thus resulting in the absence of cell clumps and allowing a comparison of the surface staining of separated cells. Second, fixation prevents the mechanical lysis of erythrocytes during centrifugation and resuspension; therefore suspensions are free of extracellular hemoglobin, avoiding non-specific staining as a result of heme peroxidase activity. Finally prior fixation prevents the redistribution of surface antigens induced by multivalent ligands in live cells; this phenomenon which has been well documented for the B-lymphocyte membrane (see below) has to be also taken in account at least for membrane antigens of nucleated erythrocyte precursors.[88] The specificity of labelling is checked by the following controls: (1) treatment of erythrocytes of unrelated group; (2) omission of first layer; (3) inhibition of staining by prior incubation of anti-A coated cells with non-conjugated anti-IgM antibody and (4) replacement of conjugated anti-IgM by HRP-conjugated normal rabbit IgG.

Surface and cytoplasmic immunoglobulins (SmIg, cyIg) of fixed B-cells

In this system a direct one-layer procedure is used, the cell pellet being resuspended in 1 ml of pure conjugated anti-Ig antibody (0.5 to 1 mg). When investigating cells from patients with unknown phenotype, a polyspecific anti-Ig conjugate is first used for detecting B-cells; monospecific conjugates for light or heavy chains are used in selected experiments to determine the precise phenotype of B-cells under study and to ascertain monoclonality, at least on the basis of light chain exclusion. Several controls are used: (1) replacement of conjugated antibody by conjugated normal rabbit IgG; (2) specific inhibition by prior incubation with appropriate non-conjugated anti-Ig antibody and finally (3) 'intrinsic' controls are represented in monoclonal samples by comparing the results given by unrelated anti-heavy or light chain conjugates.

SmIg of unfixed B-cells

In some experiments SmIg are also detected by treating live cell suspensions with conjugates at room temperature or at $+4°C$, with or without 1 per cent sodium azide, for periods of time ranging from 10 to 60 min. After extensive washes in cold PBS, antibody-reacted cells are glutaraldehyde-fixed for 30 min and further processed as indicated in Table 4.2.

RESULTS

Blood group antigens

Since the results of A and A_1 antigen detection on normoblasts, reticulocytes and erythrocytes have been extensively published[87-90] they will not be illustrated here; we will only emphasize a few points.

These IEM studies have demonstrated the synthesis of A determinants by all maturing normoblasts including early pronormoblasts. Another finding has been the variation of the staining intensity among individual cells demonstrating that a given phenotype (such as A_1, A_2, A_3 ...) comprises in fact several populations of cells according to their antigenic load. The occurrence of weak A phenotypes acquired during leukemia and preleukemic states can be interpreted in view of the physiological heterogeneity (which includes cells without detectable antigen) expressed by normal phenotypes. From a methodological point of view, the choice of an indirect two-step method for demonstrating A antigens results from a general principle in IEM technics, i.e. the necessity of coupling HRP to high amounts of purified antibody in order to obtain a good yield of specific conjugate. This implies that sufficient amounts of pure appropriate antigen should be available in order to purify antibody by the immunoadsorption procedure. Purifying anti-A antibodies from human alloantisera would have been obviously an extensive work; on the other hand the indirect method appears more appropriate since it implies conjugated anti-human Ig as the second layer. The purification of major Ig classes from human sera with monoclonal component is feasible without major technical difficulties and, therefore, permits the acquisition of large amounts of pure anti-Ig antibodies. Furthermore the latter reagents have been suitable for studying B-lymphocytes by the direct one-step procedure.

SmIg of unfixed cell suspensions

Lymphocytes from normal individuals and patients with chronic lymphocytic, acute B-lymphoblastic (Burkitt-type) and hairy-cell leukemias have been studied. Irrespective of time and temperature of incubation with conjugate, and of the presence of sodium azide (an inhibitor of capping) SmIg have been found in every case at the level of limited segments of the membrane (Fig. 4.23), the reaction product being also internalized in round or elongated vesicles; a diffuse staining of SmIg on the whole surface is very uncommon. In some sections, stained vesicles appear to be in connection with the outer wall of the cell (Fig. 4.24), thus resulting from an invagination of the stained membrane. Stained vesicles are also seen at various locations within the cell, mostly in the Golgi area, suggesting they are migrating pinocytotic vesicles. In samples reacted without sodium azide, capping is seen as a concentration of the staining at the level of the uropod membrane and also of numerous surface invaginations and pinocytotic closed vesicles. It should be noted that B-lymphocytes and cells from

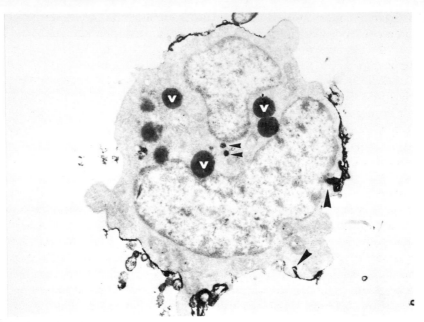

Fig. 4.23 Acute lymphoblastic leukemia (Burkitt-like) sample; detection of SmIg on unfixed cells. This blast cell contains lipids vacuoles (v). SmIg, monoclonal IgM, is revealed by anti-μ conjugate (30 min at 4°C). The surface staining is seen on limited areas leaving unstained membrane segments; invaginations of the positive membrane are also seen (single arrows) as well as some positive closed pinocytotic vesicles (double arrow). ($\times$ 7750)

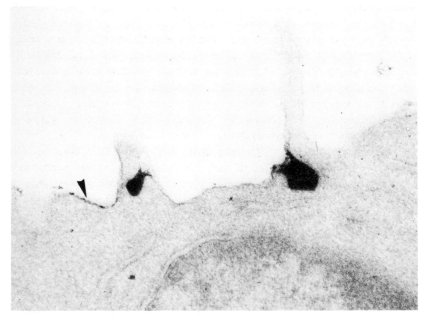

Fig. 4.24 Chronic lymphocytic leukemia sample; detection of SmIg on live cells. SmIg is a monoclonal IgM revealed by anti-μ conjugate. This high power view emphasizes the circumscribed surface staining (arrow) and the invagination of positively stained membrane, as a result of cross-linking of SmIg by divalent antibody. ($\times$ 34 850)

HCL have lost most of their surface villous architecture (see below), a finding also in accordance with the process of surface invagination leading to an alteration of the surface morphology.[91] It is known that the 'spotty' pattern of SmIg as viewed by immunofluorescence,[92] results from the redistribution of SmIg on the cell membrane induced by divalent anti-Ig antibodies. This initial passive process is followed by an active process leading to the polar concentration (capping) when viewed at the optical level or to internalization at the ultrastructural level.[85] These various phenomena (redistribution, capping, internalization) point to the fact that the antigen distribution and surface architecture are altered as a result of the interaction of live cells with ligands.

SmIg of fixed cell suspension

When cells are fixed prior to reacting with anti-Ig conjugate the reaction product outlines the entire perimeter of cells indicating that SmIg are diffusely distributed all over the cell surface[85] (Figs 4.25 and 4.26). Such a distribution pattern is at variance with previous IEM observations using autoradiography or virus, ferritin and peroxidase markers, in which SmIg appeared to be restricted to circumscribed segments of the cell membrane.[85] These previously published experiments had been carried out on live (unfixed) lymphocytes thus allowing redistribution and endocytosis of the reagent, as discussed above. It is of interest that when lymphocytes were exposed to monovalent Fab fragments of antibody, SmIg were found to be diffusely distributed.[72] The diffuse staining of SmIg has been observed on normal B-lymphocytes as well as on a variety of B-cells from immunoproliferative disorders and HCL.

Further information provided by our IEM studies is that the villous surface architecture of normal B-lymphocytes, identified by the presence of surface IgM, contrasts with the smooth or poorly villous nature of T-lymphocytes;[85] these data confirm by immunologic identification the work of Polliack et al[93] based on scanning electronmicroscopy. In some sections B-lymphocytes are found to have concentrated their microvilli at one pole, i.e. at the level of their uropod (a process independent of conjugate in this particular procedure) with a parallel accumulation of the specific staining. This observation gives additional evidence for the relationship between microvilli and SmIg (Fig. 4.25).

Much controversy exists in the literature regarding the villous nature of B-lymphocytes.[94, 95] Differences in the technics used to handle and process the cells could explain such discrepancies. In addition, they may also result from the fact that *normal* and *abnormal* B-cells have been used indistinctly in some studies of the surface architecture. In our experience microvilli are a constant feature of *normal* human B-lymphocytes; although found in a number of chronic lymphocytic leukemia samples they are a less constant feature in a wide range of B-cell proliferations. As an example cells from the prolymphocytic variant[96] express monoclonal SmIg, but are frequently smooth, with none or few short microvilli;[97] similar features are seen in cells from 'Burkitt-like' acute leukemias and in Burkitt-derived cell lines. In contrast, Sézary cells expressing T surface properties are seen with segments of villous membrane.[97] These observations suggest that although microvilli are a feature of normal B small lymphocytes (also confirmed by others),[98] they are not necessarily characteristic of other

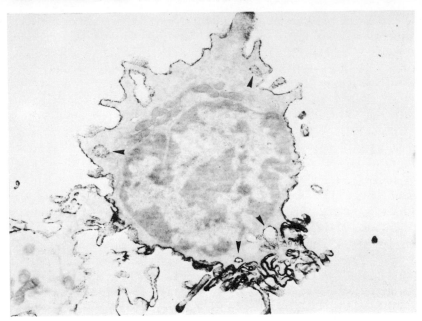

Fig. 4.25 Normal blood B-lymphocyte identified by anti-μ conjugate; SmIg detected on a fixed cell suspension. Surface IgM is revealed by a diffuse reactivity of the whole membrane; note the irregular surface architecture and the concentration of villous processes at the level of the uropod, with parallel accumulation of the staining. Stained vesicles (arrows) correspond to cross-sectioned spontaneous surface invaginations of the membrane since they are stained by anti-μ conjugate applied after fixation of the cells. Note the absence of reactivity in any cytoplasmic structures. ($\times 10\,450$)

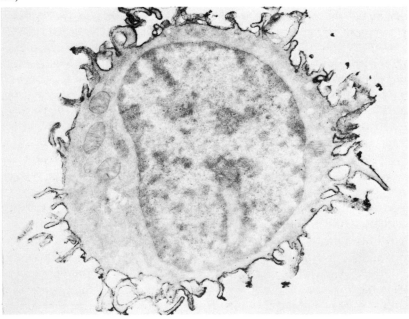

Fig. 4.26 Hairy-cell leukemia blood sample; SmIg are revealed by anti-γ conjugate on a fixed cell suspension. The diffuse surface staining of IgG outlines the typical hairy surface of the cell. ($\times 10\,050$)

monoclonal B-cell proliferations. Incidently, our IEM studies of mononuclear cell suspensions using the immunoperoxidase technic show that granulocytes and monocytes are simultaneously identified by their MPO-positive granules (reacting as HRP in the presence of diaminobenzidine). This may be useful for the recognition of contaminating monocytes which can be stained by anti-γ, κ, λ conjugates as a result of the Fc-binding of IgG extrinsic molecules. Similarly the identification of contaminating SmIg-bearing monocytes has been proposed in immunofluorescence studies by using an additional MPO counterstaining.[99]

Cytoplasmic Ig

The distribution of major Ig classes on the cell surface (IgM, IgD, IgA, IgG) and the results of specificity controls listed above[85, 97] clearly indicate that the surface staining as seen on fixed normal and leukemic B-cells does not result either from a non-specific adsorption of conjugate or from the detection of passively adsorbed Ig *in vivo*, but rather demonstrates truly synthesized SmIg. It should be noted that in our initial studies of B-lymphocytes from normal and chronic lymphocytic leukemia samples the positive staining has been restricted to the surface of cells and not found in any cytoplasmic structure. We have first interpreted the absence of intracellular staining as resulting from a limited penetration of the conjugate, as detailed above (see introduction). This was reinforced by the hypothesis that in our system SmIg could constitute, when cross-linked by glutaraldehyde fixation, an additional barrier preventing the penetration of conjugate molecules. However, as IEM studies were employed on a wider range of immunoproliferative disorders, it was soon established that HRP-conjugated whole antibody molecules did penetrate within suspended fixed cells showing in some cases a specific cyIg staining.[100]

We have detected varying amounts of cyIg in the following samples: some chronic lymphocytic leukemias with associated serum monoclonal component, Waldenström disease, myeloma, small and large cell lymphomas, pokeweed-stimulated lymphocytes and continuous B-cell lines (Burkitt and infectious mononucleosis derived).[101] Various patterns of cyIg staining have been found: (1) both SmIg and cyIg are simultaneously detected (Figs 4.27 and 4.28); (2) cyIg are demonstrated in various localizations, including strands of endoplasmic reticulum (Fig. 4.29), perinuclear space, Golgi lamellae and (3) some cyIg positive cells do not exhibit a plasmacytic pattern, i.e. endoplasmic reticulum, but rather a heavy and diffuse cytoplasmic specific staining, located outside secretory organelles (Fig. 4.30). Such Ig-synthesizing cells may represent a distinct subset of B-cells.

The results of our IEM studies suggest that the present technics may be of potential value in investigating cells from immunoproliferative disorders by providing information, on the relationship of SmIg and cyIg, the precise localization of synthesized Ig in secretory organelles and the identification of Ig-containing B-cells without plasmacytic differentiation. The latter may be of interest in large cell lymphomas since the presence of cyIg in such cells (as revealed by lightmicroscopy) could be taken as evidence of plasmacytic differentiation ('immunoblastic' lymphoma[102]). Finally the IEM technic should be useful in

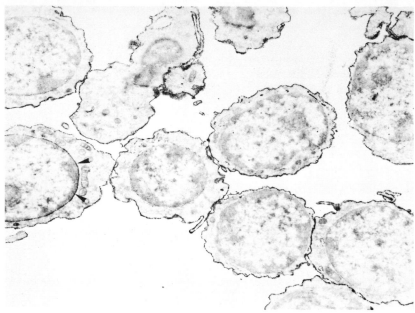

Fig. 4.27 Spleen cells of a case of lymphoma ('poorly differentiated' on histological grounds); a monoclonal surface IgM is detected on these fixed cells by anti-μ conjugate. All cells have a diffuse SmIg distribution; note that the surface morphology is intermediate between villous and smooth. In addition some SmIg positive cells exhibit a perinuclear specific staining (arrows) corresponding to newly synthesised cyIg. ($\times 4640$)

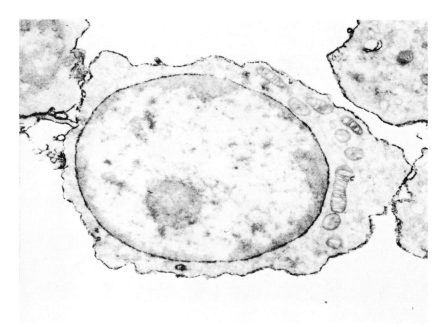

Fig. 4.28 Same sample; this enlargement emphasizes both SmIg and cyIg (perinuclear) staining. ($\times 10\,050$)

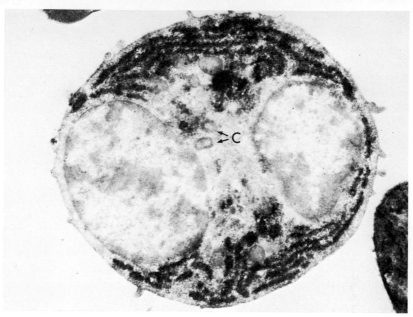

Fig. 4.29 Blood plasma cell in a case of Waldenström disease; fixed cell suspension reacted with anti-μ conjugate. Large amounts of IgM are visible in endoplasmic reticulum channels; note that no SmIg are detectable. C, centrioles; the Golgi apparatus is not clearly apparent in this section. ($\times 10\,450$)

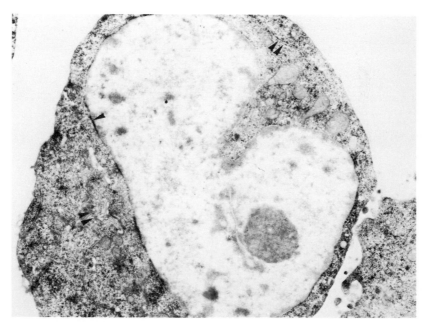

Fig. 4.30 Burkitt-derived (Raji) B-cell line; cyIg detected by anti-μ conjugate in fixed cell suspension. The cyIg are detected as a diffuse reactivity mostly located at the level of free polyribosomes; with the exception of segments of perinuclear space (single arrow) the lumen of endoplasmic reticulum and Golgi lamellae are free of reactivity (double arrow). ($\times 7350$)

discriminating among cyIg-positive cells between truly synthesized Ig (being localized in specific organelles) and ingested external Ig. This for instance may be relevant to HCL[19] and to Reed-Sternberg cells.[103]

Acknowledgments

We are indebted to Mrs Anne-Marie Dulac for secretarial work and Ph. Reboul for photographic assistance.

REFERENCES

1 Kaplow L S 1969 Buffy coat preparatory tube. American Journal of Clinical Pathology 51: 806–807

2 Hirsch J G, Fedorko F 1968 Ultrastructure of human leukocytes after simultaneous fixation with glutaraldehyde and osmium tetroxide and 'post-fixation' in uranyl acetate. Journal of Cell Biology 18: 615–627

3 Anderson D R 1966 Ultrastructure of normal and leukemic leukocytes in human peripheral blood. Journal of Ultrastructure Research, suppl 9: 5–42

4 Bainton D F, Ullyot J L, Farquhar M G 1971 The development of neutrophilic polymorphonuclear leukocytes in human bone marrow. Journal of Experimental Medicine, 134, 907–934

5 Karnovsky M J 1965 A formaldehyde-glutaraldehyde fixative of high osmolarity for use in electron microscopy. Journal of Cell Biology 27: 137A–138A (Abstract)

6 Reynolds E S 1963 The use of lead citrate at high pH, as an electron opaque stain in electron microscopy. Journal of Cell Biology 17: 208–212

7 Bessis M 1973 Living Blood Cells and their Ultrastructure. Springer-Verlag, Berlin

8 Cawley J C, Hayhoe F G J 1973 Ultrastructure of haemic cells. A cytological atlas of normal and leukaemic blood and bone marrow. W B Saunders, London

9 Tanaka Y, Goodman J R 1972 Electron microscopy of human blood cells. Harper & Row, New York

10 Hurez D, Flandrin G, Preud'homme J L 1972 Unreleased intracellular monoclonal macroglobulin in chronic lymphocytic leukaemia. Clinical and Experimental Immunology 10: 223–234

11 Bessis M, Breton-Gorius J, Binet J L 1963 Étude comparée du plasmocytome et du syndrome de Waldenström. Examen au microscope électronique. Nouvelle Revue Française d'Hématologie 3: 159–184

12 Katayama I, Schneider G B 1977 Further ultrastructural characterization of hairy cells of leukemic reticuloendotheliosis. American Journal of Pathology 86: 163–182

13 Daniel M T, Flandrin G 1974 Fine structure of abnormal cells in hairy cells (tricholeukocytic) leukemia, with special reference to their in vitro phagocytic capacity. Laboratory Investigation 30: 1–8

14 Bessis M, Breton-Gorius J 1969 Pathologic et asynchronisme de développement des organelles cellulaires au cours des leucémies aiguës granulocytaires. Étude au microscope électronique. Nouvelle Revue Française d'Hématologie 9: 245–278

15 Breton-Gorius J, Houssay D 1973 Auer bodies in acute promyelocytic leukemia. Demonstration of their fine structure and peroxidase localization. Laboratory Investigation 28: 135–141

16 Graham R C, Karnovsky M J 1966 The early stages of absorption of injected horseradish peroxidase in the proximal tubules of mouse kidney: ultrastructural cytochemistry by a new technique. Journal of Histochemistry and Cytochemistry 14: 291–302

17 Breton-Gorius J, Guichard J 1972 Ultrastructural localization of peroxidase activity in human platelets and megakaryocytes. American Journal of Pathology 66: 277–286

18 Breton-Gorius J, Guichard J 1976 Améliorations techniques permettant de révéler la peroxydase plaquettaire. Nouvelle Revue Française d'Hématologie 16: 381–390

19 Reyes F, Gourdin M F, Farcet J P, Dreyfus B, Breton-Gorius J 1978 Synthesis of a peroxidase activity by cells of hairy cell leukemia: a study by ultrastructural cytochemistry. Blood 52: 537–550

20 Roels F, Wisse E, De Prest B, Van Der Meulen J 1975 Cytochemical discrimination between catalases and peroxidases using diaminobenzidine. Histochemistry 41: 281–311

21 Anderson W A, Trantalis J, Kang Y H 1975 Ultrastructural localization of endogenous

mammary gland peroxidase during lactogenesis in the rat. Results after tannic acid-formaldehyde-glutaraldehyde fixation. Journal of Histochemistry and Cytochemistry 23: 295–302

22 Fahimi H D 1969 Cytochemical localization of peroxidatic activity of catalase in rat hepatic microbodies (peroxisomes). Journal of Cell Biology 43: 275–288

23 Novikoff A B, Goldfischer S 1969 Visualization of peroxisomes (microbodies) and mitochondria with diaminobenzidine. Journal of Histochemistry and Cytochemistry 17: 675–680

24 Novikoff A B, Novikoff P M, Davis C, Quintana N 1972 Studies on microperoxisomes. II A cytochemical method for light and electron microscopy. Journal of Histochemistry and Cytochemistry 20: 1006–1023

25 Novikoff A B, Novikoff P M, Davis C, Quintana N 1973 Studies on microperoxisomes. V Are microperoxisomes ubiquitous in mammalian cells? Journal of Histochemistry and Cytochemistry 21: 737–755

26 Breton-Gorius J, Guichard J 1975 Fine structural and cytochemical identification of microperoxisomes in developing human erythrocytic cells. American Journal of Pathology 79: 523–536

27 Breton-Gorius J, Guichard J 1975 Two different types of granules in megakaryocytes and platelets as revealed by the diaminobenzidine method. Journal de Microscopie et de Biologie Cellulaire 23: 197–202

28 Breton-Gorius J, Coquin Y, Guichard J 1978 Cytochemical distinction between azurophils and catalase-containing granules in leukocytes. I Studies in developing neutrophils and monocytes from patients with myeloperoxidase deficiency: comparison with peroxidase-deficient chicken heterophils. Laboratory Investigation 38: 21–31

29 Breton-Gorius J, Guichard J 1978 Cytochemical distinction between azurophils and catalase-containing granules in leukocytes: distribution in human promyelocytes and promonocytes. Journal of the Reticuloendothelial Society 24: 637–646

30 Thiery J P 1967 Mise en évidence des polysaccharides sur coupes fines en microscopie électronique. Journal de Microscopie 6: 987–1017

31 Breton-Gorius J, Reyes F 1976 Ultrastructure of human bone marrow cell maturation. International Review of Cytology 46: 251–321

32 Breton-Gorius J, Reyes F, Duhamel G, Najman A, Gorin N C 1978 Megakaryoblastic acute leukemia: identification by the ultrastructural demonstration of platelet peroxidase. Blood 51: 45–60

33 Chan B W B, Fleman R J, Zbinden G 1971 Acute leukemia with megakaryocytic predominance. Cancer 28: 1343–1349

34 Fabich D R, Raich P C 1977 Acute myelofibrosis. American Journal of Clinical Pathology 67: 334–338

35 Flandrin G, Daniel M T, Valensi F, Schaison G, Breton-Gorius J 1977 Leucémie aiguë à mégacaryoblastes. Étude clinique et morphologique de 11 observations. Actualité Hématologiques 11 ème série: 200–212

36 Den Ottolander G J, Te Velde J, Brederoo P, Geraedts J P M, Slee P H T, Villemze R, Zwaan F E, Haak H L, Muller H P, Bieger R 1979 Megakaryoblastic leukaemia (acute myelofibrosis): a report of three cases. British Journal of Haematology 42: 9–20

37 Bennett J M, Catovsky D, Daniel M T, Flandrin G, Galton D A G, Gralnick H R, Sultan C 1976 Proposals for the classification of the acute leukaemias. British Journal of Haematology 33: 451–458

38 Breton-Gorius J, Reyes F, Vernant J P, Tulliez M, Dreyfus B 1978 The blast crisis of chronic granulocytic leukaemia: megakaryoblastic nature of cells as revealed by the presence of platelet-peroxidase. A cytochemical ultrastructural study. British Journal of Haematology 39: 295–303

39 Marie J P, Vernant J P, Dreyfus B, Breton-Gorius J 1979 Ultrastructural localization of peroxidases in 'undifferentiated' blasts during the blast crisis of chronic granulocytic leukaemia. British Journal of Haematology 43: 549–558

40 Bain B, Catovsky D, O'Brien M, Spiers A S D, Richards H G H 1977 Megakaryoblastic transformation of chronic granulocytic leukaemia: an electron microscopy and cytochemical study. Journal of Clinical Pathology 30: 235–242

41 Catovsky D, O'Brien M, Cherchi M, Benavides I 1978 Ultrastructural, cytochemical and surface marker analysis of cells during blast crisis of chronic granulocytic leukaemia. Bolletino dell' Istituto Sieroterapico Milanese 57: 344–354

42 Bainton D F, Friedlander L M, Shohet S B 1977 Abnormalities in granule formation in acute myelogenous leukemia. Blood 49: 693–704

43 Tulliez M, Breton-Gorius J 1979 Three types of Auer bodies in acute leukemias. Visualization of their protein by negative contrast after peroxidase cytochemistry. Laboratory Investigation 47: 419–426

44 Mintz U, Djaldetti M, Rozenszajn L, Pinkhas J, De Vries A 1973 Giant lysosome-like structures in promyelocytic leukemia. Ultrastructural and cytochemical observations. Biomedicine 19: 426–430

45 Tulliez M, Vernant J P, Breton-Gorius J, Imbert M, Sultan C Pseudo Chediak-Higashi anomaly in a case of acute myeloid leukemia. Electron microscopic studies. Blood 54: 863–871

46 Bainton D F 1975 Abnormal neutrophils in acute myelogenous leukemia: identification of subpopulations based on analysis of azurophil and specific granules. Blood Cells 1: 191–199

47 Breton-Gorius J, Houssay D, Dreyfus B 1975 Partial myeloperoxidase deficiency in a case of preleukemia. I Studies of fine structure and peroxidase synthesis of promyelocytes. British Journal of Haematology 30: 273–278

48 Anteunis A, Audebert A A, Krulik M, Debray J, Robineaux R 1978 Acute eosinophilic study. An ultrastructural study. Virchows Archives B Cell Pathology 27: 237–248

49 Denegri J F, Naiman S C, Gillen J, Thomas J W 1978 In vitro growth of basophils containing the Philadelphia chromosome in the acute phase of chronic myelogenous leukaemia. British Journal of Haematology 40: 351–352

50 Bainton D F 1975 Ultrastructure and cytochemistry of monocytic leukemia. In: Mononuclear phagocytes in immunity, infection and pathology. Blackwell Scientific, Oxford. p 83–93

51 Lambertenghi-Deliliers G, Pozzoli E, Zanon P, Maiolo A T 1978 Ultrastructural study of myeloperoxidase activity in acute leukemia cells. Journal of Submicroscopic Cytology 10: 239–247

52 Bouroncle B A, Wiseman B K, Doan C A 1958 Leukemic reticuloendotheliosis. Blood 13: 609–630

53 Catovsky D, Pettit J E, Galton D A G, Spiers A S D, Harrison C V 1974 Leukemic reticulo-endotheliosis ('hairy cell leukemia): a distinct clinico-pathological entity. British Journal of Haematology 26: 9–27

54 Flandrin G, Daniel M T, Fourcade M, Chelloul N 1973 Leucémie à tricholeucocyte (hairy cell leukemia). Etude clinique et cytologique de 55 observations. Nouvelle Revue Française d'Hématologie 13: 609–640

55 Stefani S, Chandra S, Schrek R, Tonaki H, Knospe W H 1977 Endoplasmic reticulum-associated structures in lymphocytes from patients with chronic lymphocytic leukemia. Blood 50: 125–139

56 Jansen J, Schuit H R E, van Zwet Th L, Meijer C J L M, Hijmans W 1979 Hairy cell leukemia: a B lymphocytic disorder. British Journal of Haematology 42: 21–33

57 Catovsky D, Sperandio P, O'Brien M, Cherchi M, Galton D A G 1977 Phagocytic potential of leukaemic B-lymphocytes. Scandinavian Journal of Haematology 19: 211–216

58 Catovsky D, Pettit J E, Galetto J, Okos A, Galton D A G 1974 The B lymphocyte nature of the hairy cell of leukaemic reticuloendotheliosis. British Journal of Haematology 26: 29–37

59 Jaffe E S, Shevach E M, Frank M M, Green I 1974 Leukemic reticuloendotheliosis: presence of a receptor for cytophilic antibody. American Journal of Medicine 57: 108–114

60 Rieber E P, Hadam M R, Linke R P, Saal J G, Rietmüller G, van Heyden H W, Waller H D 1979 Hairy cell leukaemia: surface markers and functional capacities of the leukaemic cells analysed in eight patients. British Journal of Haematology 42: 175–188

61 Bodel P T, Nichols B A, Bainton D F 1977 Appearance of peroxidase reactivity within the rough endoplasmic reticulum of blood monocytes after surface adherence. Journal Experimental of Medicine 145: 264–274

62 Breton-Gorius J, Guichard J, Vainchenker W, Vilde J L Ultrastructural and cytochemical changes induced by short and prolonged culture of human monocytes. Journal of Reticuloendothelial Society 27: 289–301

63 Reyes F, Gourdin M F, Daniel M T, Breton-Gorius J 1978 Fine structure and ultrastructural cytochemistry of hairy cells. Abstracts, XVII Congress of the International Society of Hematology, Paris, July 1978

64 Cawley J C, Burns G F, Nash T A, Higgy K E, Child J A, Roberts B A 1978 Hairy-cell leukemia with T cell features. British Journal of Haematology 51: 61–69

65 Coons A H 1956 Histochemistry with labeled antibody. International Review of Cytology 5: 1–23

66 Sternberger L A 1967 Electron microscopic immunocytochemistry: a review. Journal of Histochemistry and Cytochemistry 15: 139–159

67 Singer S J 1959 Preparation of an electron-dense antibody conjugate. Nature (London) 183: 1523–1525
68 Rifkind R A, Osserman E F, Hsu K C, Morgan C 1962 The intracellular distribution of gamma-globulin in a mouse plasma cell tumour ($\times$5563) as revealed by fluorescence and electron microscopy. Journal of Experimental Medicine 116: 423–432
69 Sternberger L A 1974 Immunocytochemistry, Prentice-Hall, Inc, Englewood Cliffs, New Jersey. p 56–88
70 Davis W Z, Douglas S S, Petz L D, Fudenberg H H 1968 Ferritin-antibody localization of erythrocyte antigenic sites in immune hemolytic anemia. Journal of Immunology 101: 621–628
71 Hammerling U, Rajewsky K 1971 Evidence for surface-associated immunoglobulin on T and B lymphocytes. European Journal of Immunology 1: 447–451
72 De Petris S, Raff M C 1973 Normal distribution, patching and capping of lymphocyte surface immunoglobulin studied by electron microscopy. Nature New Biology 241: 257–259
73 Avrameas S 1969 Coupling of enzymes to proteins with glutaraldehyde. Use of the conjugates for the detection of antigens and antibodies. Immunochemistry 6: 43–52
74 Nakane P K, Pierce G B 1966 Enzyme-labeled antibodies: preparation and application for the localization of antigens. Journal of Histochemistry and Cytochemistry 14: 929–931
75 Bretton R, Terninck T, Avrameas S 1972 Comparison of peroxidase and ferritin labelling of cell surface antigen. Experimental Cell Research 71: 145–155
76 Leduc E H, Avrameas S, Bouteille M 1968 Ultrastructural localization of antibody in differentiating plasma cells. Journal of Experimental Medicine 127: 109–118
77 Gonatas N K, Antoine J C, Stieber A, Avrameas S 1972 Surface immunoglobulins of thymus and lymph node cells demonstrated by the peroxidase coupling technique. Laboratory Investigation 26: 253–261
78 Matter A, Lisowska-Bernstein B, Ryster J E, Lamelin J P, Vassali P 1972 Mouse thymus-independant and thymus-derived lymphoid cells. II Ultrastructural studies. Journal of Experimental Medicine 136: 1008–1030
79 Kuhlman W D, Avrameas S, Ternynck T 1974 A comparative study for ultrastructural localization of intracellular immunoglobulins using peroxidase conjugates. Journal of Immunological Methods 5: 33–48
80 Krahenbul J P, Galardy R E, Jamieson J D 1974 Preparation and characterization of an immunoelectron microscope tracer consisting of a heme-octapeptide couple to Fab. Journal of Experimental Medicine 139: 208–223
81 Avrameas S, Ternynck T 1971 Peroxidase-labelled antibody and Fab conjugates with enhanced intracellular penetration. Immunochemistry 8: 1175–1179
82 Lobo P I, Westervelt F B, Horwitz D A 1975 Identification of two populations of immunoglobulin-bearing lymphocytes in man. Journal of Immunology 114: 116–119
83 Molin S O, Nygren H, Hansson H A 1978 Binding of glutaraldehyde reacted peroxidase to cell surface. A source of error in immunochemistry. Journal of Histochemistry and Cytochemistry 26: 325–326
84 Avrameas S 1973 Enzyme markers: their linkage with proteins and use in immunohistochemistry. In: Stoward P J (ed) Fixation in histochemistry. Chapman and Hall, London. p 183–192
85 Reyes F, Lejonc J L, Gourdin M F, Mannoni P, Dreyfus B 1975 The surface morphology of human B lymphocytes as revealed by immunoelectron microscopy. Journal of Experimental Medicine 141: 392–410
86 Avrameas S, Ternynck T 1969 The cross-linking of proteins with glutaraldehyde and its use for the preparation of immunoadsorbents. Immunochemistry 6: 53–66
87 Reyes F, Gourdin M F, Lejonc J L, Cartron J P, Breton-Gorius J, Dreyfus B 1976 The heterogeneity of erythrocyte antigen distribution in human normal phenotypes: an immunoelectron microscopy study. British Journal of Haematology 34: 613–621
88 Gourdin M F, Reyes F, Lejonc J L, Breton-Gorius J, Dreyfus B 1976 The cellular distribution of erythrocyte and normoblast A antigens in normal and dyserythropoietic states. Blood Cells 2: 221–236
89 Reyes F, Lejonc J L, Gourdin M F, Ton That H, Breton-Gorius J 1974 Human normoblast A antigen seen by immunoelectron microscopy. Nature 247: 461–462
90 Cartron J P, Reyes F, Gourdin M F, Garreta M, Salmon Ch 1977 Antigen site distribution among 'weak A' red blood cell populations. Immunology 32: 233–244
91 Gourdin M F, Reyes F, Lejonc J L, Breton-Gorius J, Mannoni P, Dreyfus B 1976 Ultrastructural studies of human erythrocyte and lymphocyte series with peroxidase

conjugated antibodies. In: Feldman G, Druet P, Bignon J, Avrameas S (eds).
'Immunoenzymatic techniques'. Elsevier, North Holland. p 245–253

92 Taylor R B, Duffus N P, Raff M C, De Petris S 1971 Redistribution and pinocytosis of
lymphocyte surface immunoglobulin molecules induced by anti-immunoglobulin antibody.
Nature New Biology 233: 225–227

93 Polliack A N, Lampen N, Clarkson B D, De Harven E, Bentwich Z, Kunkel H G 1973
Identification of human B and T lymphocytes by scanning electron microscopy. Journal of
Experimental Medicine 138: 607–624

94 Alexander E L, Wetzel B 1975 Human lymphocytes: similarity of B and T cell surface
morphology. Science 188: 732–734

95 Roath S, Newell D, Polliack A, Alexander E, Lin P S 1978 Scanning electron microscopy
and the surface morphology of human lymphocytes. Nature (London) 273: 15–18

96 Galton D A G, Goldman J M, Wiltshaw E, Catovsky D, Henry K, Goldenberg G J 1974
Prolymphocytic leukaemia. British Journal of Haematology 27: 7–23

97 Gourdin M F, Reyes F, Lejonc J L, Mannoni P, Dreyfus B 1976 Surface features of cells in
human lymphoproliferative disorders. An immunoelectron microscopy study. In: Neth R,
Gallo R C, Mannweiper K, Maloney N C (eds) 'Modern Trends in Human Leukemia II'.
Lehmanns Verlag, München. p. 207–219

98 Mason D, Labaume S, Preud'homme J L 1977 The detection of membrane and
cytoplasmic immunoglobulins in human leukocytes by immunoperoxidase staining. Clinical
and Experimental Immunology 29: 413–421

99 Preud'homme J L, Flandrin G 1974 Identification by peroxidase staining of monocytes in
surface immunofluorescence tests. Journal of Immunology 113: 1650–1653

100 Reyes F, Gourdin M F, Farcet J P, Breton-Gorius J, Dreyfus B 1978 Immunoglobulin
production in lymphoma cells: an immunoelectron microscopy study. Recent
results in Cancer Research 64: 176–179

101 Preud'homme J L, Gourdin M F, Reyes F, Fellous M 1978 Human lymphoid cell lines with
pre-B cell characteristics. In: Serrou B, Rosenfeld C (eds) Human lymphocyte
differentiation: its application to Cancer. Elsevier, North Holland. p 345–352

102 Lukes R J, Collins R D 1975 New approaches to the classification of the lymphomata.
British Journal of Cancer 31 suppl II: 1–28

103 Taylor C R 1974 The nature of Reed-Sternberg cells and other malignant 'reticulum' cells.
Lancet ii: 802–807

5

Membrane Markers in Leukemia

George Janossy

INTRODUCTION

The analysis of marker characteristics of leukemic cells is a most interesting area where hematologists and immunologists have collaborated intensively during the last few years. The active involvement of immunologists originated from two factors: first, the lymphoid system is of central interest in the immunological discipline, and many leukemias derive from lymphoid cells, and second, classical morphological criteria do not distinguish between the different types of lymphoid cells. Immunological technics on the other hand can provide fine distinctions between different lymphocyte classes and subclasses. It is therefore logical that immunological technics should also be used for the analysis of lymphoproliferative malignancies.

During the sixties the main concepts about the function of the lymphoid system changed considerably. It became clear that under antigenic challenge[1] or after an exposure to certain leukoagglutinating proteins (such as Phytohemagglutinin[2] or pokeweed mitogen[3]) small lymphocytes become activated within a few hours and 'transformed' into dividing large lymphoblasts within 2 to 4 days in tissue culture. These observations suggested that the morphology of lymphoid cells could change according to the cells' functional state. Other studies have revealed that cells exhibiting small lymphocyte morphology are heterogeneous. It has been shown that some lymphocytes are educated in the thymus (T-lymphocytes) while others in the mammalian equivalent of the avian bursa (B-lymphocytes; precursors of plasma cells; reviewed in ref. 4). Important further observations have indicated that these T- and B-lymphocytes, although morphologically similar, can readily be distinguished by their membrane marker characteristics in the mouse,[5] as well as in man.[6,7] With the new concepts a novel technology arrived and a new branch of immunology (cellular immunology) emerged. Cellular immunology is primarily concerned with the analysis of cellular events and interactions which develop during immune responses.

This chapter attempts to summarize the immunological methods which have been applied in the analysis of various cell types in leukemia ('cellular immunohematology'). It is not surprising that these studies have started with the investigation of various lymphocyte membrane markers in the different forms of leukemia.[8-11] These observations showed that most cases of chronic lymphoid leukemia (CLL), and many lymphomas, derived from B-lymphoid cells, and also defined a proportion of acute lymphoid leukemias (ALL) expressing T-lymphoid markers (T-ALL). The majority of ALL cases nevertheless remained unreactive with T- and B-cell markers. An interesting further development started when some research groups developed antisera against leukemic cells[12-14] and introduced these new reagents in large studies. Although these reagents are not leukemia specific in the strict sense, some of them have been useful in diagnosis and helped to focus attention on a new class of normal cells. These cells show 'lymphoid' morphology but do not carry the characteristic membrane markers of thymocytes, mature T- or B-lymphocytes, and probably include various hemopoietic (including lymphoid-) precursor cells or stem cells.[15]

These early studies as well as later developments (reviewed in ref. 16) have delineated the primary role of membrane marker analysis in leukemia research and diagnosis. This includes the characterization of the various types of T- and B-lymphoid cells as well as their leukemic counterparts with a well established technology, although the characterization of various subsets, within the T and B categories, is still in progress. In addition, membrane marker studies give invaluable help in the analysis of hemopoietic precursor cells and their leukemic counterparts. These cells show 'lymphoid' or 'undifferentiated' morphology but lack the membrane marker characteristics of mature T- and B-lymphoid cells. This area of research is still in its infancy. The membrane marker analysis of other, including granulocytes, monocytes, megakaryocytes and erythroblasts cell types, is also possible but play a far less important role than the well established hematological technics. The exceptions are antisera which react with the earliest identifiable precursors of these cell lines (e.g. myeloblasts)[17-19] which are also useful in leukemia diagnosis.

The technical aspects of membrane marker studies fall into three parts. First, the basic methods for preparation of antibodies and detection of membrane antigens are described. Second, the individual reagents most commonly used for leukemia diagnosis are introduced. These include antibodies, analyzed mostly in immunofluorescence (IF) assays, and rosette tests (i.e. the binding of erythrocytes to various receptor sites on leukocytes). Finally, some special investigations using various reagent combinations which facilitate the phenotypic analysis of rare hemopoietic precursor cells and residual leukemic cells in patients under treatment are described.

In general, the technics described fall into two categories. The simple immunochemical methods and marker assays can easily be standardized in laboratories with limited resources—possibly with the critical use of carefully selected commercial reagents. These technics are described in detail. Other technics, such as the analysis of leukemic cells on the Fluorescence Activated Cell Sorter or preparation of monoclonal antibodies by somatic cell hydridization can only be carried out in specially equipped laboratories. Nevertheless, these technics represent fascinating new avenues in clinical research. Their description is less detailed but important because it facilitates the mutual understanding between scientists and clinicians in a rapidly developing area.

PREPARATION OF ANTIBODIES AND DETECTION OF MEMBRANE ANTIGENS

PREPARATION OF CONVENTIONAL ANTIBODIES

The analysis of the hemopoietic (including lymphoid) system revealed that functionally distinct cell populations display unique surface molecules which mediate their functions and reflect their stage of differentiation. The basic principle of membrane marker analysis is to recognize these structures by specific antisera. These unique structures are referred to as 'differentiation antigens'. An extension of this principle is the production of antisera against characteristic membrane structures on leukemic cells, i.e. the identification of 'leukemia associated' antigens.

The only practical possibility for producing clinically useful antisera against human leukemic cells is to make these reagents in animals. Antisera raised between species are known as xenogeneic or heterologous. These usually recognize species differences (i.e. species specific antigens). When distinct subpopulations of cells are used for xenogeneic immunization, the antisera also contain antibodies that recognize the particular subsets of cells—react with the tissue-specific differentiation antigens.

These differentiation antigens can only be analyzed if the species specific (anti-human) antibodies are first removed from the antiserum by absorption with human cells which do not carry the relevant differentiation antigens. Consequently, the preparation of heterologous antisera to membrane antigens almost invariably includes immunization followed by extensive absorption.

As a result of the detailed characterization of membrane antigens (e.g. differentiation antigens) by specific antisera, new possibilities arise for heterologous antibody production: these antigens can be *isolated* (either by immuno-chemical or biochemical methods) and used for immunization in a purified form. Antisera made against these purified products will require less absorptions.

It has been well documented that antisera raised between different animals within the same species (e.g. between inbred strains of mice) are particularly useful to detect differentiation and leukemia associated antigens.[20] These reagents, known as allogeneic sera, recognize the allelic polymorphism of the given antigenic moieties within the species. The particular usefulness of allogeneic antisera (as opposed to heterologous antisera) is highlighted by the observations that when a closely related animal is immunized the unique differentiation antigen may become a major foreign antigenic structure, for example when Rh⁻ individuals are immunized with Rh⁺ red cells. If rabbits are immunized, the antigens common to all human RBC will predominate. Similar situations may exist with the relatively weak 'leukemia-associated' antigens in man.[21]

Unfortunately allogeneic antisera have only limited use in human leukemia diagnosis because (1) immunization with leukemic cells in man is unethical, (2) patients do not seem to make antibodies against their own leukemic cells which could be used for diagnosing leukemia in others, and (3) it is disadvantageous to use antisera which show allo-reactivity (i.e. react with one patient's cells but not with others). In an outbred human population the analysis of leukemic cells with such a reagent would be meaningless without additional genetic analysis. Thus the use of allo-antisera in man is restricted mainly to histocompatibility testing and is applied only as a research tool, under well-defined conditions, in leukemia diagnosis[22] (see also 'Ia-like antigens' below). It is important to note, however, that a few interesting immunological manipulations have already been suggested and used to suppress the response of immunized animals against the major human species specific antigens in order to shift the immune response against minor (and more important) human differentiation antigens.

This section describes the methods for immunization of animals, the absorption of antisera and the basic manipulations (purification steps) with the antisera obtained.

Immunization

The technology of immunizing animals with protein antigens and cellular products has been described in handbooks.[23,24] A recent summary about handling of animals is given by Garvey et al.[25] The purpose of immunization for membrane marker analysis in leukemia is two-fold: (1) to immunize animals with different cell types in order to produce antisera which can be made specific for differentiation or leukemia associated antigens by suitable absorptions; and (2) to produce antisera against well-defined proteins (e.g. different immunoglobulin isotypes and Ia-like antigens) which are present on the membrane of certain normal and leukemic cells. It is convenient to consider these two procedures separately (see below).

There are no strict 'rules' for producing antisera. There are a number of factors which profoundly influence the outcome of immunization. These are: the choice of animals; the route of immunization; the immunogenic properties of the antigen used; the dose of antigen; the use of adjuvants; and the length of the immunization course.

Few attempts have been made to study the role and relative importance of these divergent factors for various reasons. First, the immune response of individual animals to purified protein antigens is variable and probably governed by genetic factors. In outbred animal colonies the analysis of the other factors would require large experimental groups. Second, the individual factors influence others. For example, the immunogenic properties of the antigen are determined not only by its chemical structure but also by the choice of animal species (depending on the phylogenetic distance between the donor and recipient); the use of adjuvants modifies the optimal dose of antigen, etc. In spite of these inherent problems some conclusions can be drawn from the observations made in different laboratories.

Immunization with cells

Many observations are available on the production of antihuman lymphocyte sera (ALS),[24] antisera reacting with human thymocytes/T cells ([26] review) and ALL blasts ([6,21] review). Most of these reagents have been produced in rabbits; goats have also been used occasionally.[27,28] Good antisera can be obtained by the intravenous (i.v.) injection of $2-5 \times 10^8$ viable cells (thymocytes or ALL blasts) into rabbits on days 0, 14 and once again around days 21 to 28. The sera can be harvested 6 to 8 days after the last injection.[14,29] No apparent additional benefit can be obtained when rabbits are immunized subcutaneously (s.c.) in addition to the i.v. injections. (The s.c. injection in these experiments contained 10^8 to 10^9 cells emulsified in complete Freund's adjuvant.)[30] It has to be emphasized, however, that the efficacy of i.v. immunization using viable cells has not been formally compared with other schedules using s.c. or intramuscular (i.m.) injections of emulsified cells administered in complete Freund's adjuvant (CFA). In a small study with low numbers of immunizing cells the i.v. route was slightly more efficient than the s.c. injection.[28]

Repeated multiple immunizations and hyperimmunizing schedules (using 5 or more monthly injections) may show rising titers in the unabsorbed antisera but the method does not seem to be convenient for producing specific antisera against membrane antigens. The main reason is that frequently vast amounts of cells are required for the absorption of these hyperimmune reagents (in order to remove species specific activity) and yield disappointingly weak specific activity against the differentiation antigens. Short immunization schedules are particulary important when the antibodies are assayed in complement-mediated cytotoxicity tests. Only early bleeds of anti-T-cell sera could be easily absorbed to yield specific reagents used in cytotoxic assay.[31]

Immunization with purified proteins
Animals most commonly used are rabbits, goats, sheep and chickens. Similar immunization schedules can be given in all of these species. These include 3 or 4 monthly immunizations, each containing 0.3 to 3 mg of antigen in complete Freund's adjuvants (CFA) according to well established principles.[23,32] The protein solution (in 1 to 1.5 ml saline) is emulsified very thoroughly in 1 to 1.5 ml CFA until the emulsion is stable and the water and oil phase do not separate.[33] Since the thick emulsion sticks to the wall of the tubes considerable losses can occur and should be taken into account during the preparation of the immunogen. A total of 3 ml emulsion is injected in equal parts into six intradermal sites (in goats and sheep) or 2 ml into 2 to 4 i.m. sites (in the hind leg of rabbits and chickens). Foot-pad injections in rabbits are also effective but painful for the animal. There are three important points which influence the course of immunization with purified protein antigens.

First, the antibody response should be monitored throughout the course. When purified antigens are used the reactivity and the titer of unabsorbed heterologous antisera give more meaningful information than similar tests performed after immunization with unpurified membrane antigens or whole cells (see above). Test bleeds are usually taken at intervals of 7 days after each immunization and tested for reactivity and titer using Ouchterlony and immunoelectrophoretic technics. Depending on the test bleed further boosts may be needed at monthly intervals (or bi-weekly intervals if the use of CFA is abandoned, see below). Once a suitable high titer has been reached large bleeds should be taken on two or three consecutive days.

Second, since the reactivity of different animals (within the same outbred species) can be highly variable, it is advisable to immunize more than one animal (4 to 5 rabbits) and select the high responder(s) on the basis of early test bleed results. Commercial companies always select the highest responders from large herds. It saves considerable effort to abandon the immunization of low responders and concentrate on the proper challenge and testing of high responders.

Third, the use of adjuvants (e.g. CFA from Difco Labs.) is important to present the protein antigens in a more immunogenic form to the animal. However, the prolonged use of CFA will give rise to adverse reactions (granuloma formation). When this occurs it might be advisable to use alternative adjuvants (e.g. Freund's incomplete adjuvant that lacks mycobacteria also available from Difco Labs.) or gelatinous aluminium hydroxide (available as Alhydrogel from Miles Labs. Ltd.).[33]

Modulation of heteroantibody production

The aim is the suppression of heteroantibody production against species specific antigens and the stimulation of antibody production to differentiation- and/or leukemia-associated antigens.

The three main possibilities are shown in Fig. 5.1. Rabbit antisera to the common non-T, non-B type of ALL are produced in a number of laboratories by injecting ALL cells incubated ('coated') with rabbit antilymphocyte serum.[14, 34] The rationale of this method is based on elegant studies in the chicken where antibodies to weak A_2 erythrocyte isoantigens are generated at late stages of the immune response, following the production of agglutinating antibodies against the stronger B_2 antigens. If erythrocytes (carrying both B_2 and A_2 antigens) coated with anti-B_2 antibodies are injected, antibody production to A_2 antigens is accelerated and to B_2 antigens is suppressed. Interestingly, erythrocytes expressing only A_2 (and no B_2) are not immunogenic.[35] Similar observations have been made in the mouse where antisera to lymphoma/leukemia associated antigens were generated by coating the immunizing cells with antilymphocyte antibodies.[36, 37]

Rabbit antisera to monkey thymocytes (MT) are excellent diagnostic reagents for human leukemias of the T-cell lineage.[29, 38] Monkey and human thymocytes/ T-cells share strong differentiation antigens,[29] but express partially different species specific antigens. Thus anti-MT sera require less absorption when used as reagents on human cells than do antihuman thymocyte sera.[26]

Finally, tolerance induction in mice against normal remission bone marrow followed by immunization with the leukemia of the same patient looks a most attractive but rather impractical method to produce antisera against leukemia.[39] In fact, this technology, used in combination with the production of 'monoclonal antibodies' in mice (see below) will almost certainly be the most useful method to produce highly specific antisera against subgroups of human leukemias and bone marrow stem cells.

Absorptions of antisera

Absorption is carried out by incubating antisera with insoluble antigens (cells or insolubilized proteins) that bind 'irrelevant' antibodies without removing antibodies intended for use. The antigens required for the absorption of various heterologous antisera include species specific and cross-reactive heteroantigens,

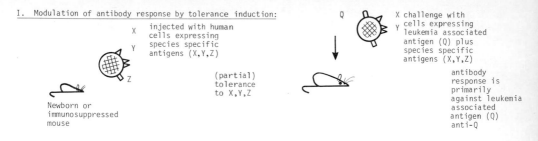

I. Modulation of antibody response by tolerance induction:

X injected with human cells expressing species specific antigens (X,Y,Z)

Y

Z

Newborn or immunosuppressed mouse

(partial) tolerance to X,Y,Z

Q   X challenge with cells expressing leukemia associated antigen (Q) plus species specific antigens (X,Y,Z)

Y

antibody response is primarily against leukemia associated antigen (Q) anti-Q

II. Modulation of antibody response by injecting antibody coated cells:

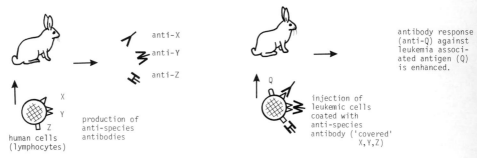

anti-X

anti-Y

anti-Z

human cells (lymphocytes)

X

Y

Z

production of anti-species antibodies

injection of leukemic cells coated with anti-species antibody ('covered' X,Y,Z)

Q

antibody response (anti-Q) against leukemia associated antigen (Q) is enhanced.

III. Injection of cells (from another species) which express the same differentiation antigens but different species specific antigens:

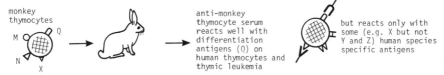

monkey thymocytes

M

N

Q

X

anti-monkey thymocyte serum reacts well with differentiation antigens (Q) on human thymocytes and thymic leukemia

but reacts only with some (e.g. X but not Y and Z) human species specific antigens

Fig. 5.1 Modulation of heteroantibody production. The production of heteroantibodies against 'irrelevant' (species specific-, etc.) antigens (X, Y, Z) can be suppressed and against unique leukemia associated- or differentiation-) antigens (Q) enhanced. I. Mice made partially tolerant against the individual patients' remission leukocytes make antibodies against leukemia associated antigens (AML or ALL) present on the leukemic blasts.[39] II. Rabbits injected with ALL cells which had been coated with human antilymphocyte serum produce antibodies to ALL-associated membrane antigens[14] III. Rabbits injected with rhesus monkey thymocytes make strong antibodies against thymic/T-lymphoid differentiation antigens shared between rhesus monkey and man. These antisera require less absorption because certain species (monkey) specific antigens are absent on human cells. Antibodies against the rhesus specific antigens are irrelevant in human diagnosis.

alloantigens, differentiation antigens expressed on more than one cell lineage, various serum proteins, immunoglobulin isotypes, etc.

The preparation of appropriate immunoabsorbents embraces a variety of methods. Some of these are simple but need collaboration between different branches of medicine (Table 5.1) while others require bulk tissue culture facilities.

An elegant method for the absorption of antisera, to react against certain types of leukemic cells (e.g. thymic ALL), is to prepare large quantities of continuously growing B-lymphoid cells (B-LCL) from the same leukemic patients (by transforming B-cells with Epstein-Barr virus) and to use these B-LCL' for absorption. These absorptions will remove most heteroantibodies, alloantibodies and common lymphoid differentiation antigens.[40–42]

Further absorptions with other (myeloid) cell populations might also be needed but these are unlikely to be extensive. If facilities for this method are not available in the laboratory, then various cell types and purified proteins are lined up for absorption (Table 5.1). The wide range of cellular absorbents needed explains the scarcity of well characterized heterologous antisera.

The importance of appropriate absorptions is not always fully appreciated. For example, many reports claim to have standardized antisera to human T-cells/thymocytes[26] or to B-lymphocytes, and a number of commercial firms produce 'antilymphocyte sera'. It is frequently unclear from these communications

Table 5.1 Immunoabsorbents used for preparation of reagents in leukemia analysis.

1. **Normal cells**
   Cadaver liver,[a] kidney[a] (sometimes spleen[b])
   AB red cells[a]
   Tonsil lymphocyte suspensions (from tonsillectomy)[b, d]
   Infant thymocytes (from elective cardiac surgery)[c, d]
   Bone marrow (from ribs recovered during thoracic surgery)[b, e]

2. **Lymphoid cell lines**[f] expressing the phenotye of
   Common-ALL (NALM-1, Reh, KEM)
   Thymic-ALL (MOLT-4, CCRF-CEM, HPB-ALL)
   B-lymphoid cells (RAJI, Bristol-7, other EBV transformed lines[g])

3. **High count leukemias**
   CGL (chronic phase)[b, c, e]
   High count CLL (B-type)[b, d, e]
   Thy-ALL[b, d, e]
   AML[b, e]

4. **Protein antigens** (glutaraldehyde treated or bead-bound)
   Fetal calf serum[a]
   Normal human serum[a]
   Cord serum[h]
   Agammaglobulinemic serum[h]
   Myeloma proteins[h]
   Bence-Jones proteins[h]

[a] All heterologous antisera.
[c] Anti-Ia serum.
[e] Anti-thymocyte/T-cell serum.
[g] See text.

[b] Anti-ALL serum.
[d] Anti-myeloid serum.
[f] See Table 5.4.
[h] Various anti-Ig reagents.

whether these reagents have been tested for antibody binding on 'irrelevant' non-lymphoid cells such as myeloid and erythroid bone marrow cells in general and on the various subsets of these populations (myeloblasts, erythroblasts, etc.) in particular. It would be unwise to recommend these reagents, on the basis of the information available, for leukemia diagnosis or for the treatment of patients (e.g. in aplastic anemia).

Even if the absorption of antisera is properly controlled in the laboratory, it can be difficult to produce specific reagents which react with virtually all cells within the 'relevant' population but show no reactivity with subpopulations of other cell types. After a few absorptions (e.g. with liver powder, red cells, a few cases of high count leukemias and selected cell lines) an antiserum (e.g.

an antithymocyte serum) may show almost perfect specificity, except that it might still react with a small subset of myeloid cells in the bone marrow. At this stage it is important to screen many cases of acute myeloid leukemias (AML) and find one which still reacts with the antiserum. The absorption with this particular leukemic sample may be essential to make the serum useful.

The absorption of antisera with intact cells is carried out as follows:

1. One vol. of cells is washed three times in 10 vol. of PBS (10 min, 4°C; leukocytes: 400 g; red cells: 1000 g). After the final wash remove supernate as completely as possible
2. Add 3 vol. of serum to 1 vol. cell pellet. Resuspend cells in the serum with a Pasteur pipette. Add proteolytic inhibitor (e.g. Trasylol 1000 K.I.U. per ml serum, Bayer Ltd) and seal tube
3. Rotate the cell/serum mixture for 30 min to 1 h at 4°C or in a cold room
4. Spin for 15 min, 2000 g at 4°C. Keep serum and discard cells.

Similar absorption procedure can be carried out with liver extracts,[43] cells fixed with formalin,[44] proteins cross-linked with glutaraldehyde[45] and with various antigens coupled to Sepharose beads. A convenient method for linking proteins to Sepharose 4B beads is the cyanogen bromide method.[46,47] Since the use of cyanogen bromide is unpleasant and hazardous, the use of CNBr activated Sepharose 4B (Pharmacia Fine Chemicals Ltd) is recommended.

It is important to point out that antisera made against purified antigens may also contain irrelevant antibodies which interfere with the intended use. These antibodies can be generated during immunization (representing cross-reacting antibodies or antibodies against impurities in the immunizing protein antigen) or could be heteroantibodies against foreign proteins and heterocytotropic antibodies which had been present in the serum prior to immunization. During recent years the quality of commercially available reagents has improved considerably and information about their specificity and cross-reactivity with immunoglobulins of other species is frequently provided. It is nevertheless unreasonable to expect that these reagents can be totally specific in all the different test systems. Thus, simple absorption technics should be available in the laboratory even if commercially available reagents are used.

Manipulations with antibodies

Immune complexes and immunoglobulin (Ig) aggregates interfere with the membrane marker analysis of cells. Absorbed antisera are therefore cleaned up with the following methods: (1) removal of complexes by ultracentrifugation; (2) preparation of F(ab)$_2$ fragment of Ig from whole serum; (3) preparation of gammaglobulin fraction and (4) elution of pure antibodies from immunoadsorbent columns.

In general, most complexes and Ig aggregates can be removed from antisera (including specific antisera conjugated to fluorochromes) by ultracentrifugation at 100 000 to 150 000 g for 30 min to 1 h. Antisera should therefore be ultracentrifuged and sterile filtered before distribution into small aliquots and stored frozen at −20°C. When these samples are thawed they should be centrifuged again in a small high-speed bench centrifuge (Beckman or Eppendorf) for 15 to 30 min immediately before use.[7]

The preparations described below are important in sensitive immunological assays, e.g. in the analysis of monoclonality of B-lymphoid cells in leukemia and lymphoma, etc. The use of pure antibodies (e.g. fluorochrome labelled second layers) is essential if the antigens studied are weakly expressed.

Preparation of F(ab)$_2$ fragments

Principle. A convenient and easy method for preparation of F(ab)$_2$ fragments requires an acid pH to precipitate the majority of proteins in the antisera and enzymatic digestion of the remaining molecules using high activity pepsin which destroys the Fc region leaving the F(ab)$_2$ antigen binding fragment intact.[48]

Materials

1. Antiserum
2. Pepsin 1:60 000 (Sigma Chemical Co. Ltd.)
3. 0.005 mol/l phosphate buffer pH 7.4
4. 0.3 mol/l hydrochloric acid
5. Visking tubing (for dialysis, Scientific Instrument Centre Ltd).

Method

1. 2 mg of pepsin are added to 1 ml aliquots of antiserum
2. Adjust solution to pH 4 using 0.3 mol/l hydrochloric acid
3. Incubate mixture for 16 h at 37°C
4. Centrifuge 10 000 r/min for 20 min; discard precipitate
5. Dialyze supernatant overnight against 0.005 mol/l phosphate buffer (pH 7.4)
6. Centrifuge 10 000 r/min for 20 min
7. Discard any precipitate
8. Use supernatant directly as the F(ab)$_2$ fragment of the antiserum.

Note: Rabbit IgG binds particularly strongly to human Fc$_{IgG}$ receptors. It is therefore important to prepare F(ab)$_2$ fragments from rabbit antisera. Goat, sheep and chicken IgM binds human Fc$_{IgG}$ less avidly and therefore the preparation of F(ab)$_2$ fragments is frequently not essential.

Preparation of gammaglobulin fraction of antisera
A gammaglobulin fraction of the crude antiserum is required before further purification steps (see below) can be undertaken. This can be precipitated by 50 per cent ammonium sulfate.[49]

Adsorption and elution of pure antibody
Principle. The gammaglobulin fraction can be purified by adsorption to and elution from immunoadsorbent columns. The immunoadsorbent column is an insoluble matrix to which the relevant antigen has been coupled.[46,47] The material eluted consists of pure antibodies without irrelevant serum Ig and other proteins. The immunoadsorbent column can only be made if the pure antigen

is available in large quantity; for this reason this elegant technic is most extensively used to prepare various antiimmunoglobulin reagents (e.g. second layers in indirect IF test, etc.). In a number of sensitive IF tests high titer pure antibodies are essential to decrease non-specific background staining so commonly encountered with crude antisera.

The elution of pure antibodies from an immunoadsorbent column does not guarantee that the reagent is specific. The complementary role of immunoabsorbent columns and the elution of pure antibodies (from an immunoadsorbent column) can be illustrated with the following example. Pure specific antibodies to human IgM (μ chain specific) are required. The anti-IgM serum, made against, for example, IgM (κ) myeloma is first absorbed on four sequential Sepharose bead columns coated with: hypogammaglobulinemic serum, Bence-Jones protein (κ), IgG (κ or λ) myeloma, and IgA (κ or λ) myeloma. This antiserum now appears to be specific for μ chain in Ouchterlony tests and membrane marker studies. *Pure antibodies* are then eluted from an IgM (λ) column.[50] These can be coupled to flurochromes (see below) and provide a powerful and clean reagent for meticulous studies. Similarly, when pure antibodies to rabbit IgG are prepared (in order to be used as a second layer in indirect IF test) the antiserum is first absorbed on a Sepharose bead column coated with human serum and then eluted from a rabbit IgG column.

PREPARATION OF MONOCLONAL ANTIBODIES

Conventional heterologous antisera to different human cell types require extensive absorptions. It is frequently impractical to prepare large quantities of standard antisera with this technology and is therefore important to pay attention to a new technic by which large amounts of standard reagents can be produced (Table 5.2).

This new technic combines conventional immunological methods with somatic cell hybridization and the selection of appropriate hybrids (Fig. 5.2). Hybrids formed by the fusion of myeloma cell lines and single B-lymphocytes have useful properties. They inherit the ability of the myeloma cells to grow indefinitely in culture (and in serial passage through inbred strains of mice), and in addition, the ability of B-lymphocytes to synthesize one single antibody with a given immunological specificity. Thus a clone of cells synthesizing only one single type of antibody can be produced and propagated. Under the tissue culture conditions used (after hybridization), only the B-lymphocyte-myeloma cell hybrids survive and grow while the non-hybridal B-lymphocytes and myeloma cells die.

The technic was originated by Milstein and his associates.[51] Whilst studying the expression of Ig light and heavy chains, they fused a non-secreting, light chain variant of the mouse myeloma MOPC 21 with spleen cells from a mouse that had been immunized against sheep red cells (SRBC). They found that a large proportion of the clones of hybrid cells secreted the mouse anti-SRBC antibody, whilst none of the myeloma light chain was released. Intraspecies hybrids are fairly stable. Interspecies hybrids show higher incidence of gene deletion and are therefore rarely used for Ig production.

The original mouse *myeloma* MOPC 21 variant is called P3 and secretes IgG_1 (κ). The most commonly used myeloma for hybridization is a sub-line of this: P3-NS1. This is a non-secreting variant which synthesises κ light chain but does not secrete it. The P3–NS1 line has been adapted to grow in medium containing $20\,\mu g/ml$ 8-azaguanine for the reasons outlined below.[52] This line, P3-NS1/1 Ag4-1, is available from Flow Labs, Scotland. Other mouse and rat myeloma lines are also of use.

Standard immunization methods can be used to produce antibody-secreting spleen cells: 15 to 25 Balb/c mice are immunized with cells bearing the relevant surface antigen and boosted at 4 to 6 week intervals until a good serum titer against the immunizing cell is achieved. A final boost is given i.v. 3 to 5 days before hybridization.

Table 5.2 Steps required for producing reagents for leukemia diagnosis by conventional immunization and by mouse B-cell-myeloma hybrids.

Conventional antisera	Monoclonal antibodies
Repeated immunization of large animals	Immunization of small animals (mice or rats)
Repeated absorptions of crude antisera with large amounts of cells (cell lines; bulk leukemias)	Fusion of B-lymphocytes with myeloma cells
Specificity testing	Preliminary screening of large numbers of clones (using a few established cell lines or well characterized leukemias)
Further absorptions with selected leukemias	Selection, cloning and propagation of interesting clones
Further specificity testing	Very extensive testing of the few useful clones on a large panel of normal and leukemic cells (frequently a collaborative effort between different laboratories)
The final reagent is available in limited quantity; in spite of extensive testing it is not a standard reagent; the limited quantity and range of cells available for absorption may restrict production	The final reagent is available in large quantity; it is a standard reagent; no absorption is required

The mouse giving the highest titer of serum antibody against the immunizing cells is sacrificed. Spleen cells are teased out with forceps into RPMI medium containing 2 to 5 per cent FCS under sterile conditions.

Myeloma cells are fused with mouse spleen cells in the presence of concentrated polyethylene glycol (PEG) as *fusogen*.[53] PEG of 1000 to 1500 M.W. produce the highest yield of fusion.[54]

The principle of growing myeloma-B-cell hybrids is as follows. The presence of 8-azaguanine in the medium (see above) selects for myeloma cells that are deficient in an enzyme of the purine salvage pathway (hypoxanthine, guanine phosphoribosyl transferase: HGPRT). Cells which contain the enzyme incorporate the toxic azaguanine into the DNA and die; mutant cells deficient in HGPRT do not incorporate azaguanine and survive by synthesizing nucleo-

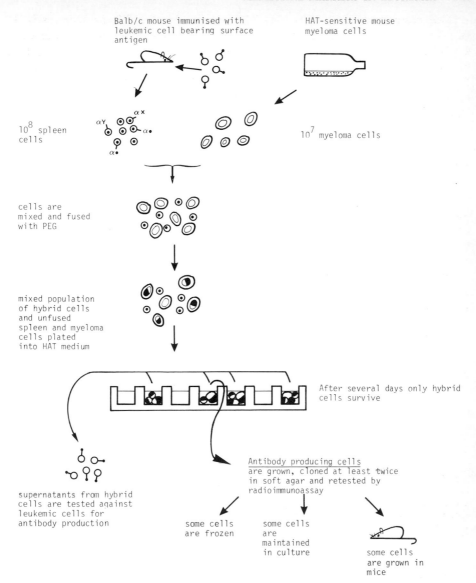

Fig. 5.2 Preparation of monoclonal antibodies. For details see text.

tides *de novo*. Clearly, these mutant cells loose their chance of survival when they are transferred to HAT medium (a normal growth medium lacking 8-azaguanine but supplemented with 10^{-4} mol/l hypoxanthine, 4×10^{-7} mol/l aminopterin and 1.6×10^{-5} thymidine) since aminopterin blocks *de novo* nucleotide synthesis (by competitive inhibition of dihydrofolic reductase). Hybrids of the HAT sensitive mutant myeloma and normal spleen B-lymphocytes, on the other hand, continue to grow because these hybrids inherit the HGPRT enzyme from their B-lymphocyte parents and operate the purine salvage pathway.[51-53] As normal (non-hybrid) B-lymphocytes are 'mortal' short-lived cells *in vitro* and die off within 4 to 6 days in culture, only the hybrids survive in HAT medium. The individual clones of myeloma-B-lymphocyte hybrids can later be isolated from others by conventional 'cloning' procedures in soft agar.[55] All cells of one single clone synthesize the same single antibody.

The analysis of monoclonal antibodies proceeds in several stages.

The first stage of investigation is the analysis of antibody production by the small clumps of hybrid cells 7 to 10 days after fusion. This is a screening procedure studying supernates from 50 to 100 wells on a limited number of cell types. These include the immunizing antigen (or cell type) and a few well characterized cell lines, leukemic cells and/or normal hemopoietic cells. Clearly, the purposeful selection of these cell types during screening is very important and varies according to the aims of the investigator. The most convenient method at this stage is a radioimmunoassay (RIA) using I^{125} labelled goat anti-mouse Ig as a second layer.

It is important to keep in mind that since the cultures have not yet been cloned at this stage certain wells may contain more than one antibody producing clone (i.e. antibody mixtures), and that antibodies showing low or intermediate counts in the binding assay should not be ignored because these can be as interesting as antibodies showing high counts. For example, ALL associated antigens are present in relatively low density on leukemic cells when compared with Ia-like or HLA-A,B,C antigens. A monoclonal antibody recognizing ALL-associated antigen would therefore almost certainly give lower counts than antibodies against the core determinants of Ia-like or HLA-A,B,C, antigens.

The second stage of investigation is carried out after successful cloning of selected antibody-producing cultures. In addition to RIA, further test systems (analysis of binding by IF method using the fluorescence microscope; see below) and a collection of cell types, including normal and leukemic cells, are used.

Third stage. This is to compare the activity of the new reagent with other well established markers in double marker systems using antiserum combinations labelled with different fluorochromes. There are a variety of studies which can easily be performed in double marker assays: e.g. it is possible to study whether the antibody reacts with B- or T-lymphocytes or their subsets. Various types of normal bone marrow cells can be studied in combination with anti-Ia-like reagents, etc. These investigations can lead to observations about the specificity of the monoclonal antibodies and also about the characteristics of the various cells studied.

DETECTION OF MEMBRANE ANTIGENS

It is difficult to label membrane antigens with antibodies on cells spread on slides: the cell membrane is distorted and intracellular staining also occurs. Membrane antigens ('markers') are therefore studied by labeling the cells in suspension. The first part of this section describes the preparation of leukocyte suspensions (red cell free) from blood and bone marrow.

The binding of antibodies to cell membranes can be detected in a number of test systems (Fig. 5.3) which can be used for analyzing leukemic cells. Each

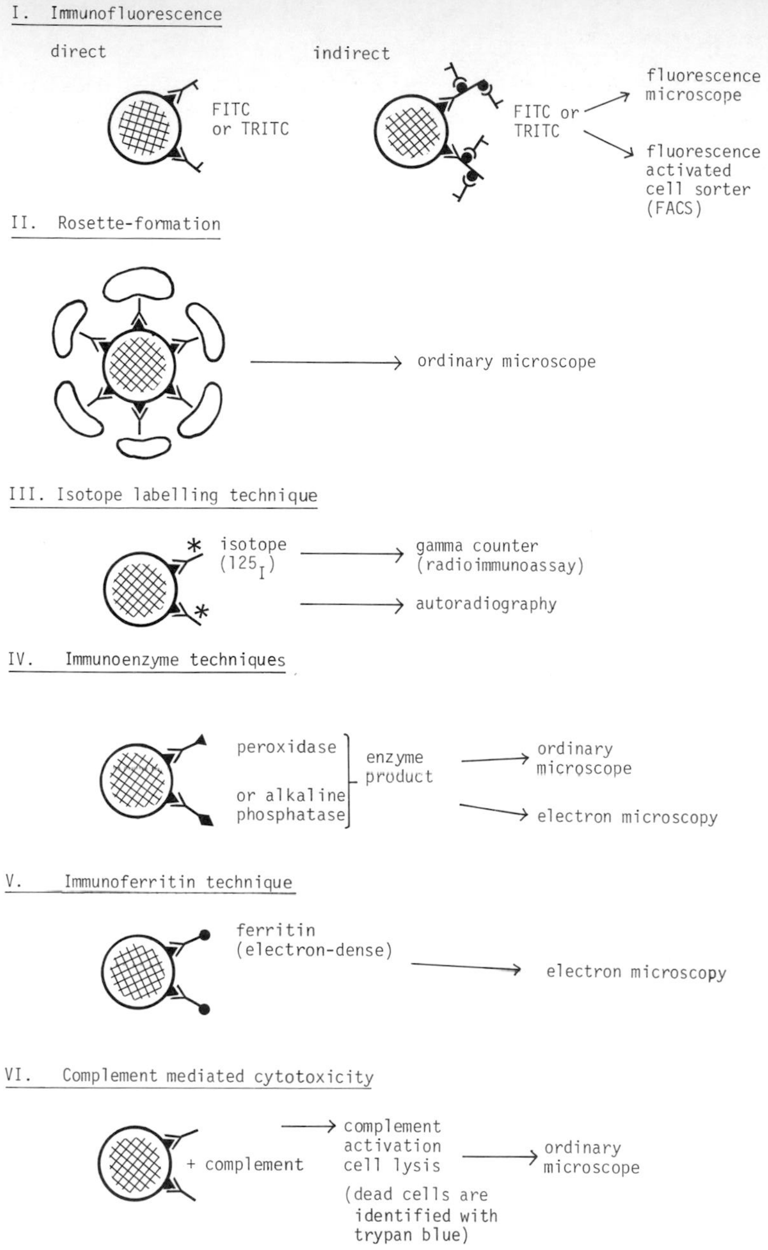

I. Immunofluorescence

direct   indirect

FITC   FITC or   fluorescence
or TRITC   TRITC   microscope

                                           fluorescence
                                           activated
                                           cell sorter
                                           (FACS)

II. Rosette-formation

→ ordinary microscope

III. Isotope labelling technique

* isotope   →   gamma counter
  (125_I)   (radioimmunoassay)

              →   autoradiography

IV. Immunoenzyme techniques

peroxidase ⎤
           ⎥ enzyme   → ordinary
           ⎦ product   microscope
or alkaline
phosphatase⎦   → electron microscopy

V. Immunoferritin technique

ferritin
(electron-dense)   → electron microscopy

VI. Complement mediated cytotoxicity

              → complement
                activation   → ordinary
+ complement   cell lysis   microscope

              (dead cells are
               identified with
               trypan blue)

Fig. 5.3 Detection of antibody binding to cell membranes. Antibodies can be labeled with various 'identity tags' which are recognized in the different detection systems. *Immunofluorescence* gives sharp image and good resolution when used on cell suspensions; it is combined with phase contrast on the immunofluorescence microscope or with rapid quantitative cell population studies and cell separation of the Fluorescence Activated Cell Sorter (FACS). Indirect fluorescence (sandwich technic) is more sensitive than direct fluorescence. *Rosette formation* can be carried out with erythrocytes coupled to specific antibody: a very sensitive method. *Radioimmunoassay* gives numerical (printed) information on antibody binding to cell populations (but no information on individual cells): a quick method for **analyzing** large numbers of samples. *Autoradiography* can combine morphological analysis with membrane marker studies and is an elegant but time-consuming analytical technic.[18,58,59] *Immunoenzyme and immunoferritin technics* used mainly for electronmicroscopy, are not discussed in this chapter.[60] *Complement-mediated cytotoxicity* detects complement fixing antibodies which initiate cell lysis.

system has certain advantages and disadvantages which influence its application. In earlier years complement mediated lysis was used most extensively; in recent years IF has been favoured.[21,56]

When the specificity of antisera is analyzed the following criteria should be applied in all detection systems.[7] First, serial two-fold dilutions of the antiserum should be made and the percentage of positive cells (or the counts detected on isotope counter) recorded. It should be possible to titrate the reagents to a plateau which defines a distinct population of reactive cells in the positive sample, while showing negligible values in the negative samples. Two to four times the concentration of reagent required to reproduce the plateau value should be used in subsequent tests. Second, combined tests on various mixed populations should be performed in order to analyze the range of reactivity of different reagents in relation to each other. These combined single cell assays provide invaluable information about the reactivity of antisera to leukemia associated antigens on normal hemopoietic stem cells[57] and can detect 'undesired' antibodies against minority cell populations in antisera which, by other criteria, may appear to be fully specific.

Removal of RBC on Ficoll-Isopaque

Principle. When anticoagulated diluted blood or bone marrow is layered on top of a mixture of Ficoll-Isopaque (FI) and centrifuged at 20°C, erythrocytes and granulocytes sediment to the bottom, while lymphocytes, monocytes, mononuclear bone marrow elements and leukemic cells remain on the top of FI at the interphase.[61]

Materials

1. Separation fluid: 10 parts Isopaque (33.9 per cent density 1.200 g/ml Triosil, Vestric Ltd) are mixed with 24 parts Ficoll (9 per cent, Pharmacia Ltd). Final density is 1.077 g/ml. Various companies supply separation fluid but it is cheaper to prepare it in the laboratory
2. Collect blood into Lithium-Heparin vials (10 ml, Seward Lab.). Alternatively, use 10 IU preservative-free heparin per each ml blood. Collect bone marrow into similar heparinized vials and add 2 to 4 ml of Hanks, TC-199 or other tissue culture medium
3. PBS (containing 1 to 2 per cent bovine serum albumin)
4. Tubes (14 to 15 ml total capacity)
5. Hemocytometer.

Method

1. Dilute blood with PBS if $<20 \times 10^9/1$ twice; if $>20 \times 10^9/1$ four times. Mix sample
2. Place 4 ml FI into a 14 ml tube and carefully layer on 10 ml diluted blood without disturbing the interphase
3. Spin at 1800 r/min (400 g) for 25 min at 20°C (not at 4°C)

4. Discard top portion of supernate and transfer the layer of leukocyte around the interphase into another tube ('trimming around')
5. The suspension should be diluted at least five times and centrifuged at 400 g (10 min at 20°C). Since this sample still contains some FI leukocyte losses would occur at lower speeds
6. Remove supernatants, wash cells again in 10 ml PBS and resuspend in 2 to 5 ml PBS. Count cells in hemocytometer. Adjust cell concentration to 1 to 2×10^7/ml PBS.

Notes. See ref. 7 for the vagaries of the technic. A modification of the method for analyzing small samples is as follows. Smaller polyethylene tubes (with caps, volume: 1.5 ml, W. Sarstedt Ltd) and a microcentrifuge (e.g. Eppendorf) are used. 0.5 ml FI is placed into the tube and 1.0 ml cell suspension is layered on it. Tubes are spun for 1 min (approx. 600 g, fixed speed).

Acetate wash of cells (to remove cytophilic proteins)
Principle. Serum immunoglobulin and other proteins attach to leukocytes and interfere with the analysis of surface membrane Ig (SmIg). It is possible to denude the cell surface of existing Ig molecules by exposing the cells to trypsin, incubate them *in vitro* and allow the resynthesis of a 'clean membrane'.[62] This technic is difficult and recommended only for special studies. The bulk of passively absorbed protein can be eluted with a simpler, gentle method which satisfies stringent criteria for monoclonality testing in malignant B-cell disorders. Cells are incubated at pH 5.5 for 10 min and then in medium (pH 7.2, 37°C) for 2 h.[63]

Materials
1. Acetate buffer: solution 1—glacial acetic acid 12.0 ml/l
   solution 2—anhydrous sodium acetate 16.4 g/l
   Mix 8.8 ml of solution 1 to 41.2 ml of solution 2 and make up to 200 ml with dist. water. To each 200 ml add 1.8 g NaCl and 0.2 g anhydrous $CaCl_2$. Store 10 ml aliquots at $-20°C$
2. Medium (TC-199, or Dulbecco modified MEM or RPMI with 10 per cent FCS)
3. Water bath, 37°C
4. Cell suspension (1 to 2×10^7/ml)
5. Bench centrifuge.

Method
1. Resuspend cells in acetate buffer and incubate at 37°C for 10 min with occasional shaking
2. Wash cells twice and resuspend in medium. Put cells into water bath 37°C and incubate for 2 h with occasional mixing
3. Wash cells twice and resuspend in medium.

Note. After wash, minimal dot-like polyclonal Ig staining on myeloid cells is still observed. The staining of malignant B-lymphocytes seems to be stronger than before wash and shows genuine monoclonality (see below).

Membrane immunofluorescence (IF)

Principle. Antibodies react with membrane marker determinants of viable cells in suspension. In order to prevent extensive movement of the membrane protein-antibody complexes (which can lead to 'cap-formation' and shedding of caps)[64] 0.02 per cent sodium azide, a metabolic inhibitor, is added. Antibodies are either directly labeled with fluorochromes (direct IF test) or the cells are incubated with unlabeled antibody (first layer), washed and reincubated with labeled antibodies (second layer) directed against the first layer (indirect IF test). The indirect test is more sensitive than the direct test. Afterwards, wash cells are viewed with a fluorescence microscope either in suspension under a sealed coverslip or in freshly prepared fixed smears.

Materials

1. Cells (1 to 2×10^7/ml) in PBS + 2 per cent bovine serum albumin + 0.02 per cent azide
2. Antisera (of known specificity and strength) and normal control serum (from the same species)
3. PBS containing 2 per cent bovine serum albumin and 0.02 per cent azide
4. Plastic tubes (volume: 2 ml, LP3, Sterilin Ltd)
5. Eppendorf pipette (50 μl) and tips
6. Bench centrifuge
7. Glass micropipettes (1, 2 and 5 μl volume)
8. Fine Pasteur pipettes
9. Ice bucket with chips
10. 8 per cent formalin.

Method

1. Dispense 50 μl of cell suspension (0.5 to 1×10^6 cells/tube) with the Eppendorf pipette into LP3 tubes according to the number of antisera tested. Include controls for staining with normal serum
2. Add antibody with glass pipettes, mix well by tapping and incubate for 30 min at 4°C (on ice). Agitate samples once or twice during incubation
3. Top up tube with PBS, spin (3 min, 400 g), discard supernate and wash resuspended cells twice
4. If indirect test is used, leave approximately 50 μl fluid on the cells after the last wash. Add second antibody with glass pipettes. Repeat incubation and washings as above
5. Keep the tubes on ice while slide-preparations are made. Resuspend cells in 25 to 30 μl volume, place one small drop of cells on slide, cover with coverslip and press gently. Finally seal with nail varnish
6. Study cells immediately. If cells cannot be analyzed with 30 min add one drop of 8 per cent formalin (approximately 2 per cent final concentration) in order to fix cells as soon as possible (before preparing the slides).

Notes. It is important to wash samples well. Residual traces of the first antibody in the supernate can form soluble complexes with the second antibody and bind to Fc receptors on irrelevant cells. The fine morphology of membrane staining is informative. If azide is omitted and the samples are left on the bench for a long period the binding of antibodies (i.e. the crosslinking of membrane antigens) will result in active membrane movement. This leads to 'cap-formation' and to shedding and/or endocytosis of membrane receptors (Fig. 5.4E). Obviously this must be prevented and the tests are therefore performed on ice in the presence of azide. Nevertheless minimal membrane movement (patch formation) (Fig. 5.4B–C) does occur even in the presence of azide, and in fact helps to recognize genuine membrane staining. This staining pattern is distinct from the binding of Ig-aggregates or complexes to cells that express strong Fc receptors. In the latter case little 'lumps' seem to be lifted out from the plane

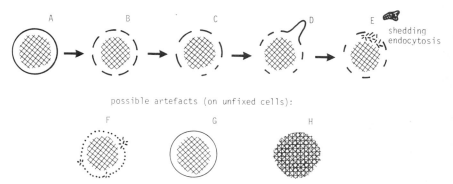

Fig. 5.4 Fine morphology of membrane staining. Under normal conditions membrane antigens are evenly distributed on the cell surface. This can be shown by the staining of cells pre-fixed (e.g. with formalin) prior to membrane staining (A). If, however, viable cells are incubated with antibodies, the cross-linking of membrane antigens leads to patch formation (B, C), cap formation (D) and, finally, to shedding and endocytosis of the membrane elements (E). This is an energy dependent process which is, to a certain extent, inhibited by azide (0.02 per cent) and cold (4°C). Under these conditions only patch-formation occurs (B).

Soluble aggregates or complexes can bind to Fcγ receptors on certain cells and give a characteristic 'dot-like' staining pattern (F). Weak but perfect ring staining (G) on unfixed cells is most frequently an artefact. Dead cells frequently show homogeneous stain all over the cell (H). In preparations properly stained for membrane antigens B and C are seen. F, G and H are likely to be artefacts.

of the membrane, and do not tend to show a linear apposition (Fig. 5.4F). Also, rarely, viable cells can show a weak but perfect ring-staining (Fig. 5.4G) which is an artefact. Some overconjugated commercial reagents can give this non-specific staining pattern. Dead cells in the suspension homogeneously stain with labeled antibodies (Fig. 5.4H). Some investigators prefer to read the results of membrane staining in viable (or formalin fixed) suspension of cells. It requires only a minimal effort to perfect this analysis along the line of phase contrast studies described by Bessis.[65] Others resuspend cells in a droplet of buffered glycerol.[66] An important point is to avoid excessive amount of fluid on the slides under the coverslip. This results in a 'halo' effect around the cells when viewed under phase. Apply a gentle pressure on the coverslip. This slightly flattens the cells and facilitates photography by preventing their movement. Other investigators prefer to spread droplets of cells on slides, let them dry on the bench, fix for 5 min in ethanol, wash in PBS and mount in glycerol.[67] Interestingly the intensity of fluorescence staining increases when the stained cells are smeared, but cells can shrink as they dry out. Finally, one can prepare fixed preparations of stained cells on a cytocentrifuge. The quick elimination of fluid by this process prevents the shrinkage of cells and optimal morphology is obtained. Nevertheless, the investigator has to be aware of the fact that smaller cells can sometimes be selectively lost during this process. Clearly, cytocentrifuge preparations are particularly suitable when the membrane labeled preparations are to be re-stained for cytoplasmic or nuclear antigens (see Fig. 5.9).

Fluorochrome labeling of antisera

Principle. Fluorochromes are dyes which absorb radiation. The excited molecules generated during this process emit light of a different wavelength. This effect is called fluorescence. Certain fluorochrome derivatives contain chemically active groups, e.g. isothiocyanates, which can be readily coupled with protein. Thus immune serum can be labeled with a firmly attached tracer which becomes conspicuous when excited by u.v. light. The labeled immune serum, i.e. the conjugate, if properly prepared should retain its immunological reactivity and therefore the site of antigen-antibody interaction appears fluorescent.

There are two major flurochromes commonly in use: fluorescein isothiocyanate (abbreviated as FITC and commonly referred to as fluorescein) which on excitation by u.v. light emits visible yellow-green light, and tetramethyl-rhodamine-isothiocyanate (abbreviated as TRITC and commonly referred to as rhodamine) which emits a red-orange light.

There are two essential requirements for a flurochrome conjugated antiserum: (1) it should contain potent antibody activity (2) the fluorochrome to protein ratio should be such that good specific staining is obtained and unwanted fluorescence is avoided.[68, 69]

Materials

1. Gammaglobulin or IgG fraction of antiserum
2. Sephadex G-25 column
3. Phosphate buffered saline (PBS)
4. Fluorescein isothiocyanate Isomer I (FITC; BDH Chemicals Ltd)
5. Tetramethyl rhodamine-isothiocyanate (TRITC; Nordic Immunological Labs. Ltd or Baltimore Biological Labs.)
6. Celite, analytical (BDH Chemicals Ltd)
7. 1 mol/l sodium hydroxide
8. u.v. Spectrophotometer.

Method

1. Adjust antiserum (gammaglobulin fraction) to pH 9.5 using 1 mol/l sodium hydroxide
2. Mix FITC and celite using 1 part FITC to 9 parts celite
3. Add FITC/celite mixture to the antiserum using 1 mg mix per 3 mg protein
4. Stir solution for 20 to 25 min at room temperature

5. Spin out any celite remaining in solution 2000 g for 3 min at room temperature

6. Pass conjugated antiserum over a G25 column equilibrated with PBS to separate the bound from the free FITC

7. The FITC conjugate will be found in the first fraction from the column

8. Concentrate this fraction and store either in PBS or a borate buffer at 4°C ready for testing

9. If there is an unacceptable degree of non-specific staining even after absorption with liver powder it may be necessary to fractionate the conjugate by ion exchange chromatography using an elution gradient of increasing ionic strength

10. The fluorochrome: protein ratio should be calculated every time a new conjugate is made. The presence of the fluorochrome interferes with the O.D. of the protein at 280 nm and this is allowed for in the formula:

$$\text{FITC: protein ratio} = \frac{2.87 \times \text{O.D. 495 nm}}{\text{O.D.}_{280\,nm} - 0.35 \times \text{O.D.}_{495\,nm}}$$

Notes. Conjugation with TRITC can be done under similar conditions. Select a batch of TRITC which is soluble. It is advisable to add TRITC/celite mix to the antiserum using 1 mg mix to 10 mg protein. Also it is necessary to double the length of the G25 column normally used for fractionation procedures.

$$\text{TRITC: protein ratio} = \frac{\text{O.D. 515 nm}}{\text{O.D. 280 nm}}$$

The fluorochrome to protein ratio should be low 1.5:1 if the conjugate is to be used to stain fixed material, e.g. cytoplasmic staining. However, for cell surface staining of viable cells higher fluorochrome: protein ratio (up to 3:1) can be used. Finally, the conjugate should be distributed in small aliquots and stored at −20°C.

Use of the fluorescence microscope

Recent developments in the design of microscopes and in the quality of filter sets have led to major advances in fluorescence microscopy.

Modern fluorescence microscopes use incident-light excitation (epi-illumination or epi-fluorescence)[70] instead of transmitted light excitation. The advantages of the epi-fluorescence system are considerable. First, the exciting light passes through the specimen downwards and is lost without interfering with the fluorescence image. The fluorescence image, on the other hand, passes directly upwards through an ingeniously designed chromatic beam splitter into the eye-pieces. Second, when the epi-fluorescence system is used the design of the reflector housing (containing the filters and beam splitters) is compact and may contain up to four filter sets on larger microscopes or two filter sets (one for FITC and one for TRITC) on smaller microscopes. The switch from one set to another is rapid. Thus epi-fluorescence microscopy and the design of reflector-housing facilitate the routine application of double labeling technics with combinations of antisera labeled with FITC and TRITC, respectively. A further advantage of the new development is that the compact epi-fluorescence condensers are easily fitted to all microscopes of the standard line (produced by the same firm) which instantly converts a bench microscope into a most efficient fluorescence microscope. This decreases the cost of the investment required. In fact, the smaller epi-fluorescence condensers (using HBO high pressure mercury lamp, HBO 50) give higher total energy yield in the specimen plane (and somewhat brighter image) than most larger, more expensive photomicroscopes. Filters for narrow band FITC and TRITC excitation are available as standard sets.

The brightest objectives (suitable for analyzing samples labeled with FITC and TRITC) are the Planapochromatic 63 Ph3 oil objectives (numerical aperture 1.40). Membrane marker studies can also be performed with cheaper 100 Ph3 oil objectives (numerical aperture: 1.25 to 1.30). It is important to emphasize, however, that fluorescence studies should always be combined with a most careful analysis of the cells under phase contrast. Although this image does not provide as much detail as conventional hematological preparations, the identification of distinct subpopulations (e.g. granulocytes, promyelocytes, myeloblasts with multiple nucleoli, normoblasts, cells of lymphoid appearance sometimes showing variable sizes, etc.) is possible and a meaningful comparison with the hematological morphology is feasible. This extra information is so valuable that the analysis of FITC or TRITC labeled cells on a good microscope is preferable to the quicker and more quantitative analysis carried out on a Cytofluorograph or Fluorescence Activated Cell Sorter.

Use of the Fluorescence Activated Cell Sorter

Principle. The binding of fluorochrome (FITC or TRITC) labeled antisera to cell membranes can be quantitated by the Fluorescence Activated Cell Sorter (FACS).[71] The FACS measures the fluorescence light and scattered light of individual cells as they flow through a laser illumination system coupled to a set of detectors. The fluorescence signal is roughly proportional to the amount of antibodies bound and the scatter signal to the cell size. These signals are displayed as a histogram which show numbers of cells versus fluorescence brightness or numbers of cells versus scatter (size). Even more informative is the display of two dimensional spot diagrams in which each cell is recorded as a spot. The distance of this spot from one axis represents the cell's brightness and from the other axis represents its size (Fig. 5.5). From these analytical data subpopulations of cells are identified which the machine can then be programed to separate.

Clearly, the FACS is a versatile instrument which can be used as a sensitive analytical tool and, in addition, as a cell separator. FACS is made by Becton Dickinson Inc, Mountain View, California. If the interest in the laboratory is *entirely* analytical then a new family of cheaper cytofluorographs can provide an equally satisfactory service.

The use of FACS in leukemia. The FACS can not substitute for a careful analysis of cells by conventional light microscopy or by immunofluorescence

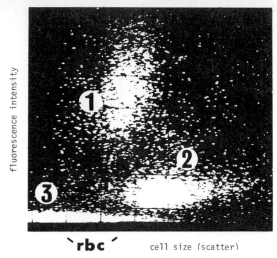

Fig. 5.5 Definition of subset heterogeneity on the Fluorescence Activated Cell Sorter (FACS). Cells were incubated with an FITC-labeled antibody and analyzed on the FACS. Each cell is recorded as a spot. The distance of this spot from the Y axis represents the cell's brightness and from the X axis the light scatter (cell size). This particular antibody distinguishes three populations: (1) small bright cells; (2) larger dull cells and (3) small to intermediate negative cells. Subsequent cell sorting and morphological analysis revealed that population 1 had lymphoid morphology; population 2 consisted of myeloid-granulocytic cells and population 3 contained erythrocytes (RBC) and precursors.

microscopy. Nevertheless, the FACS can supplement these observations in three different ways.[72]

First, the quantitative aspects of antibody binding are important. Some antisera can bind very strongly to one cell type, moderately strongly to another cell type and very weakly to a third cell type. These observations can be documented on the FACS, which then helps to define the diagnostic use and limitation of antisera.

Second, the FACS provides an elegant way to combine immunological membrane marker analysis with classical hematological analysis. The different populations defined by the fluoresence-scatter spot diagrams are separated on the FACS and stained in smears by May-Grünwald-Giemsa or by histochemical technics. These studies confirm the impression of investigators obtained by the combined fluorescence-phase contrast studies (see above) and give valuable information on the morphology of leukemic cells and the normal cell types reactive with individual antisera (Figs 5.6 and 5.7).

Probably the most important potential application of the FACS is the separation of cells for further functional studies (e.g. in colony forming assays *in vitro*). This technic has already been used to analyze cells expressing leukemia associated antigens in normal and regenerating bone marrow samples.[72] A major problem, however, is that at the present time methods for analyzing functional characteristics of human pluripotential stem cells and early lymphoid stem cells are not yet fully established (see Ch. 8). It may be important to combine cell separation studies (using antibodies and the FACS) with newly developed tissue culture methods an *in vitro* diffusion chamber experiments.[73]

The use of RBC coated with antibodies to leukocyte membrane antigens

Various methods are available for coupling proteins (i.e. antibodies) to the erythrocyte surface, and chromium chloride as a coupling agent has proved the most reproducible.[74] Even this recent improved method requires very careful standardization in the laboratory. The essential problem is to establish a chromic chloride concentration that will adequately bind the protein to the cells without forming excess chromic ion cross-linking on the cell surface that leads to hemagglutination. The optimum chromic chloride concentration should therefore be established for each experiment using standard protein, such as gammaglobulin from the same species in which the antibody was produced.

Ox RBC are recommended. Human RBC are also suitable. The method is apparently very sensitive for detecting various immunoblobulin isotypes on CLL cells.[75] A further advantage of the rosette method is that rosette-forming cells can be isolated from other mononuclear or leukemic cell populations.[76,77] On Ficoll-Isopaque(FI) gradient (see above) rosetted cells sediment to the bottom of the tube together with RBC. Non-rosetted cells remain in the interphase. This technic is applicable for all rosette methods, including those which are described below. Rosette-forming cells can then be 'freed' by lysing the RBC with ammonium chloride as follows:

1. Layer the suspended rosettes over FI and centrifuge at $400\,g$ for 10 min
2. Take off cells at the interface (non-rosetted cells)
3. Tip of the FI from the red cell button and resuspend in $0.17\,mol/1\,NH_4Cl$. Spin immediately and resuspend in NH_4Cl again. Leave this at room temperature for 10 to 15 min
4. When the RBC are lysed, layer the suspension over undiluted fetal calf serum and spin at $100\,g$ for 7 min. Discard the interphase containing the RBC stroma and analyze the free leukocyte population in the pellet.

Radioimmunoassay (RIA) for membrane antigens

Principle. When large numbers of samples are analyzed (e.g. for testing antibody activity in supernatants of B-cell-myeloma cultures after hybridization; see above) RIA is the most practical method.[44] Frequently, this is an indirect antibody binding test where the second layer of antibody is labeled with I^{125} using the chloramine-T method.[78]

The disadvantage of the method is that it does not provide information about the heterogeneity of antibody binding on the individual cells in the populations studied. The relevant results obtained with this technic should therefore be followed up by further simple cell studies using immunofluorescence or other assay tests.

Complement-mediated cytotoxicity

Principle. Certain immunoglobulin classes (primarily IgM) can fix cytolytic complement (C') when attached to cell membranes. Cytotoxic tests analyze the permeability of cell membranes after incubation with antibody and C'. If cytolytic C' is bound to the cell membrane, an increased permeability can be detected by adding a solution of eosin (or trypan blue). The dye penetrates into dead cells (positive reaction) but fails to stain viable cells (negative reaction). This technic is routinely used in histocompatibility testing to detect cytotoxic alloantisera with a micromethod in Terasaki plates.[79] The advantage of this technic is its speed and suitability for large scale studies: no centrifugation is involved. The test is very economical (on cells and reagents) and is read on an inverted microscope.

Materials

1. Hanks' solution (or veronal buffered saline, VBS)
2. Cell suspension (2×10^6/ml Hanks)
3. Rabbit complement: fresh serum allowed to clot for 30 min at 37°C; screened for the presence of natural toxins against human cells; titrated but may be used undiluted. Suitable sera are pooled, aliquoted and kept in liquid N_2 until use
4. Eosin: 5 per cent solution in distilled water (pre-spun and filtered)
5. Formalin (20 per cent adjusted to pH 7)
6. Terasaki plates (60 wells; Falcon Plastics or similar product)
7. Hamilton microsyringes (2 with 50 μl capacity; 2 with 250 μl capacity) and Hamilton repeating dispenser
8. Inverted microscope
9. Doubling dilutions of antisera in Hanks or VBS
10. Liquid paraffin.

Method

1. Terasaki tray is flooded with liquid paraffin and 1 μl antisera (1 push with 50 μl microsyringe in dispenser) are dispensed to the bottom of wells
2. 1 μl cell suspension is added to each (using another 50 μl syringe) and incubated at 20°C for 30 min
3. 5 μl complement is added into each well (1 push with 250 μl syringe) and incubated for a further 60 min
4. Add 5 μl eosin to each well, allow the tray to stand for 2 min and then add 5 μl formalin. This fixes the cells and the results can be read when convenient
5. Count the proportion of dead (red) cells on an inverted microscope.

Notes. If the laboratory is not equipped for the microtest, the assay can be stepped up 10-fold in tubes or microplates and evaluated in hemocytometer using Trypan blue (1 per cent solution in water, diluted with saline 1/10 before use) instead of eosin and formalin. It is important to have controls with no antibodies. If an antibody titration is carried out the titer is the dilution which kills 50 per cent of relevant cells (i.e. leukemic blasts).

Comparison of C′-mediated cytotoxicity with other tests

The cell lysis in the C′-mediated test is dependent upon the presence of antibodies to membrane antigens, on the C′-fixing properties of these antibodies and to what extent the target cells are sensitive to C′-lysis. Thus the test can

Table 5.3 Main leukemia groups distinguished by antisera to membrane antigens, rosette tests and the TdT enzyme assay.[g]

	ALL antigen	Ia-like antigen	HuTLA	My antigen	SmIg (monoclonal)	Rosette tests E	Rosette tests M	TdT enzyme test
1. Non-T, non-B ALL[a]	+	+	−	−	−	−	−	+
lymphoid blast crisis[b,f]	+	+	−	−	−	−	−	+
2. Thy-ALL[c]	−	−	+	−	−	+	−	+
3. CLL,[d] PLL and B-ALL	−	+	−	−	+	−	+[d]	−
4. AML[e]	−	+(−)[e]	−	+	−	−	−	−
myeloid blast crisis[f]	−	+(−)[e]	−	+	−	−	−	−

[a]Some heterogeneity in group. Some cases are ALL⁻, Ia⁺, TdT⁺ or, rarely, ALL⁺, Ia⁺, TdT⁻.[85] Approx. 30% of cases exhibit cytoplasmic IgM (pre-B ALL).[86-88]

[b]Ph[1] positive cases which can present as CML or, rarely, as Ph[1] positive All.[89] Cell populations are frequently heterogeneous and exhibit mixture of ALL⁺, Ia⁺, TdT⁺ ('lymphoid') and ALL⁻, Ia⁺, TdT⁻ (myeloid) blast cells (Fig. 5.6).

[c]Invariably HuTLA⁺, Ia⁻[47] but some are E⁻ and/or ALL⁺ (pre-thymic ALL?). Some cases EAC⁺ (see Rosette tests).

[d]Only CLL, and a few hairy-cell leukemias form M-rosettes; prolymphocytic leukemia (PLL) and lymphomas are M⁻ (see Table 5.8) The Ig expression is monoclonal (either κ or λ).

[e]Some cases of AML and most promyelocytic leukemias are Ia⁻.[91] Cases with monocytic differentiation strongly express Fcγ EA receptors (see Rosette tests).

[f]Acute phase of Ph[1] positive CML.

[g]Approx. 7% of acute leukemias remain unclassifiable with this panel of markers.[85]

be sensitive to certain antibody classes (e.g. IgM) but the results are not directly comparable to the observations obtained in IF tests or RIA. In fact, antisera found specific to certain cell types by C'-mediated cytotoxicity most frequently prove to be not specific by the IF assay. On the other hand, reagents specific by IF are frequently not cytotoxic in the C'-mediated assay.

The great advantage of the C'-mediated test is that it can be performed on large numbers of sera and cells.[80] This is offset by the disadvantages that the cells reacting with the antibody are destroyed by the lysis and are not amenable for further analysis, and that the sensitivity of the test is hampered by the presence of dead cells in the initial starting sample. Thus the C'mediated cytotoxic test is unlikely to reliably detect < 10 per cent genuine positive cells in the cell suspension.

IMMUNOLOGICAL REAGENTS FOR LEUKEMIA DIAGNOSIS

These include antisera and erythrocyte reagents for rosette tests.

ANTISERA

During the last few years a consensus has been reached regarding the diagnostic use of certain antisera.[81] These reagents have been standardized independently in a number of laboratories and seem to recognize normal gene products on cells at various stages of hemopoietic (lymphoid) differentiation (see below). Three of these reagents define differentiation markers that are present on cells committed to one of the three main cell lineages. Anti-HuTLA reagents detect *thymocyte and T-lymphoid antigens*, various anti-immunoglobulin sera react with surface membrane *immunoglobulin (SmIg) on B-lymphocytes*, and anti-myeloid sera detect *myeloid antigens*.

Two other antisera recognize differentiation antigens on relatively *immature cells*.[15] The anti-ALL serum weakly reacts with bone marrow precursor cells of unknown function (with its main expression on the common non-T, non-B form of ALL). The other antiserum, referred to as anti-'Ia-like' serum, also reacts with precursor cells including myeloid precursors and, in addition, with B-lymphocytes. Finally, the enzyme terminal deoxynucleotidyl transferase

Table 5.4 Lymphoid cell lines.[a]

Non-T, non-B ALL cell types
REH, KM-3, NALL-1

Non-T, non-B ALL line with pre-B ALL features
NALM-6, NALM-1[b]

Thymic (Thy-ALL) type
CCRF-CEM, CCRF-HSB-2, MOLT-4, RPMI-8402, HPB-ALL, HPB-MLT, T-ALL-1

B-cell type
DAUDI, BALL-1, U-698-M, Burkitt lymphoid cell lines (RAJI, RAMOS, Bristol-7, Bristol-8, etc)

[a] For further reading see ref. 92 and Table 5.3 for phenotypic details.
[b] Ph[1] positive cell line.

(TdT), detected by a biochemical assay (see Ch. 7) or by a specific antibody,[82] is expressed in bone marrow precursor cells and in cortical thymocytes.[83,84] Thus this enzyme can be considered as a third marker for immature cells. These introductory notes already indicate that the various antisera (together with certain rosette tests and TdT enzyme determinations) play complementary roles in the classification of leukemias (Table 5.3) and various lymphoid cell lines (Table 5.4).

Anti-ALL serum

This antiserum is prepared by injecting non-T, non-B ALL blasts (coated with rabbit antilymphocyte serum, ALS; Fig. 5.1) into rabbits.[14,34,38,93-95] The fully absorbed antisera react with antigenic determinant(s) on a single glycosylated polypeptide with a mol. wt. of 95 000 to 100 000.[34,96] The reactivity pattern on normal and leukemic cells is shown in Table 5.5.

Immunization

1. First prepare ALS by intravenous injection of 10^8 tonsil lymphocytes into a rabbit on days 0 and 14. Bleed on day 21. The unabsorbed serum is used to 'coat' leukemic blasts prior to injection
2. Resuspend $1-3 \times 10^8$ prewashed non-T, non-B ALL blasts in 2 ml ALS. Wash in saline and inject intravenously into another rabbit on days 0 and 14. Bleed on days 21, 22 and 23.[14] Alternatively inject cells *plus* ALS (without washing) on days 0 and 14. Bleed around day 28.[34,94]

Absorption

The following absorption schemes have been reported: red cells ($3 \times$), tonsil lymphocytes ($4-5 \times$), normal bone marrow ($4 \times$), AML cells ($1 \times$), infant thymocytes ($1 \times$) by Greaves et al;[14] red cells, B-lymphoid line ($4 \times$), K-562 line ($4 \times$), CLL cells ($3 \times$) by Koshiba et al.[95] Less absorption may be required if ALS is also injected into the rabbits together with the unwashed immunizing cells.[34,94]

Test systems

Indirect IF is used most frequently, sometimes in various combinations with other antisera.[21] Some positive cells express ALL antigen only weakly and it is important to compare observations with cells incubated with normal rabbit Ig controls (absorbed twice with tonsils). $F(ab)_2$ reagents are strongly recommended. Only exceptional anti-ALL reagents are cytolytic in complement-mediated cytotoxicity.[34]

   Notes. The antiserum reacts with 71 to 83 per cent of childhood ALL (including cases with good prognosis)[97] and 51 to 66 per cent of adult ALL cases.[85,98] In these positive cases frequently a large proportion of blasts are cALL$^+$. In other cases there is a heterogeneity in ALL antigen expression within the lymphoblast cell population and many blasts are cALL$^-$. Some cases of acute undifferentiated leukemias (AUL) and 'lymphoid' blast crisis (LyBC) of Ph^1 positive CML or Ph^1 positive ALL are also cALL$^+$. The reactive cells in LyBC most frequently exhibit 'lymphoid' morphology and can occur in the company of cALL⁻ myeloblasts and differentiating myeloid cells. Other leukemias (including AML and B-lymphoid disorders) are almost invariably cALL⁻. Rare cases of Thy-ALL are weakly positive with anti-ALL serum (see below).

Normal T- and B-lymphoid cells as well as various myeloid cells are cALL⁻. In some non-leukemic neonatal and juvenile bone marrow samples a few (usually <10 per cent) cALL⁺ cells can be observed. These cells express cALL antigen very weakly and have small lymphocyte morphology but fail to express thymocyte, T-cell or B-cell markers. Adult bone marrow contains very few (<1 per cent) cALL⁺ cells. In some conditions, however, the proportion of cALL⁺

Table 5.5 Reactivity of anti-ALL serum[a]

Normal cells[b]
Negative populations (<0.1%):
  Lymphocytes, thymocytes and stimulated lymphoblasts (T and B)[21]
  Bone marrow cells: erythroid and myeloid cells, including myeloblasts, most adult bone marrow lymphocytes

Positive populations:
  A subpopulation of normal infant bone marrow 'lymphocytes' (BM Ly); BM Ly population in neonatal BM lymphocytosis and during BM regeneration after cessation of cytotoxic therapy[b]

Leukemic cells[c]

| Thy-ALL | cALL | AML | AUL | Ph¹ (+) leukemia | | Lymphoma | CLL |
				Blast Cr.	CML		
36/0[d]	252/187	81/3	18/9	45/22	19/1	23/6	10/0

[a] Tested by indirect immunofluorescence.
[b] Weakly positive small cells.[15, 99]
[c] From ref. 98: samples tested/samples positive. Immunoabsorption indicates that the same antigenic group(s) are expressed on the positive leukemic cells.[96,98]
[d] In a more recent analysis 9 out of 100 cases were weakly ALL⁺ (Fig. 5.7)[85, 92]

cells can be higher (10 to 20 per cent). These are fetal bone marrows, cases of neonatal anemia and transient bone marrow lymphocytosis, early phases of bone marrow regeneration following allogeneic bone marrow transplantation, and regeneration following drug induced bone marrow hypoplasia. The latter group includes most patients studied after the cessation of chemotherapy given for various diseases such as solid malignancy (e.g. neuroblastoma), lymphoma, AML as well as common-ALL.[15] Although in most of these cases the cALL⁺ population consists of small cells which express the cALL antigen very weakly, the reagent is clearly not suitable to predict relapse of common-ALL in patients off treatment.[99] The cALL⁺ normal cells are likely to be hemopoietic (lymphoid?) precursor cells. Functional tests are not yet available to assess their developmental potential. These cells do not form myeloid colonies in agar.[93, 100]

Antisera to human Ia-like (p28,33) antigens

The major histocompatibility gene complex (HLA in man) controls the expression of two groups of polymorphic cell surface glycoproteins. One group represents major transplantation antigens (coded by the HLA-A, HLA-B and HLA-C loci) which are present on all cell types (except erythrocytes and thymocytes). The second group comprises the *Ia* (immune-associated) antigens. These were described in mice as gene products of the I region within the H-2 gene complex: I region controls immune responsiveness to certain antigens. Murine Ia antigens are a complex of two glycoproteins of 33 000 and 28 000 mol. wt. (p28,33). Similar p28,33 glycoprotein structures exist on human cells[102] which are probably controlled by the HLA-DR locus. These p28,33 structures are referred to as Ia-like antigens. The polymorphic allotypic determinants of Ia-like antigens are identified by human allo-antisera to HLA-D locus governed antigens; these are used in histocompatibility testing. The core determinants

Table 5.6 Reactivity of anti-Ia-like serum. (Reviewed.[16,81] Ia-like antigens seem to have a differentiation linked expression: They are retained on B-lymphocytes until the plasma cell stage (myelomas are Ia⁻) and on myeloid/erythroid cells during earliest stages of development, but not expressed on thymocytes/T-cells until late stages of T-effector cell development.)

1. Normal tissues

Positive populations:
    B-lymphoid cells including pre-B cells, B-lymphocytes, B-lymphoblasts and lymphoid cell lines and plasmablasts
    Subset of monocytes (variable expression from strong to undetectable) tissue macrophages, dendritic reticular cells. Strongest expression is on interdigitating reticular cells.[106]
    Non-T, non-B bone marrow cells of small lymphocyte morphology, myeloblasts and few promyeloblasts. Myeloid CFUc cells (variable expression); erythroid BFU (weak)
    A subset of peripheral T-lymphocytes (weak)
    Epithelial cells, in the thymus
Negative or very weakly positive populations:
    Thymocytes and most T-lymphocytes
    Subset of monocytes and tissue macrophages (e.g. sinus histiocytes).
    Myeloid cells from promyelocytes to granulocytes
    Erythroid cells (except early precursors)
    Other tissues

2. Leukemias

Positive populations:
    Common-ALL, lymphoid blast crisis of CML
    60–70% of AML cases, proportion of blasts in myeloid crisis of CML
    CLL, PLL, B-lymphomas, B-ALL
    A few peripheral T-CLL and T-lymphoma (mostly weak)
Negative or very weakly positive populations:
    Thy-ALL, lymphoblastic lymphoma of Thy-type, most cases of T-lymphomas and T-CLL
    Some AML, CML in chronic phase
    Other malignancies (e.g. anaplastic carcinoma).

of the same molecules (common to all individuals) are recognized by heterologous anti-Ia-like sera. These are made in rabbits or chicken and used in leukemia testing. The peculiar tissue distribution of Ia-like antigens is interesting (Table 5.6).

Since Ia-like antigens are very immunogenic many research groups have succeeded in producing heteroantisera to various Ia-positive cell types. These reagents show the same 'Ia-like' reactivity pattern, irrespective of whether they have been made against B lymphocytes, CLL, human B-lymphoid lines,[103–105] lymphosarcoma cells,[106] papain digests from AML and ALL[13,107] or purified Ia-like antigens.[42,48,108–110] In these studies Ia-like antigens are frequently referred to as B-cell associated-, leukemia associated- or p28,33 antigens.

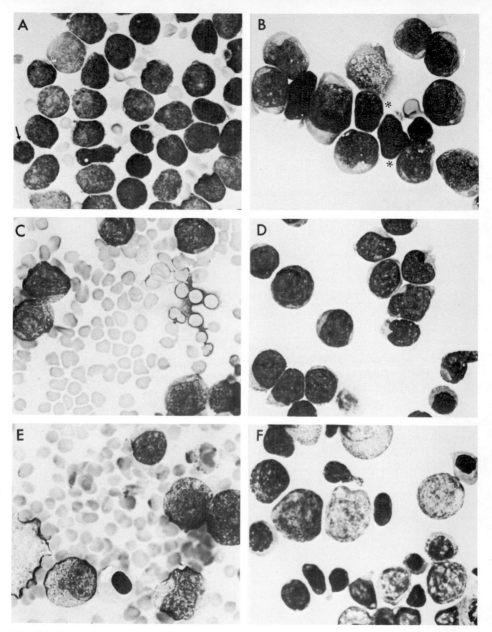

Fig. 5.6 Morphology of Ia$^+$ and Ia$^-$ leukemic cells. (A) Bone marrow sample from a patient during Ph^1 positive lymphoid blast crisis. 80 per cent of cells were Ia$^+$. These cells, also positive with anti-ALL serum (ALL$^+$), were labeled in indirect IF test and separated on the FACS. The film was made from a suspension containing >90 per cent Ia$^+$, ALL$^+$ cells. The morphology of blast cells is similar to typical ALL. (B) Peripheral blood film from a patient presenting in Ph^1($+$) blast crisis. Virtually all blasts (88 per cent of cells) are Ia$^+$ but only 40 per cent of blast cells, including the smaller lymphoid blasts (asterisk), are ALL$^+$. The blast cell population is clearly heterogeneous; myeloid blast cells are also seen. The transition from lymphoid to myeloid morphology is continuous. (C) Ia$^+$ blast cells separated from an AML sample; the cells are typical myeloblasts. (D) Ia$^+$ blasts separated from a bone marrow sample of a case of Ph^1($+$) CML in myeloid blast crisis. (E) Ia$^-$ cells separated from an AML sample. One myeloblast, five large promyelocytes and one normoblast are shown. (F) Ia$^-$ cells separated from a Ph^1($+$) myeloid blast crisis. Samples A, C and E contain sheep red cells. From ref 112 (with permission).

Immunization

1. Papain extract of B-lymphoid cells (e.g. RAJI or Daudi B-cell lines or CLL cells) prepared by the method of Mann et al[111] is recommended as immunogen. Alternatively, purified Ia-like antigens can be prepared by the method of Snary et al[110] except that the plasma membrane should be solubilized in Triton instead of sodium deoxycholate
2. Inject rabbits (at multiple sites, intramuscularly) with 0.2 to 0.4 µg glycoprotein per 1 ml PBS emulsified with equal volume of complete Freund adjuvant on days 0, 28 and bleed on days 41, 42, 43.[107,110]

Absorption

Antisera may require no absorption[107] or only minimal absorptions with AB erythrocytes (2 ×), formalin fixed CML cells (2 ×, in chronic phase), thymocytes or Thy-ALL (2 ×).

Test systems

Anti-Ia-like antisera are used in complement-mediated cytotoxicity[107] or in indirect IF test.[42,108,112] Chicken anti-Ia-like sera can be used in double fluorescence systems in combination with rabbit antibodies to other antigens.

Notes. Anti-Ia-like antisera strongly react with B-lymphoid malignancies including CLL, B-lymphomas, B-ALL and PLL. In contrast, they fail to react with Thy-ALL and most T-cell derived CLL and lymphoma. Recently, however, a few Ia$^+$ peripheral T-cell malignancies have been described.[85,114] Blasts in common-ALL and lymphoid blast crisis of CML are mostly strongly positive. Many AML and myeloid blast crisis of CML are also Ia$^+$ but show a somewhat weaker and more variable Ia expression. Some AML and most promyelocytic leukemias[91] are Ia$^-$ (Fig. 5.6). Cells in the chronic phase of CML, megakaryocytic and erythro-leukemias are Ia$^-$.[42,91,108,112]

The reactivity of leukemic cells with anti-Ia sera in most leukemias seems to reflect the characteristics of normal equivalent cells (Table 5.6). For example, early normal myeloid precursors (myeloblasts and myeloid colony-forming cells) tend to be Ia$^+$ while most promyelocytes and all myelocytes to granulocytes are Ia$^-$.[100,107,108,115] This largely explains the similar pattern of Ia expression on myeloid leukemias.[116]

Anti-human T-lymphocyte antigen (HuTLA) sera

These antisera are prepared by injecting human thymocytes or human T-lymphoid cell lines or monkey thymocytes into rabbits. Anti-monkey thymocyte sera require less absorption than anti-human thymocyte sera (Fig. 5.1[26,29]). The absorbed antisera react with multiple different antigenic determinants. Some of these are thymus specific[42,117] and may be similar to TL (thymus leukemia) allo-antigens in mice;[118] others are present on thymocytes as well as peripheral T-lymphocytes.[119]

Immunization and absorption

1. Inject suspension of human T-lymphoblastic cell lines or thymocytes or

monkey thymocytes $(1-3 \times 10^8$ in 1 ml) intravenously into rabbits on days 0, 14 and 21. Bleed on days 27, 28 and 29

2. Absorb with liver homogenate $(2-4 \times)$, AB red cells $(2-4 \times)$, B-lymphoid cell lines and B-CLL(<5 per cent T-cell contamination; $3-5 \times$) and formalin fixed CML cells $(1-3 \times)$

3. At this stage the antiserum is likely to discriminate between thymocytes/T-cells versus B-lymphoid cells but might still react with subsets of myeloid cells in normal bone marrow and with some AML. The latter can be used for a final absorption.

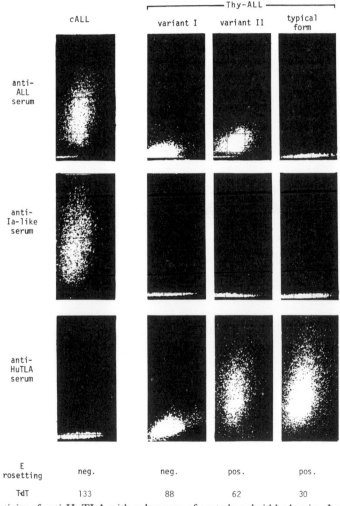

Fig. 5.7 Reactivity of anti-HuTLA with subgroups of acute lymphoid leukemias. Leukemia cell populations were stained with various antisera in indirect IF test and quantitative assessment of antibody binding was made on the FACS (x axis: cell size; y axis: fluorescence intensity). Note that anti-Ia-like and anti-HuTLA sera discriminate between non-T, non-B ALL (Ia$^+$, HuTLA$^-$) and the different forms of Thy-ALL (Ia$^-$, HuTLA$^+$) in spite of the fact that a few cases in the latter group weakly express ALL antigen, fail to form E-rosettes and do not show localized acid phosphatase activity.[122] From ref 85 (with permission).

Notes. Anti-HuTLA serum reacts with Thy-ALL (Fig. 5.7) and leukemias/lymphomas expressing peripheral T-cell characteristics (T-CLL, Sézary syndrome and mycosis fungoides).[120] Some of these HuTLA$^+$ Thy-ALL and T-CLL/lymphoma cases fail to form E-rosettes.[41,85,45] A number of anti-HuTLA antisera described in the literature are unreactive with Ia$^+$ non-T, non-B ALL and AML.[38,41,42,90] The anti-HuTLA/anti-Ia-like reagent combination provides the most precise distinction between Thy-ALL (HuTLA$^+$/Ia$^-$) and cALL (HuTLA$^-$/Ia$^+$; Fig. 5.7).

Multiple marker analysis suggests that all HuTLA$^+$ normal cells belong to the thymocyte/T-cell pathway. The vast majority of strongly HuTLA$^+$ cells in normal bone marrow are Ia$^-$ and lack TdT enzyme. These are bone marrow T-lymphocytes.[57] Anti-HuTLA antisera do not inhibit the growth of myeloid colony forming cells (CFUc[121]).

Anti-myeloid reagents

Since the purpose of membrane marker analysis is to study the phenotype of immature forms of hemopoietic malignancies, the requirements for anti-myeloid antisera are reactivity with myeloid heteroantigens present on myeloid blast cells and negativity with ALL blast cells. Only a handful of reagents produced so far satisfy these criteria.[18,19,123]

Immunization and absorption

1. Inject 2×10^8 viable AML or AMoL cells into rabbits intravenously on days 0, 14 and 42. Bleed two weeks later and collect serum.[19] Jäger et al[18] injected granulocytes in complete Freund's adjuvant subcutaneously on days 0, 14, 15, 16 and 23 and bled rabbits 7 days later
2. Absorb serum with kidney homogenate ($2 \times$), AB red cells ($3 \times$) and tonsil lymphocytes (4–$8 \times$). Ultracentrifuge and prepare F(ab)$_2$ fragments. Only some of the absorbed antisera contain sufficient reactivity against myeloid blasts and in the few instances tried the success rate could not be increased by injecting myeloblasts 'coated' with anti-lymphocyte serum (Roberts, M.; unpublished).

Test systems

Investigations have been carried out in cytotoxicity and indirect IF tests (combined with cell sorter analysis)[19] and by immunoperoxidase analysis.[18]

Notes. Anti-myeloid serum reacts with AML, AMML, AMoL, myeloid blast crisis (BC) of CML and some cases of AUL which were found to be negative with the anti-ALL serum. On the other hand, only 2 out of 32 cases of ALL and lymphoid BC of CML tested were positive.[19] There is no convincing evidence that the antisera produced in rabbits,[124] mice[39] or Rhesus monkeys[80] react with myeloid leukemia specific antigens. All of these reagents, when tested, were found to be reactive with normal human myeloid precursors (myeloblasts, myeloid CFUc). The antisera made in rabbits react rather weakly with normal myeloblasts and promyelocytes while they react strongly with mature granulocytic and monocytic cells;[18,19] absorptions with granulocytes remove the activity against AML and myeloblasts. Antisera made against monocytes extensively cross-react with granulocytic cells.[125,126]

The use of anti-immunoglobulin antibodies

Surface membrane immunoglobulin (SmIg) detected by immunofluorescence (IF) is the most reliable marker for B-lymphoid cells, and a clonal marker for malignant B-cell proliferations when antisera specific for various Ig isotypes (e.g. κ and λ light chains) are used.

Principle. Individual B-lymphoid cells (and plasma cells) synthesize only one type of light chain, κ or λ. The ratio of κ^+ and λ^+ B-lymphoid cells in normal populations is 2:1. B-lymphoid malignancies derive from one cell (κ^+ or λ^+) and all members of the clone express the same light chain. Residual normal populations are 'diluted' with these malignant cells. Cell suspensions showing higher than 10:1 or lower than 1:5 ratios of $\kappa^+ : \lambda^+$ can safely be considered as 'monoclonal', i.e. they represent mainly malignant cells derived from κ^+ or λ^+ 'ancestors', respectively. These conclusions are not invalidated by the simultaneous presence of μ, δ, γ or α heavy chains on the same B cells: these cells express the same antigenic recognition site (i.e. the light chain and heavy chain variable regions) attached to different heavy chain, constant region. B cells can switch their predominant heavy chain type during normal physiological clonal evolution.[127] This 'switch' is sometimes also observed during the clinical progression of a malignant B-cell clone (e.g. μ^+ monoclonal cells can give rise to a γ^+ population but still express the same light chain and idiotype;[56]). These considerations clearly indicate that in monoclonality testing emphasis has to be given to κ and λ light chain analysis, and that the study of heavy chain expression is only used as additional evidence to characterize the uniformity or clonal progression of the malignant disease.

There are two technical difficulties. First, Ig molecules can passively attach to membranes (Table 5.7), and these Ig molecules have to be eluted from the cell surface prior to testing. Second, the density of SmIg on different B-cells

Table 5.7 Pitfalls of detecting surface membrane immunoglobulin (SmIg) on B-lymphocytes and leukemias.

In vivo artefacts[a]

Circulating immune complexes (present in the patient's blood) attach to Fc_{IgG}, Fc_{IgM} and complement receptors on cells

The membrane bound IgM has anti-IgG activity (rheumatoid factor)

Antibodies made against leukemia associated antigens (by the patient) attach to leukemic cells

In vitro artefacts[b]

IgG aggregates present in the animal antiserum (e.g. rabbit IgG) attach to Fc_{IgG} receptors[b,d]

The antiserum used is not fully specific[c]

---

[a] Remedy: wash cells in acetate buffer (see Detection of membrane antigens[67]).

[b] Remedy: use F(ab)$_2$ fragment of rabbit antisera, ultracentrifuge reagents (see Preparations of reagents).

[c] It is assumed that the anti-Ig reagents are specific for the given Ig isotypes when tested by immunoprecipitation technics. Further specificity checks should be performed in the following tests: (1) membrane marker analysis using SmIg$^-$ cell types; e.g. peripheral T-lymphocytes and ALL blasts; (2) test for cytoplasmic immunoglobulin (e.g. on myelomas expressing κ or λ[67]); (3) membrane marker tests on cells expressing large amounts of SmIg (e.g. prolymphocytic leukemia or malignant B-lymphoid cell lines of κ and λ variety; see Table 5.8); (4) beads coated with pure myeloma proteins, Bence-Jones proteins, etc. can also be used as Ig-coated 'cells' to test reagent specificity.[130] If non-specific staining is identified absorb antisera (with cells or protein coated beads; see Absorption of antisera).

(and on different types of B-leukemias) is widely variable. Strong reagents with minimal or no non-specific reactivity are required.

Reagents and cell preparations

Animals are immunized with purified myeloma proteins. (See Preparation of antibodies.) The quality control of prepared and commercial antisera is shown in Table 5.7. Anti-Ig reagents are most frequently used in direct IF test. Sometimes, when very weakly $SmIg^+$ populations (e.g. CLL) are studied, indirect IF test can also be attempted, after thorough washing, and with proper controls (normal sera plus second layer; testing the same conditions on well characterized κ^+ and λ^+ cell lines, etc.). It is essential to wash the cells in acetate buffer (see Acetate wash); this procedure eliminates non-specific staining on lymphoid cells and frequently increases the intensity of specific staining.[106]

The investigation to follow can vary depending on the proportion of leukemic cells in the sample. If it is >50 per cent, the anti-Ig $(\kappa + \lambda)$, anti-κ, and anti-λ staining can be carried out in separate tubes with FITC conjugated reagents. If, however, the number of leukemic B-cells is <50 per cent, it is important to use reagent combinations. These might be essential in the analysis of the bone marrow involvement of lymphomas, etc. The following combinations can be used:

1. Anti-κ-TRITC mixed with anti-λ-FITC. It is advisable to use reagents made in the same species. The proportion of red:green cells in the sample gives the $\kappa:\lambda$ ratio. This is also an excellent method to test the specificity of antisera and the quality of washing! Double-stained (non-specific) cells are not welcomed but can be recognized and ignored
2. In three separate tubes direct staining with goat-anti-Ig $(\kappa + \lambda)$-FITC, goat-anti-κ-FITC and goat-anti-λ-FITC can be individually combined with indirect staining for rabbit-anti-Ia-like (first layer) followed by goat-anti-rabbit-Ig-TRITC (second layer). Counting of Ig^+, κ^+ and λ^+ cells is then focused on the Ia^+ cells. These include all B-lymphoid cells (but not all Ia^+ cells are B-cells; see Ia-like-antisera). The rest of the population (which could be as high as 95 per cent) is ignored. These tests enable us to perform monoclonality testing in minor B-cell populations but require good reagents.

Notes. Staining of SmIg on malignant B-cells can be easy or difficult, depending on the intensity of specific and background staining and on the proportion of B-cells versus myeloid/monocytic cells in the sample.

In B-CLL the Ia^+ lymphoid cells express SmIg weakly; in some cases the SmIg is not readily detectable (Table 5.8). In a high proportion of these cases the leukemic B-cells form mouse RBC(M) rosettes which help the immunological diagnosis (see Rosettes). In contrast, prolymphocytic leukemia cells have large quantities of SmIg but do not form M-rosettes. Lymphomas exhibit SmIg with variable intensity. Interestingly, in Waldenström macroglobulinemia a high proportion of the circulating B lymphocytes show light chain restriction in the absence of high WBC counts. This suggests that these cells belong to the proliferating malignant clone, which are, unlike most cases of CLL, able to undergo interrupted maturation from B lymphocyte to IgM secreting plasma

Table 5.8 M-rosettes and SmIg in B-lymphoproliferative diseases. (From Catovsky et al.[131])

Disease	No of cases	M-rosettes			SmIg		
		$<30\%$	30–49%	$>50\%$	Negative	Weak to moderate	Strong
Chronic lymphocytic leukemia (CLL)	115	1	21	93	22	87	6
Prolymphocytic leukemia (PLL)	20	16	4	0	0	2	18
Hairy-cell leukemia (HCL)[a]	23	14	8	1	1	12	10

[a] Leukemic reticuloendotheliosis.
[b] Intensity of membrane fluorescence.

cells. Similarly, immunological phenotyping can establish the common clonal B-cell origin of morphologically dissimilar cell types in 'histiocytic' lymphomas supervening on CLL or macroglobulinemia and in those of CLL in transformation.[8,128] It is worth noting that these acute forms of B malignancies (including the rare B-ALL) are different from the so-called pre-B type ALL cases. The former are SmIg+, terminal transferase negative. The latter are SmIg , mostly terminal transferase positive leukemias which contain only cytoplasmic Ig[87,88] (see below and Table 5.3).

All these cases can be further analyzed by antisera to heavy chains and by rosette tests; the predominant heavy chain class in them is IgM and IgD. Small amounts of IgG (monoclonal; κ or λ) can be picked up on a number of CLL cases by rosetting with anti-Ig-coated red cells.[75] Some lymphomas and occasional CLL cases express dominant IgG. With a panel of rosette test 'receptor-profiles' of B-leukemias and lymphomas can be established which probably reflect the phenotypic characteristics of the normal B-lymphocytes at the corresponding stage of maturation.[63,129]

The analysis of bone marrow involvement in lymphomas is difficult but possible when the multiple marker combinations described above are used. In these studies it is helpful if the phenotype (κ or λ; strong or weak staining) of the malignant population is first established in an involved sample (e.g. in a lymph node or leukemic blood) and one can then search for the rare cells which exhibit the same surface phenotype as the lymphoma cells.

ROSETTE TESTS

Leukocytes can bind RBC when brought into close contact *in vitro*. The leukocyte surrounded by adherent RBC gives the appearance of a rosette when viewed under the microscope and the term 'rosette-formation' has become accepted for these tests.

The percentage of rosetted leukocytes in the total leukocyte populations can be counted in unstained preparations under phase contrast. The count is more reliable when the leukocytes are stained with acridine-orange,[132] or methylene-blue, toluidine blue or, as a test for viable cells, with diacetyl fluorescein.[133]

In most cell suspensions there is a great deal of variability in the number of RBC which bind to the individual rosette-forming cells. Only leukocytes binding three or more RBC are counted as 'rosettes'. Typical rosettes are surrounded by 6 to 12 RBC. Interestingly, some leukocytes can bind so many RBC that the leukocyte in the middle may not be visible under phase contrast ('morula'). These preparations have to be stained in order to distinguish rosettes from RBC clumps.

Types of rosettes

Formation of rosettes between certain lymphocytes and heterologous RBC is a fortuitous phenomenon which does not have obvious physiological significance ('spontaneous' rosettes). Sheep RBC (E) bind to human T-lymphoid cells (E-rosetting).[7] Mouse RBC (M), on the other hand, bind to a subpopulation of human B-lymphocytes and their leukemic counterparts (M-rosetting).[134] The avidity of spontaneous binding between leukocytes and RBC is low in both tests. In order to enhance the avidity of binding in most laboratories the RBC are pre-treated with neuraminidase,[135] or papain[136] or with the sulphydryl compound 2-5-aminoethyl isothiourium (AET).[137] Furthermore, extra care has to be taken to avoid the disruption of these weak rosettes when the cell suspensions are resuspended prior to counting. These tests are described below in further detail.

In other types of rosette tests the RBC (E) are pre-treated with various types of antibodies and complement factors. The sensitivity of these tests is increased when ox RBC are used which can be heavily coated with antibody without agglutination.[138,139] E can be coated with anti-RBC antibodies of IgG class (EA_{IgG}) in order to detect leukocytes which express receptors for the Fc part of the IgG molecules (Fc_γ receptor) in rosette tests.[63,138,140,141] If an anti-RBC antibody of IgM class is used the coated RBC (EA_{IgM}) will form rosettes with cells which exhibit receptors for the Fc portion of the IgM molecule (Fc_μ receptor[63,140,142]). When EA_{IgM} are further incubated with serum or purified complement components (C) these bind to EA_{IgM} and EAC complexes are formed. These bind to the various complement receptors on leukocytes.[63,116,143,144] All these receptors are present on various subsets of B-lymphocytes and are therefore useful in the classification of B-lymphomas.[63,144] Nevertheless, neither of these receptors are restricted to B-lymphocyte subsets. Thus these tests have only a limited use in leukemia diagnosis. The salient points are summarized in Table 5.9 and for further details we refer to the original publications.

Sheep RBC (E) rosette test for T-lymphoid cells

Principle. T-lymphoid cells (i.e. thymocytes, T-lymphocytes, T-lymphoblasts as well as leukemias of thymocyte and T-cell origin) form 'spontaneous' rosettes with sheep RBC (E).[7] The E-rosette formation requires active metabolism; metabolic inhibitors in the medium such as azide should be avoided. The E-rosettes are of low avidity but their formation is facilitated by pre-treatment of the RBC with neuraminidase[135] and by the presence of serum (e.g. fetal or inactivated, human or horse serum) in the medium during the incubation period.

Materials

1. Sheep RBC (E) less than 14 days old in Alsever solution
2. Neuraminidase (Behringwerke or Sigma, Type VI. Cl. perfringens)
3. Fetal calf serum (FCS)
4. Culture medium or balanced salt solution (BSS; pH 7.0 to 7.2, e.g. Eagle's or Hanks' solution)
5. Acridine-orange (0.001 per cent) or diacetyl-fluorescein (Sigma; 5 mg/ml in acetone diluted 10 000 times in PBS) or methylene blue (0.01 per cent).

Preparation of reagents

1. Absorb 4 volumes of FCS with 1 volume of E twice (see Absorption of antisera). Absorbed FCS (FCS-A) can be stored in small aliquot at $-20°$ until use
2. Make 2 per cent suspension of E in BSS (0.2 ml packed E + 10 ml BSS). Wash three times
3. Incubate E suspension with 15 U/ml neuraminidase for 30 min at 37°C. Wash three times in BSS and reconstitute to the original 2 per cent v/v concentration. The neuraminidase treated E-cells (E-neur.) can be kept for at least 7 days at 4°C
4. Separate leukocytes on Ficoll-Isopaque (see above) and adjust to 10^7 WBC/ml BSS.

Test

1. Mix 50 μl leukocytes (5×10^5 cells) + 100 μl 2 per cent E-N + 50 μl FCS-A in plastic tube of approx. 2.5 ml capacity (LP3)
2. Centrifuge 150 g (around 700 r/min) for 5 min at 20°C
3. Leave pelleted suspension on the bench for 60 min (some investigators leave the pellets in the refrigerator overnight)
4. Resuspend pellet by very gentle tapping
5. Add 1 or 2 drops of stain (methylene-blue or acridine-orange or diacetyl-fluorescein). Place sample into hemocytometer. Observe methylene-blue stained preparation under ordinary light.

   Alternatively, observe acridine-orange or diacetyl-fluorescein stained rosettes with low transmitted light superimposed upon the incident u.v. light (FITC filters). Acridine-orange brilliantly stains the nucleus. Diacetyl-fluorescein diffusely stains the cytoplasm of the viable leukocytes
6. Count the proportion of rosettes within the leukocyte population and assess the size of the rosetting cells (small lymphocytes or blast cells?). Calculate the per cent of rosette-forming (E) cells.

Interpretation of results

More than 95 per cent of human thymocytes and the vast majority of T-lymphocytes form E-rosettes while no other cell types are E-positive. Thus E-rosetting is a reliable marker for the T-cell lineage. In approximately 90 per cent of Thy-ALL cases large proportions (>60 to 90 per cent) of blasts form E-rosettes. Most frequently these blasts show high avidity for E, which is also characteristic

Table 5.9 Reactivity pattern observed in rosette tests to assess similarity between certain normal cells and their malignant counterparts.
++ = strong reactivity in most cells; + = majority of cells (not necessarily all) form rosettes; − = <10–15% cells form rosettes; ++/+
and −/+ show heterogeneous populations.

	Sheep erythrocyte (E-rosette)	Mouse erythrocyte (M-rosette)	EA_IgG (Fc_γ receptor)[d]	EA_IgM (Fc_μ receptor)	EAC rosette[q]
Normal cells					
1. Thymocyte	++	−			Fetal thymocytes +[r]
2. T-lymphocytes	++/+[a]	−	Some T-cells (Tγ cells)[e]	Some T-cells (Tμ cells)[e]	−
3. B-lymphocytes	−	+[b]	+[f]	+[f]	Mostly + some −[s]
4. Blood 'null' (non-T, non-B) cell population	−	−[b]	++[g]	?	Mostly −[t]
Monocytes	−	−	++[g]	[l,m]	+
Myeloblasts	−	−	−	−	−[x]
5. Myelocytes	−	−		−[l]	+
Immature neutrophils	−	−	+/++[h]		+
Mature neutrophils	−	−	++		−[s]
Malignant cells					
0. Common-ALL	++/+	−	−[i]	Conflicting results[n]	Conflicting results[u]
1. Thy-ALL	++/+	−			40–80% of cases +[v]
2. T-lymphoma, Sézary syndrome, mycosis fungoides, T-CLL	++/+	−	−/+	−/+	+ or −[s,w]
B-CLL	−	+[c]	+[j]	+[k,l]	++/+[s]
Lymphoma	−	+/−	mostly −[j]	B-lymphoid line +[o]	or −[p]
3. B-PLL	−	+ or −	+	?	20%[p]
HCL	−	−	++[k]	+[k]	weak[k]
4. Acute monocytic leukemia	−	−	++[k]	−[k]	50% of cases +[k]
5. Acute myeloblastic leukemia	−	−	−/+	−	−[x]

[a] For heterogeneity of E-rosettes ('active' and 'non-active') see Hockland P, Heron I 1979 Scand J Immunol 9: 333.

[b] Only a subpopulation of B-lymphocytes forms M-rosettes. The test is nevertheless B-cell specific—monocytes and most 'null' cells are negative.[148,149]

[c] 'Specific' marker for CLL (unreactive with PLL; see text).

[d] Identical reactivity pattern is seen when Fc_γ receptor is detected by tests using aggregated human IgG (Dickler H B 1974 J exp Med 140: 508) or rabbit IgG b4/anti-b4 complexes (Winfield J B et al 1977 J Immunol 119: 1778), or EA_{IgG} test (Clements P J, Levy J 1977 Clin Exp Immunol 34: 281). The latter two papers are particularly informative about the quantitative aspects of Fc-receptor heterogeneity on various cell types.

[e] EA_{IgG}-rosetting and EA_{IgM}-rosetting T-cells are different cells ($T\gamma$ and $T\mu$, respectively), but do not represent entirely different T-cell lineages (ref 140, p. 1540). These cells have different functions: $T\mu$ cells help and $T\gamma$ cells suppress immunoglobulin synthesis by stimulated human B-lymphocytes (Moretta L et al 1977 J Exp Med 134: 200; Heijnen C J et al 1979 Cell Immunol 43: 282). In order to detect EA_{IgM}-rosetting on T-cells overnight incubation at 37°C and washing (elution of IgM from the lymphocyte surface) is necessary prior to testing.

[f] The same B-cells express both EA_{IgG} and EA_{IgM} receptors.[140]

[g] When Rh^- red cells sensitised with incomplete anti-Rh IgG (EA_{Ripley}) the test system is less sensitive and detects only the strongly $Fc_\gamma +$ monocytic cells.[7]

[h] Dickler H B 1976 Adv Immunol: 167.

[i] Two cases (out of ~40) are EA_{IgG}: Esber E C et al 1978 Clin Exp Immunol 32: 523.

[j] Only half of CLL cases (Ferrarini M et al 1975 Eur J Immunol 5: 89) and <10% of lymphomas tested are EA_{IgG} positive (Habeshaw J et al 1979 Brit J Cancer 40:11).

[k] Burns G F et al 1977 Brit J Haemat 36: 71, Cawley J et al 1978 Scand J Haem 21: 233.

[l] Ref 141.

[m] Monocytes are negative; a subset (~30%) exposes EA_{IgM} receptor after incubation with neuraminidase (Haegert D G et al 1979 Clin Exp Immunol 35: 484).

[n] 6 out of 6 Thy-ALL cases $EA_{IgM}+$ (Moretta L et al 1977 Clin Immunol Immunopath 7: 405); in contrast, 10 out of 10 Thy-ALL cases $EA_{IgM}-$ (Kaplan J, personal communication).

[o] Pichler W J 1978 Eur J Immunol 8: 274.

[p] Buskard et al 1978 Hämatologie und Bluttransfusion 18: 237.

[q] For detailed technology, see Ross G D 1979 Blood 53: 799 and Habeshaw et al 1979 Brit J Cancer 40: 11.

[r] Infant thymocytes are EAC^+; many fetal thymocytes are EAC^- (Gatien J G et al 1975 Eur J Immunol 5: 312).

[s] Habeshaw et al 1979 Brit J Cancer 40: 11.

[t] Niaudet P et al 1979 Scand J Immunol 9: 387.

[u] Compare Jaffé E S et al 1978 Blood 48: 213 and Kadin M F, Billing R J 1977 Blood 50: 771.

[v] Ref 159 and Kadin M F, Billing R J 1977 Blood 50: 771.

[w] Ross G D et al 1973 J Clin Invest 52: 377.

[x] Ross G D et al 1978 J exp Med 147: 730.

of normal thymocytes and mitogen stimulated lymphoblasts. Ten per cent of Thy-ALL cases fail to express E-receptor but react with anti-T (HuTLA) serum and show other features of Thy-ALL (Ia⁻, TdT⁺).[16,41,85,90,122] T-cell lymphomas, cases of CLL of T-type, and malignant cases in Sézary syndrome also form E-rosettes, sometimes of weak avidity. Occasional cases fail to form E-rosettes but, again, react with anti-HuTLA serum.[145]

The interpretation of observations can be difficult if the proportion of blast cells in the sample is low and normal T-lymphocytes are present (e.g. residual T-cells in the blood). Close examination of the size of rosetting cells (blasts?) using acridine-orange staining or analysis of the morphology of rosetted cells in stained cytocentrifuge preparations can be helpful. (Nevertheless, in cytocentrifuge smears artefacts can develop.) Additional studies (e.g. analysis of TdT levels) or the analysis of further bone marrow samples are sometimes essential to settle the question.

In contrast to Thy-ALL, blast cells of the common non-T, non-B ALL type[11,21] and other non-T-leukemias (including B-CLL) are invariably negative for E-rosettes.[16] Thus E-rosetting remains one of the most reliable and simplest markers for classifying leukemias. A disadvantage of E-rosette test is that T-lymphocytes gradually lose rosetting capacity and the test can perform poorly in samples taken 2 to 3 days before testing.

Notes. If only few cells are available the test can be scaled down (10 μl cells + 10 μl FCS + 20 μl E). E-rosetting can be performed in combination with EAC (complement receptor) test[59,146] and with a modified IF assay for SmIg (in the absence of azide the assay for SmIg is shorter: 15 min incubation at 4°C).[147]

Mouse RBC (M) rosette test for B-lymphoid cells

Principle. A subset of B-lymphocytes (~50 per cent of blood B-cells and 15 to 30 per cent of tonsil cells) forms 'spontaneous' rosettes with mouse RBC. Thymocytes, T-cells, monocytes as well as non-T, non-B 'null' lymphoid cells of peripheral blood appear to be all negative.[148–150] Myeloid cells in the bone marrow also fail to form M-rosettes.

Materials
These are described in the E-rosette test (see above), except that fresh mouse RBC are used.

Preparations of reagents
See E-rosette test, except that mouse RBC are treated with neuraminidase (M-neur.). (Some investigators use neuraminidase-treated leukocyte suspensions in the diagnosis of CLL: 1 μg neuraminidase Type VI, Sigma, per 2.5 × 10⁶ cells for 45 min at 37°C, washed three times.)[151]

Test
See E-rosetting.

Interpretation of results
Twenty-five to 90 per cent of CLL cells (of B-type) form M-rosettes in virtually all cases so far studied.[134,150–152] Since CLL cells express particularly small

amounts of membrane Ig (and in some cases the existing methods fail to detect any Ig) the confirmation of B-cell origin with an additional independent marker is important. Hairy-cell leukemia (HCL) is the only other malignancy where >25 per cent M-rosettes were detected in ~40 per cent of cases.[151] Other B-lymphoid malignancies including cases of prolymphocytic leukemia (Table 5.8), Waldenström macroglobulinemia, poorly differentiated and well differentiated lymphomas are usually M-rosette negative. These findings may have prognostic significance. AML and ALL are also M-rosette negative.

These observations may indicate that CLL cells (and some cases of HCL) express the characteristics of a special subpopulation of B-lymphocytes (M^+, SmIg—weak) while other B-lymphoid disorders involve other B-cell populations.

INTERPRETATION OF MEMBRANE MARKER OBSERVATIONS

PHENOTYPES OF LEUKEMIC CELLS

Leukemias

It has been pointed out above that membrane markers are relevant for the analysis of leukemias which derive from 'early' undifferentiated hemopoietic precursors and lymphoid cells. Most of the observations can be interpreted in the light that the antisera used detect differentiation antigens present during various stages of hemopoietic cell development, rather than tumor specific antigenic changes. Membrane marker correlates of leukemia specific chromosome aberrations have not yet been identified.

The four major types of leukemias are shown in Table 5.3. In the following discussion some observations with the enzyme terminal transferase (TdT; see Ch. 7) are also mentioned since the levels of TdT contribute to the phenotypic analysis of leukemia, and because anti-TdT sera[82] can be used in combination with membrane markers.[57]

Acute lymphoblastic leukemia (ALL) subgroups
The major subdivision is between ALL with a non-T, non-B phenotype (common-ALL: ALL^+, Ia^+, TdT^+, E^-, $HuTLA^-$, $SmIg^-$, My^-) and with thymic phenotype (Thy-ALL: ALL^- or $ALL^\pm$, Ia^-, TdT^+, E^+, $HuTLA^+$, $SmIg^-$, My^-; Table 5.3). Some Thy-ALL cases carry receptors for complement (EAC^+). The distinction between common- and Thy-ALL has a prognostic significance. Children with Thy-ALL relapse quickly and their survival is short when compared to cases with common-ALL.[97,120,153]

Although >60 to 70 per cent of cases in each ALL group show the typical phenotype, variants have also been observed. In the Thy-ALL group some cases fail to form E-rosettes (Fig. 5.7). In the common-ALL group 10 to 15 per cent of childhood ALL cases and 29 to 50 per cent of adult ALL cases fail to react with anti-ALL serum in spite of Ia^+, TdT^+ expression.[85,98] Furthermore, a proportion of leukemias within the common-ALL subgroup show weak to variable cytoplasmic IgM expression ($cyIgM^+$; without cell membrane Ig: $SmIg^-$).[86-88] Many of these so-called pre-B-ALL cases respond well to therapy[86,88] and should therefore be distinguished from the rare ALL cases of B-cell type (B-ALL: SmIg[+], Ia[+], TdT[-], E[-], HuTLA[-], My[-]) which show distinctive 'Burkitt-like' morphology (though they are Epstein-Barr virus negative). B-ALL has the worst prognosis amongst ALL cases.[154] It is important to note that 5 to 10 per cent of acute leukemias appear to be 'undifferentiated' or unclassifiable by morphological criteria but show distinctive membrane markers of ALL and may respond to therapy given in adult ALL.[85]

Acute myeloid leukemia (AML)
The marker characteristics of AML and some 'undifferentiated' acute leukemias are My[+], frequently Ia[+], ALL[-], TdT[-], E[-] and HuTLA[-]. For details of Ia-expression see Table 5.6 and Fig. 5.6. These leukemias are heterogeneous by morphological and cytochemical criteria. Some blast cells in AML and more in acute monocytic leukemia (AMoL) appear to be SmIg[+] (κ plus λ) due to passive cytophilic adsorption of IgG to the strongly expressed Fc_γ receptors.[141,155]

Blast crisis of CML (Ph[1] positive)
Blast cells in the acute phase of Ph[1] positive leukemia are heterogeneous. 'Lymphoid' blast cells are similar to common-ALL blasts whilst myeloid blast cells are similar to AML. Frequently, a mixture of 'lymphoid' and myeloid blasts is present in the same sample (Fig. 5.5). Patients in 'lymphoid' blast crisis respond to regimens including vincristine and prednisolone (although frequently only transiently), while patients in myeloid crisis do not respond.[156,157]

Chronic lymphocytic leukemia (CLL) and lymphoma
Most CLL cases (>90 per cent) are characterised by B-lymphocyte phenotype (SmIg[+], Ia[+], M-rosetting[+], ALL[-], E[-], HuTLA[-], My[-]) with weak expression of monoclonal SmIg (κ or λ; Table 5.8). A subgroup of B-leukemia, PLL, is strongly SmIg[+] (M-rosette[-]) and shows poor prognosis. Rare cases of CLL and PLL express markers of peripheral T-lymphocytes (E[+], HuTLA[+], TdT[-], SmIg[-]); these may show skin involvement and include various forms of generalized cutaneous lymphomas (mycosis fungoides; Sézary syndrome).[114,158]

A substantial proportion of non-Hodgkin lymphomas also derive B-lymphoid cells. Many of these can be subdivided by classical morphological criteria and markers for SmIg, EA_{IgG} (Fc_γ) and EAC rosetting (C receptor) and show surprisingly homogeneous groups with fairly uniform survival time.[63] T-lymphoblastic lymphomas show Thy-ALL characteristics;[159] a few peripheral T-cell lymphomas (well differentiated) have also been observed.[160] It is important to note that membrane marker analysis of T- and B-lymphoid cells can be carried out in tissue sections of frozen lymphoma biopsies.[32]

Relation of leukemias to normal (precursor) cells
Consistent phenotypes are characteristic of the various subgroups of normal hemopoietic cells and reflect the maturation status of the malignant clone or dominant subclone. In many cases the malignant transformation arise in cell

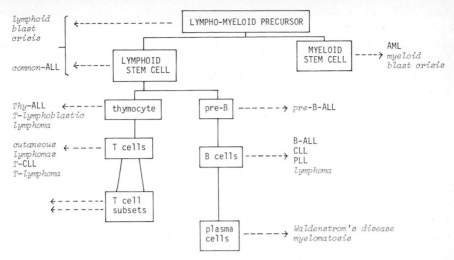

Fig. 5.8 Phenotypic 'map' of human lymphoid malignancies (from ref 15). Leukemias and lymphomas are represented in italics at positions equivalent to normal cells they appear to have the closest relationship. (Such comparisons do not directly identify the 'target' cell for any particular malignancy; see text.)

types which are less mature than the leukemic cell types which dominate the clinical picture. For example, CML arises in (pre-)myeloid stem cell(s),[161] and Waldenström macroglobulinemia arises in B-lymphocytes.[62, 129] Thus the phenotype of leukemic cells represents either the phenotype of the cell in which the malignant transformation has taken place ('target cell') or the phenotype of cells at the maturation level which has been attained by the dominant sub-clone.[15] This concept explains that in some leukemias the malignant populations apparently contains mixtures of cells with variable degrees of maturation (which in fact mimics, to a certain extent, the maturation of the corresponding normal cell types).[102, 129] Figure 5.8 suggests the position of the phenotypes of lymphoid malignancies in relation to normal cell lineages.

REAGENT COMBINATIONS

Analysis of rare cells
Figure 5.8 implies that in non-T, non-B ALL (including pre-B ALL) and Ph[1] positive 'lymphoid' blast crisis early hemopoietic precursor cell types are involved which express the ALL$^+$, Ia$^+$, TdT$^+$, HuTLA$^-$, SmIg$^-$ phenotype. This hypothesis can be directly proven in single cell assays using combinations of reagents labeled with different fluorochromes[57] (Fig. 5.9). Non-T, non-B cells with common-ALL phenotype are present in various non-leukemic tissues such as normal fetal and neonatal bone marrow, and regenerating hemopoietic tissues (after bone marrow transplantation for aplastic anemia or after cessation of chemotherapy for various non-leukemic and leukemic malignancies).[15] Thus the technology is suitable to characterize rare normal precursor cells but might be inadequate to distinguish these precursors from early stages of leukemic relapse.[15, 99]

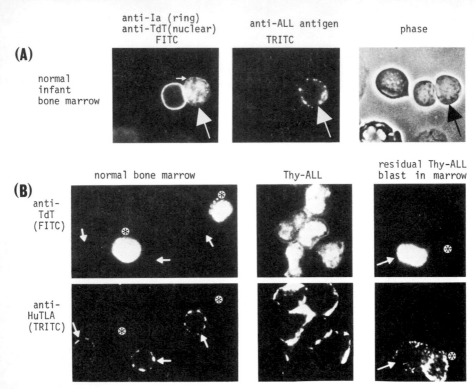

Fig. 5.9 (A) TdT $^+$, ALL $^+$, Ia $^+$ bone marrow cell from a normal infant (large arrow). The same field was photographed with phase contrast and selective filters for FITC (nuclear TdT stain + ring membrane Ia stain: small arrow) and TRITC (ALL antigen). The membrane staining was performed in suspension. Smears were made and stained for nuclear TdT. From ref 57 (with permission). (B) Combination staining for membrane HuTLA (TRITC; in suspension) and nuclear TdT (FITC; in smear). In the normal bone marrow putative precursor cells are TdT $^+$, HuTLA $^-$ (asterisks) and T lymphocytes are HuTLA $^+$, TdT $^-$ (small arrows) but no TdT $^+$, HuTLA $^+$ cell is seen. In contrast, Thy-ALL blast cells are TdT $^+$, HuTLA $^+$ corresponding to the thymocyte phenotype. Thus residual Thy-ALL blast cells can be recognized in the bone marrow (arrow). From Janossy et al (Ref. 170).

Similar combined analyses can be carried out on thymocyte subpopulations or in bone marrow samples with small numbers of lymphoma cells (see The use of anti-immunoglobulin reagents), etc.

Heterogeneity and anomalous gene expression in leukemia

Reagent combinations are the method of choice in the detailed analysis of leukemia heterogeneity. One reagent (e.g. anti-TdT antibody) can be used to label most leukemic cells, and then the expression of the ALL antigen can be studied within the TdT $^+$ population. The characterization of leukemia heterogeneity is important. These studies may throw light on the development of distinct drug-resistant subclones from minority populations.[99, 163, 164] Reagent combinations can also detect abnormal gene expression in leukemia. Although the antisera available recognize normal gene products, the expression of these products can be 'deranged' in leukemic cells. Two examples are mentioned.

Some cases of Thy-ALL show certain characteristics of fetal thymocytes: they form E-rosettes and EAC rosettes.[59,159] Interestingly, however, normal fetal thymocytes in most species studied[165] (including man[166]) express TdT very weakly, while Thy-ALL blasts are strongly TdT$^+$. The E$^+$, EAC$^+$, TdT$^+$ phenotype is probably unique for Thy-ALL; these cells in normal fetal or infant thymus are extremely rare, if they exist at all. Similarly pre-B ALL blasts may simultaneously express nuclear TdT and detectable cytoplasmic IgM. Less than 1 to 3 per cent of cells within the normal pre-B cell population of the bone marrow (<0.1 per cent of the total population) has a similar TdT$^+$ (weak) cyIgM$^+$ (weak) phenotype.[57]

CONCLUDING REMARKS

Membrane marker analysis can be used for characterizing leukemias at presentation. The type and heterogeneity of leukemic cells can be assessed. This gives prognostic indications and may influence treatment. New therapeutic regimes are being developed for types of leukemia (e.g. Thy-ALL) which show bad prognosis with conventional treatment.

The recognition of individual leukemic cells (e.g. in remission bone marrow) can be difficult since the methods described may not distinguish between normal precursor cells or leukemic blasts. This is not too disappointing if one considers that antibodies originally made against leukemia will help in characterizing normal hemopoietic stem cells, particularly if the analysis is combined with the physical separation of rare reactive cells on the FACS. In spite of this the anatomical site may suggest that a cell is in fact malignant: e.g. even one single ALL$^+$ (or TdT$^+$) cell in the cerebrospinal fluid indicates central nervous system involvement.[167] Similarly the cell which exhibits thymocyte features in the bone marrow is probably a Thy-ALL blast.[168] Furthermore, leukemic cells may show an abnormal ('deranged') expression of normal gene products which can be detected with convenient marker combinations.[169]

Finally it is important to point out that the field of leukemia analysis with membrane markers is rapidly developing. New monoclonal antibodies are being standardized in combination with other markers on both normal and leukemic cell populations (Table 5.10). These pure antibodies may ultimately assist in the removal of residual leukemic cells (e.g. Thy-ALL or lymphoma cells) from a remission bone marrow prior to autologous marrow transplantation.[170] Antibodies against T lymphocytes may also assist in the prevention of graft versus host disease; i.e. they might remove T lymphocytes from allogeneic bone marrow.[171]

The new monoclonal antibodies will generate a wealth of information on the phenotypic patterns of various hemopoietic cells and on the putative differentiation pathways during hemopoietic development. This development will press for the establishment of further functional stem cell assays *in vitro* (Ch. 8). A caveat for the use of pure monoclonal antibodies in leukemia analysis is that they react with single antigenic determinants. Thus, the lack of reactivity with leukemic cell populations indicates that the cells fail to express this particular antigenic determinant but it is not known whether the malignant cells express

Table 5.10 Examples of monoclonal antibodies which have been extensively tested in leukemias/lymphomas.

Monoclonal antibody reacting with			
normal cells	leukemic cells	Designation	References*
?	non-T, non-B ALL	J-5	1
thymocytes + T cells (so-called pan-T reagents)	Thy-ALL, T malignancies	OKT3, OKT11, T101	2,3
cortical thymocytes	some Thy-ALL (weak reactivity)	NA1/34	4,5
'inducer' T cells, thymocytes	some Thy-ALL, most peripheral T leukemia	OKT4	2,6,7
'suppressor' T cells, thymocytes	some Thy-ALL, a few peripheral T leukemia	OKT8	2,6,8
Ia-like antigens	see Table VI	several monoclonal antibodies, e.g. ref 9	
B-lymphocytes	CLL, PLL	HC11 A (new name: FMC-1)	10
myeloid cells	study in progress	OKM-1	2
leukocytes (T + B lymphocytes strongly, myeloid cells weakly)	lymphomas (in tissue section; see ref 12)	2DZ	11,12

1. Ritz J et al 1980 Nature 283: 583.
2. Goldstein G, Kung P (OK Series by ORTHO Immunosciences Division; personal communication).
3. Royston I et al 1979 Blood 54 (supplement): 106a.
4. McMichael A J et al 1979 Eur J Immunol 9: 205.
5. Bradstock K F et al 1980 J Natl Cancer Inst 65: 33.
6. Kung et al 1979 Science 206: 347.
7. Reinherz E L et al 1979 J Immunol 123: 2894.
8. Reinherz E L et al 1980 Proc Nat Acad Sci 77: 1588.
9. Zola H et al 1980 Immunology in press.
10. Brooks D A et al 1980 Clin Exp Immunol 39: 477.
11. Beverley P C L 1980 in Proc IXth Intern Course on Transpl Clin Immunol in press.
12. Pizzolo G et al 1980 Cancer in press (used in tissue sections for differential diagnosis of lymphomas and anaplastic carcinomas).

* Some firms show interest in selling monoclonal antibodies. Two examples: Ortho Pharmaceutical Corporation, Raritan, New Jersey, 08869, USA; Sera-Lab Ltd, Crawley Down, Sussex, UK.

the rest of the molecule. In contrast, conventional antisera contain mixtures of antibodies, reacting with different antigenic determinants (which are frequently present on a number of different membrane proteins); lack of reactivity with conventional antisera may therefore suggest that whole molecules are absent. For this reason in leukemia diagnosis more weight should be given to negative observations made with conventional antisera than to those made by individual monoclonal antibodies. In the future the optimal panel for hematological membrane marker analysis will most probably include a wide range of reagents each containing mixtures (blends) of well characterized monoclonal antibodies reactive against chemically characterized differentiation antigens.

Acknowledgments

Ms Sylvia Granger (Immunology Department, Royal Free Hospital, London) contributed to the description of immunochemical methods. Dr Alison Goodall (Immunology Department, Royal Free Hospital, London) helped to summarize the technics for monoclonal antibody production and testing.

REFERENCES

1 Permain G, Lycette R R, Fitzgerald P H 1963 Tuberculin induced mitosis in peripheral blood leucocytes. Lancet i: 637
2 Nowell P C 1960 Phytohaemagglutinin: an initiator of mitosis in cultures of normal human leucocytes. Cancer Research 20: 462
3 Chessin L N, Börjesson J, Welsh P D, Douglas S D, Cooper H L 1966 Studies on peripheral blood lymphocytes in vitro II. Transformation of lymphocytes by pokeweed mitogen. Journal of Experimental Medicine 124: 873
4 Möller G (ed) 1969 Antigen sensitive cells. Transplant Reviews 1
5 Raff M C 1971 Surface antigenic markers for distinguishing T and B lymphocytes in mice. Transplant Reviews 6: 52
6 Greaves M F, Owen J J T, Raff M C 1973 T and B lymphocytes, origins, properties and roles in immune responses. America Elsevier, New York
7 WHO/IARC Workshop 1974 Identification, enumeration and isolation of B and T lymphocytes from human peripheral blood. Scandinavian Journal of Immunology 3: 521
8 Brouet J C, Preud'homme J L, Seligmann M 1975 The use of B and T membrane markers in the classification of human leukaemias with special reference to acute lymphoblastic leukaemia. Blood Cells 1: 81
9 Kersey J, Nesbit M, Hallgreen H, Sabad A, Yuris E, Gajl-Peczalska K 1975 Evidence for origin of certain childhood acute lymphoblastic leukemias and lymphomas in thymus derived lymphocytes. Cancer 36: 1348
10 Catovsky D, Frisch B, Van Noorden S 1975 B, T and null cell leukaemias Electron microscopy and surface morphology. Blood Cells 1: 115
11 Brown G, Greaves M F, Lister T A, Rapson N, Papamichael M 1974 Expression of T and B lymphocyte surface markers on leukaemic cells. Lancet ii: 273
12 Metzger R S, Mohanakumar T, Miller D S 1972 Antigens specific for human lymphocytic and myeloid leukemia cells: detection by non-human primate antiserums. Science. 178: 986
13 Billing R, Terasaki P J 1974 Human leukaemia antigen. Production and characterization of antisera. Journal of the National Cancer Institute 53: 1635
14 Greaves M F, Brown G, Rapson N T, Lister T A 1975 Antiserum to acute lymphoblastic leukaemia cells. Clinical Immunology and Immunopathology 4: 67
15 Greaves M F, Janossy G 1978 Patterns of gene expression and the cellular origins of human leukaemias. Biochimica Biophysica Acta 516: 193
16 Thierfelder S, Rodt H, Thiel E (eds) 1977 Immunological diagnosis of leukaemias and lymphoma. Springer, Berlin
17 Mahmoud A A F, Kellermeyer R W, Warren K S 1974 Monospecific antigranulocyte sera against human neutrophils, esinophils, basophils and myeloblasts. Lancet ii: 1163
18 Jäger G, Hoffmann-Fezer G, Rodt H, Huhn D, Thiel E, Thierfelder S 1977 Myeloid antigens and antigen densities in mice and man. In Immunological Diagnosis of Leukaemias and Lymphomas. Springer-Verlag, Berlin, Heidelberg, New York. p 109–116
19 Roberts M M, Greaves M F 1978 Maturation linked expression of a myeloid cell surface antigen. British Journal of Haematology 38: 439
20 Cantor H, Boyse E A 1977 Lymphocytes as models for the study of mammalian cellular differentiation. Immunological Reviews 33: 105
21 Greaves M F 1975 Clinical applications of cell surface markers. Progress in Hematology 9: 255
22 Fu S M, Winchester R J, Kunkel H H 1975 The occurrence of the HL-B allo-antigens on cells of acute lymphoblastic leukaemias. Journal of Experimental Medicine 142: 1334
23 Williams C A, Chase M W 1967 Methods in Immunology and Immunochemistry. Volume I. Chapter 2. Academic Press, New York, London
24 James K 1973 Preparation of anti-lymphocyte antibodies. In: Weir D M (ed) Handbook of Experimental Immunology. Blackwell Scientific Publications
25 Garvey J S, Cremer N E, Sussdorf D H 1977 Methods in Immunology. Part IV Isolation of immunoglobulins, antibodies and their subunits. W A Benjamin Inc
26 Greaves M F, Janossy G 1976 Antisera to human T lymphocytes. In: Bloom B R, David J R (eds) In Vitro Methods in Cell Mediated and Tumor Immunity. Academic Press, New York. p 89
27 Bobrove A, Strober S, Herzenberg L, De Pamphilis 1974 Identification and quantitation of thymus-derived lymphocytes in human peripheral blood. Journal of Immunology 112: 520
28 Touraine J I, Touraine F, Kiszkiss D F, Choi Y S, Good R A 1974 Heterologous specific

antiserum for identification of human T lymphocytes. Clinical and Experimental Immunology 16: 503

29 Balch C M, Dougherty P A, Dagg M K, Diethelm A G, Lawton A R 1977 Detection of human T cells using anti-monkey thymocyte antisera: tissue distribution and heterogeneity. Clinical Immunology and Immunopathology 8: 448

30 Ades E W, Gordon D S, Phillips D J, Martin L H, LaVia M F, Reimer C B 1978 Antiserums for immunofluorescent enumeration of human T lymphocytes utilizing fluoresceinated staphylococcal protein A. American Journal of Pathology 92: 619

31 Smith R W, Terry W D, Buell D N, Sell K W 1973 An antigenic marker for human thymic lymphocytes. Journal of Immunology 110: 884

32 Levy R, Warnke R, Dorfman R F, Haimovich J 1977 The monoclonality of human-B cell lymphomas. Journal of Experimental Medicine 145: 1014

33 Herbert W J 1978 Mineral oil adjuvants and the immunization of laboratory animals. In: Weir D M (ed) Handbook of Experimental Immunology; Vol. 3. Blackwell Scientific, Oxford. p A3.1–A3.5

34 Billing R J, Minowada J, Cline M, Clark W, Lee K 1978 An acute lymphocytic leukemia-associated membrane Ag. Journal of the National Cancer Institute 61: 423

35 McBride R A, Schierman L W 1970 Hapten-carrier relationship of isoantigens. A model for immunological maturation based on the conversion of haptens to carriers by antibody. Journal of Experimental Medicine 131: 377

36 Smith P J, Robinson C M, Reif A E 1974 Specificity of anti-leukemia sera prepared by immunization with leukaemia cells admixed with normal antigen-blocking sera. Cancer Research 34: 169

37 Levy R, Dilley J 1971 In vitro antibody response to cell surface antigens I. Xenogeneic response to human leukaemia cells. Journal of Immunology 119: 387

38 Janossy G, Greaves M F, Sutherland R, Dirrant J, Lewis C 1977 Comparative analysis of membrane phenotypes in acute lymphoid leukaemia and in lymphoid blast crisis of chronic myeloid leukaemia. Leukaemia Research 1: 289

39 Baker M A, Ramachander K, Taub R N 1974 Specificity of hetero-antisera to human acute leukaemia associated antigens. Journal of Clinical Investigation 54: 1273

40 Minowada J, Tsubota T, Nakazawa S, Srivastava B I S, Huang C C, Oshimura M, Sonta S, Han T, Sinks L F, Sandberg A A 1977 Establishment and characterization of leukaemic T-cell lines, B-cell lines, and Null-cell line: a progress report on surface antigen study of fresh lymphatic leukaemia in man. In: Theirfelder S, Rodt H, Thiel E (eds) Immunological Diagnosis of Leukaemias and Lymphomas. Springer-Verlag, Berlin. p 241

41 Kaplan J, Ravindranath Y, Peterson W D 1977 T and B lymphocyte antigen positive null cell leukemias. Blood 49: 371

42 Schlossmann S F, Chess L, Humphreys R E, Strominger J L 1976 Distribution of Ia-like molecules on the surface of normal and leukaemic human cells. Proceedings of the National Academy of Sciences of USA 73: 1288

43 Tupchong L, Maclennan I C M 1978 Surface antigens in AML: a study using heteroantisera. British Journal of Cancer 38: 481

44 Morris R J, Williams A F 1975 Antigens on mouse and rat lymphocytes recognized by rabbit antiserum against rat brain: the quantitative analysis of a xenogeneic serum. European Journal of Immunology 5: 274

45 Avrameas S 1969 Coupling of enzymes to proteins with glutaraldehyde. Immunochemistry 6: 43

46 March S C, Parikh I, Cuatrecasas P 1974 A simplified method for cyanogen bromide activation of agarose for affinity chromatography. Analytical Biochemistry 60: 149

47 Axen R, Porath J, Ernback S 1967 Chemical coupling of peptides and proteins to polysaccharides by means of cyanogen halides. Nature 214: 1302

48 Welsh K I, Turner M J 1976 Preparation of antisera specific for human B cells by immunization of rabbits with immune complexes. Tissue Antigens 8: 197

49 Heide K, Schwick H G 1978 Salt fractionation of immunoglobulins. In: Weir D M (ed) Handbook of Experimental Immunology. Blackwell, Oxford

50 Gathings W E, Lawton A R, Cooper M D 1977 Immunofluorescence studies of the development of pre-B cells, B lymphocytes and Ig Isotype diversity in humans. European Journal of Immunology 7: 804

51 Köhler G, Milstein C 1975 Continuous cultures of fused cells secreting antibody of predefined specificity. Nature 256: 495

52 Köhler G, Howe S C, Milstein C 1976 Fusion between immunoglobulin-secreting and nonsecreting myeloma cell lines. European Journal of Immunology 6: 292

53 Galfre G, Howe S C, Milstein C, Butcher G W, Howard J C 1977 Antibodies to major histocompatibility antigens produced by hybrid cells. Nature 266: 550
54 Steplewski Z, Koprowski H, Leibovitz A 1976 Polyethylene glycol-mediated fusion of human tumour cells with mouse cells. Somatic Cell Genetics 2: 559
55 Cotton R G H, Milstein C 1973 Fusion of two immunoglobulin-producing myeloma cells. Nature 244: 42
56 Seligmann M, Preud'homme J L, Brouet J C 1973 B and T cell markers in human proliferative blood diseases and primary immunodeficiencies, with special reference to membrane bound immunoglobulins. Transplant Reviews 16: 85
57 Janossy G, Bollum F J, Bradstock K F, McMichael A, Rapson N, Greaves M F 1979 Terminal transferase positive human bone marrow cells exhibit the antigenic phenotype of non-T, non-B acute lymphoblastic leukemia. Journal of Immunology 123: 1525
58 Thiel E, Dormer P, Rodt H, Thierfelder S 1975 Quantitative immunoautoradiography at the cellular level. 1. Design of a microphotometric method to quantitate membrane antigens on single cells using ^{125}I-labelled antibodies. Journal of Immunological Methods 6: 317
59 Thiel E, Dormer P, Rodt H, Huhn D, Bauchinger M, Kley H P, Thierfelder S 1977 Quantitation of T antigenic sites and Ig determinants on leukaemic cells by microphotometric immunoradioautography. In: Immunological Diagnosis of Leukaemias and Lymphomas. Springer-Verlag, Berlin, Heidelberg, New York. p 131–146
60 Andres G A, Hsu K C, Seegal B C 1978 Immunologic techniques for the identification of antigens or antibodies by electron microscopy. In: Weir D M (ed) Handbook of Experimental Immunology. Blackwell, Oxford
61 Boyum A 1968 A one stage procedure for isolation of granulocytes and lymphocytes from human blood. Scandinavian Journal of Clinical Laboratory Investigations 21: Suppl 97: 51
62 Preud'homme J L, Seligmann M 1972 Surface bound immunoglobulins as a cell marker in human lymphoproliferative diseases. Blood 40: 777
63 Habeshaw J A, Catley P F, Stansfield A G, Brearley R L 1979 Surface phenotyping, histology, and the nature of non-Hodgkin lymphoma in 157 patients. British Journal of Cancer 40: 11, and personal communication.
64 Taylor R B, Duffus W P H, Raff M C, De Petris S 1971 Redistribution and pinocytosis of lymphocyte surface immunoglobulin molecules induced by anti-immunoglobulin antibody. Nature New Biology 233: 225
65 Bessis M 1973 Living blood cells and their ultrastructure. Springer, Berlin
66 Vossen J M, Hijmans W 1975 Membrane associated immunoglobulin determinants on bone marrow and blood lymphocytes in the pediatric age group and on fetal tissues. Annals of the New York Academy of Sciences 254: 262
67 Preud'homme J L, Labaume S 1976 Detection of surface immunoglobulins on human cells by direct immunofluorescence. In: Bloom B R, David J R (eds) In vitro Methods in Cell Mediated and Tumour Immunity. Academic Press, New York. p 155
68 Johnson G D, Holborow E J, Dorling J 1978 Immunofluorescence and immunoenzyme techniques. In: Weir D M (ed) Handbook of Experimental Immunology. Blackwell, Oxford
69 Amante L, Ancona A, Forni L 1972 The conjugation of immunoglobulins with tetramethyl rhodamine isothiocyanate. Journal of Immunological Methods 1: 289
70 Ploem J S 1967 The use of a vertical illuminator with interchangeable dichroic mirrors for fluorescence miscroscopy with incident light. Zeitschr Wiss Mikroskopie 681
71 Herzenberg L A, Herzenberg L A 1978 Analysis and separation using the fluorescence activated cell sorter (FACS). In: Weir D M (ed) Application of Immunological Methods, 3rd Edn. Blackwell, Oxford. p 22
72 Janossy G, Roberts M M, Capellaro D, Greaves M F, Francis G E 1978 Use of the Fluorescence Activated Cell Sorter in human leukaemia. In: Knapp W, Holubar K, Wick G (eds) Immunofluorescence and Related Staining Techniques. Biomedical Press, Elsevier, North Holland. p. 111
73 Jäger G, Lau B, Packmann K, Rodt H, Netzel B, Thiel E, Huhn D, Thierfelder S, Dörmer P 1979 Cell surface differentiation of acute lymphoblastic cALL-type leukaemias in diffusion chambers. Blut 38: 165
74 Ling N R, Bishop S, Jefferis R 1977 Use of antibody coated red cells for the sensitive detection of antigen and in rosette tests for cells bearing surface Ig-s. Journal of Immunological Methods 15: 279
75 Dhaliwal H S, Ling N R, Bishop S, Chapel H 1978 Expression of IgG on blood lymphocytes in CLL. Clinical and Experimental Immunology 31: 226
76 Parish C R, Hayward J A 1974 The lymphocyte surface I relation between Fc receptor, C_3 receptors and surface immunoglobulin. Proceedings of the Royal Society of London B 187:47

77 De Gast G C, Platts-Mills T A E 1979 Functional studies on lymphocytes in adult human bone marrow II Isolated surface IgM-positive cells. Journal of Immunology 122: 285
78 Hunter W M 1978 Radioimmunoassay. In: Weir D M (ed) Handbook of Experimental Immunology. Blackwell, Oxford
79 Mittal K K, Mickey M R, Singal D P, Terasaki P I 1968 Serotyping for bone transplantation XVIII. Refinement of microdroplet lymphocyte toxicity test. Transplantation 6: 913
80 Mohanakumar T, Metzgar R S, Miller D S 1974 Human leukaemia cell antigens: serologic characterization with xenoantisera. Journal of the National Cancer Institute 52: 1435
81 WHO/IUIS Technical Report 1978 Immunological diagnosis of leukaemia and lymphoma. British Journal of Haematology 38: 85
82 Bollum F J 1975 Antibody to terminal deoxynucleotidyl transferase. Proceedings of the National Academy of Sciences of USA 72: 4119
83 Gregoire K E, Goldschneider I, Barton R W, Bollum F J 1977 Intracellular distribution of terminal deoxynucleotidyl transferase (TdT) in rat bone marrow and thymus. Proceedings of the National Academy of Sciences of USA 74: 3993
84 Barton R, Goldschneider I, Bollum F J 1976 The distribution of terminal deoxynucleotidyl transferase among subsets of thymocytes in the rat. Journal of Immunology 116: 462
85 Janossy G, Hoffbrand A V, Greaves M F, Ganeshaguru K, Pain C, Bradstock K F, Prentice H G, Kay H E M 1980 Terminal transferase enzyme assay and immunological membrane markers in the diagnosis of leukaemia—a multi-parameter analysis of 300 cases. British Journal of Haematology 44: 221
86 Vogler L B, Crist W M, Bockman D E, Pearl E R, Lawton A R, Cooper M D 1978 Pre-B cell leukaemia: a new phenotype of childhood lymphoblastic leukaemia. New England Journal of Medicine 298: 872
87 Brouet J C, Preud'homme J L, Perit C, Valensi F, Rouget P, Seligmann M 1979 Acute lymphoblastic leukemia with pre-B cell characteristics. Blood 54: 269
88 Greaves M F, Verbi W, Hoffbrand A V, Janossy G, Vogler L, Cooper M D, Bollum F J 1979 Phenotypic characteristics of pre-B cell leukaemia. Leukemia Research 3: 353
89 Catovsky D 1979 Ph¹ positive leukemia and CGL. British Journal of Haematology 42: 493
90 Andersson J K, Moore J O, Falletta J M, Terry W F, Metzgar R S 1979 Acute lymphoblastic leukaemia: classification and characterization with antisera to human T cell and Ia antigens. Journal of the National Cancer Institute 62: 293
91 McVerry B A, Goldstone A H, Janossy G 1979 Acute promyelocytic: further evidence of the differentiation-linked expression of Ia-like (p 28, 33) antigens on leukaemic cells. Scandinavian Journal of Haematology 22: 53
92 Minowada J, Janossy G, Greaves M F, Tsubota T, Sahai Srivastavia B I, Morkawa S, Tatsumi E 1978 Expression of an antigen associated with acute lymphoblastic leukemia in human leukaemia-lymphoma cell lines. Journal of the National Cancer Institute 60: 1269
93 Rodt H, Netzel B, Thiel E, Jager G, Huhn D, Haas R, Gotze D, Thierfelder S 1977 Classification of leukaemic cells with T- and O-ALL-specific antisera. In: Thierfelder S, Rodt H (eds) Immunological diagnosis of Leukaemias and Lymphomas. Springer-Verlag, Berlin. p 87
94 Billing R, Clark B, Guidera K, Minowada J 1978 Heteroantiserum against acute lymphocytic leukaemia raised to the lymphoblastoid cell line Nalm-1. International Journal of Cancer 22: 694
95 Koshiba H, Minowada J, Pressman D 1978 Rabbit antiserum against a non-T, non-B leukaemia cell line that carries the Ph¹ chromosome (NALM-1). Journal of the National Cancer Institute 61: 987
96 Sutherland R, Smart J, Niaudet P, Greaves M F 1978 Acute lymphoblastic leukaemia associated antigen II. Isolation and partial characterization. Leukemia Research 2: 115
97 Chessels J M, Hardisty R M, Rapson N T, Greaves M F 1977 Acute lymphoblastic leukaemia in children: classification and prognosis. Lancet ii: 1307
98 Roberts M, Greaves M, Janossy G, Sutherland R, Pain C 1978 Acute lymphoblastic leukaemia (ALL) associated antigen. I. Expression in different haematopoietic malignancies. Leukemia Research 2: 105
99 Greaves M F, Paxton A, Janossy G, Pain C, Johnson S, Lister A T 1980 Acute lymphoblastic leukaemia associated antigen III. Alteration in expression associated with treatment and relapse. Leukemia Research 4:1
100 Janossy G, Francis G, Capellaro D, Goldstone A H, Greaves M F 1978 Cell sorter analysis of leukaemia-associated antigens on human myeloid precursors. Nature 276: 176

101 Janossy G, Woodruff R K, Paxton A, Greaves M F, Capellaro D, Kirk B, Innes E M, Eden O B, Lewis C, Catovsky D, Hoffbrand A V 1978 Membrane marker and cell separation studies in Ph¹ positive leukaemia. Blood 51: 861

102 Humphreys R E, McCune J M, Chess L, Herrman H C, Malenka D J, Mann D L, Parham P, Schlossman S F, Strominger J L 1976 Isolation and immunological characterization of a human B lymphocyte specific cell surface antigen. Journal of Experimental Medicine 144: 98

103 Greaves M F, Brown G 1973 A human B lymphocyte specific antigen. Nature New Biology 237: 36

104 Billing R, Rafizadeh B, Drew I, Hartman G, Gale R, Teraski P 1976 Human B lymphocyte Ag-s expressed by lymphocytic and myelocytic leukaemia cells. 1. Detection by rabbit antisera. Journal of Experimental Medicine 144: 167

105 Durante A, Zighelboim J, Gale R P 1976 Leukaemia associated antigens detected by heterologous antisera. Journal of the National Cancer Institue 56: 1217

106 Hsu C C S, Marbi G E, Mittal K K 1977 Antisera against leukaemia associated antigens on human lymphocytes. Clinical and experimental Immunology 27: 487

107 Cline M J, Billing R 1977 Antigens expressed by human B lymphocytes and myeloid stem cells. Journal of Experimental Medicine 146: 1143

108 Winchester R J, Ross G D, Jarowski C L, Wang C Y, Halper J, Broxmeyer H 1977 Expression of Ia-like antigen on human granulocytes during early phases of differentiation. Proceedings of the National Academy of Sciences of USA 74: 4012

109 Klareskog L, Tragardh L, Lindblom J B, Peterson P A 1978 Reactivity of a rabbit antiserum against highly purified HLA-DR antigens. Scandinavian Journal of Immunology 7: 199

110 Snary D, Barnstable C J, Bodmer W F, Goodfellow P N, Crumpton M J 1977 Cellular distribution, purification and molecular nature of human Ia antigens. Scandinavian Journal of Immunology 6: 439

111 Mann D L, Rogentine G N, Fahey J L, Nathenson S 1969 Human lymphocyte membrane (HL-A) alloantigens: isolation, purification and properties. Journal of Immunology 103: 282

112 Janossy G, Goldstone A H, Capellaro D, Greaves M F, Kulenkampff J, Pippard M, Welsh K 1977 Differentiation linked expression of p 28, 33 (Ia-like) structures on human leukaemic cells. British Journal of Haematology 37: 391

113 Fu S M, Chiorazzi N, Wang C Y, Montazeri G, Kunkel H G, Ko H S, Gottlieb A B 1978 Ia-bearing T lymphocytes in man. Journal of Experimental Medicine 148: 1423

114 Reinherz L E, Nodler L M, Rosenthal D S, Moloney W C, Schlossman S 1979 T cell subset characterization of human T-CLL. Blood 53: 1066

115 Kaplan J, Inoue S, Offenbreit M J 1978 Myeloid colony-forming cells express human B lymphocyte antigens. Nature 271: 458

116 Ross G D, Jarowski C I, Rabellino E M, Winchester R J 1978 The sequential appearance of Ia-like antigens and 2 different complement receptors during the maturation of human neutrophils. Journal of Experimental Medicine 147: 730

117 Mills B, Sen L, Borella L 1975 Reactivity of anti-human thymocyte serum with acute leukaemic blasts. Journal of Immunology 115: 1038

118 Aoki T, Hammerling U, De Harven E, Boyse E A, Old L J 1979 Antigenic structure of cell surfaces. An immunoferritin study of the occurrence of H-2 and TL alloantigens on mouse cells. Journal of Experimental Medicine 130: 979

119 Owen F L, Fanger M W 1974 Studies on the human T lymphocyte population II. The use of a T cell specific antibody in the partial isolation and characterization of the human lymphocyte receptor for sheep red blood cells. Journal of Immunology 113: 1138

120 Kersey J, Coccia P, Bloomfield C, Nesbit M, McKenna R, Brunning R, Hallgren H, Gajl-Peczalska K 1977 Surface markers define human lymphoid malignancies with differing prognoses. In: Thierfelder S, Rodt H, Thiel E (eds) Immunological Diagnosis of Leukaemias and Lymphomas. Springer-Verlag, Berlin. p 17

121 Rodt H, Thierfelder S, Thiel E, Gotze D, Netzel B, Huhn D, Eulitz M 1975 Identification and quantification of human T-cell antigen by antisera purified from antibodies cross-reacting with haemopoietic progenitors and other blood cells. Immunogenetics 2: 411

122 Catovsky D, Cherchi M, Greaves M F, Janossy G, Pain C, Kay H E M 1978 Acid-phosphatase reaction in acute lymphoblastic leukaemia. Lancet i: 749

123 Brutuel A, Verhoef K P R, Bosma A, Bourne A E, Engelfriet P 1976 Specific antisera against human blood cells applicable in the direct immunofluorescence technique. Scandinavian Journal of Immunology 5: 1965

124 Tupchong L, Maclennan I C M 1978 Surface antigens in AML: a study using heteroantisera. British Journal of Cancer 38: 481

125 Stuart A E, Young G A, Grant P F 1976 Identification of human mononuclear cells by anti-monocyte serum. British Journal of Haematology 34: 457
126 Greaves M F, Falk J A, Falk R E 1975 A surface antigen marker for human monocytes. Scandinavian Journal of Immunology 4: 555
127 Cooper M D, Lawton A R, Kincade P W 1972 A two-stage model for development of antibody producing cells. Clinical and Experimental Immunology 11: 143
128 Enno A, Catovsky D, O'Brien M, Cherchi M, Kumarau T O, Galton D A G 1979 'Prolymphocytic' transformation of chronic lymphocytic leukaemia. British Journal of Haematology 4: 9
129 Salmon S E, Seligmann M 1974 B cell neoplasia in man. Lancet ii: 1230
130 Hayward A R, Ezer G 1974 Development of lymphocyte populations in the human fetal thymus and spleen. Clinical and Experimental Immunology 17: 169
131 Catovsky D, Pittman S, O'Brien M, Cherchi M, Costello C, Foa R, Pearce E, Hoffbrand A V, Janossy G, Ganeshaguru K, Greaves M F 1979 Multiparameter studies in lymphoid leukemias. American Journal of Clinical Pathology 72: 736
132 Brostoff J 1974 A simple technique for counting rosettes using acridine orange. Journal of Immunology 5: 303
133 Ramasamy R 1974 A fluorescent stain for viable rosette forming cells. Journal of Immunological Methods 5: 305
134 Stathopoulos G, Elliott E V 1974 Formation of mouse or sheep red-blood-cell rosettes by lymphocytes from normal & leukaemic individuals. Lancet i: 600
135 Weiner M S, Bianco C, Nussenzweig V 1973 Enhanced binding of neuraminidase treated sheep erythrocytes to human T lymphocytes. Blood 42: 939
136 Wilson A B 1975 Increased sensitivity of the rosette forming reaction of human T lymphocytes with sheep erythrocytes afforded by papain treatment of the sheep cells. Clinical and Experimental Immunology 22: 177
137 Kaplan M E, Woodson M, Clark C 1976 Detection of human T lymphocytes by rosette formation with AET treated sheep red cells. In: Bloom B R, David J R (eds) In Vitro Methods in Cell Mediated and Tumor Immunity. Academic Press, New York
138 Hallberg T, Gurner B W, Coombs R R A 1973 Opsonic adherence of sensitized ox red cells to human lymphocytes as measured by rosette formation. Int. Arch. Allergy Appl. Imm. 44: 500
139 Johnson H E, Madsen M 1978 Lymphocyte subpopulations in man: ox erythrocytes as indicators in the EA and EAC rosette tests: Serological and technical aspects. Scandinavian Journal of Immunology 8: 247
140 Pichler W J, Broder S 1978 Fc_{IgM} and Fc_{IgG} on human circulating B lymphocytes. Journal of Immunology 121: 887, and 1540
141 Burns G F, Cawley J C, Baker C R 1979 Characterization of the receptor for IgM present on human B ly-s. Immunology 36: 569
142 Moretta L, Ferrarini M, Durante H L, Mingari M C 1975 Expression of a receptor for IgM by human T cells in vitro. European Journal of Immunology 5: 565
143 Ross G D, Polley J 1976 Assay for the 2 different types of lymphocyte complement receptors. Scandinavian Journal of Immunology 5: 99
144 Stein H, Siamssen U, Lennert K 1978 Complement receptor subtypes C3b and C3d in lymphatic tissue and follicular lymphoma. British Journal of Cancer 37: 520
145 Janossy G, McVerry B A, Goldstone A H, Souhami R L, Cawley J C, Thompson D S 1977 Atypical surface marker characteristics in a T-cell lymphoma. Scandinavian Journal of Haematology 19: 411
146 Mendes N F, Miki S S, Peixinho Z F 1974 Combined detection of human T and B lymphocytes by rosette formation with sheep erythrocytes and zymosan-C3 complexes. Journal of Immunology 113: 531
147 Brown G, Greaves M F 1974 Cell surface markers for human T and B lymphocytes. European Journal of Immunology 4: 302
148 Gupta S, Good R A, Siegel F P 1976 Rosette formation with mouse erythrocytes II. A marker for human B and non-T lymphocytes. Clinical and experimental Immunology 25: 319
149 Niaudet P, Greaves M F, Horwitz D 1979 Phenotypes of 'null' cells in human blood. Scandinavian Journal of Immunology 4: 387
150 Gupta S, Good R A 1971 Rosette formation with mouse erythrocytes V. Clinical Immunology and Immunopathology 8: 520
151 Catovsky D, Cherchi M, Okos A, Hegde U, Galton D A G 1976 Mouse red cell rosettes in B lymphoproliferative disorders. British Journal of Haematology 33: 173

152 Forbes I J, Zalewski P D 1976 A subpopulation of human B lymphocytes that rosette with mouse erythrocytes. Clinical and Experimental Immunology 26: 99
153 Sen L, Borella L 1975 Clinical importance of lymphoblasts with T-markers in childhood acute leukemia. New England Journal of Medicine 292: 828
154 Flandrin G, Brouet J C, Daniel M D, Preud'homme J L 1975 Acute leukaemia with Burkitt's tumor cells. A study of six cases with special reference to lymphocyte surface markers. Blood 45: 183
155 Gordon D S, Hubbard M 1977 Surface membrane characteristics and cytochemistry of the abnormal acute leukemia. Blood 51: 681
156 Marks S M, Baltimore D, McCaffrey R 1978 Terminal transferase as predictor of initial responsiveness to vincristine-prednisolone therapy in blastic chronic myelogenous leukemia. New England Journal of Medicine 298: 812
157 Janossy G, Woodruff R K, Pippard M J, Prentice H G, Hoffbrand A V, Paxton A, Bunch C, Greaves M F 1979 Relation of 'lymphoid' phenotype and response to chemotherapy incorporating vincristine-prednisolone in the acute phase of Ph[1] positive leukemia. Cancer 43: 426
158 Edelson R L, Kirkpatrick C H, Svehach E M, Schein P S, Smith R W, Green I, Lutzner M 1974 Preferential cutaneous infiltration by neoplastic thymus derived lymphocytes. Morphologic and functional studies. Annals of International Medicine 80: 685
159 Stein H, Peterson N, Gaedicke G, Lennert K, Landbeck G 1976 Lymphoblastic lymphoma of convoluted or acid phorphatase type—a tumour of T precursor cells. International Journal of Cancer 17: 292
160 Gajl-Peczalska K J, Bloomfield C D, Coccia P F, Sosin H, Brunning R D, Kersey J H 1975 B and T cell lymphomas: analysis of blood and lymph nodes in 87 patients. American Journal of Medicine 59: 674
161 Fialkow P J 1974 The origin and development of human tumors studied with cell markers. New England Journal of Medicine 291: 26
162 Bradstock K F, Janossy G, Pizzolo G, Hoffbrand A V, McMichael A, Pilch J R, Milstein C, Beverley P, Bollum F J 1980 Subpopulations of normal and leukaemic human thymocytes: an analysis using monoclonal antibodies. Journal of National Cancer Institute 65: in press
163 Borella L, Casper J T, Lauer S J 1979 Shifts in expression of cell membrane phenotypes in childhood lymphoid malignancies at relapse. Blood 54: 64
164 Goldstone A H, McVerry B A, Janossy G, Walker H 1979 Clonal identification in ALL. Blood 53: 892
165 Bollum F J 1980 Terminal deoxynucleotidyl transferase as a hematopoietic cell marker. Blood 54: 1203
166 Janossy G, Thomas J A, Bollum F J, Granger S, Pizzolo G, Bradstock K F, Ganeshaguru K, Hoffbrand A V 1980 The human thymic microenvironment: an immunohistologic study. Journal of Immunology 125: 202
167 Bradstock K F, Papageorgiou E S, Janossy G, Hoffbrand A V, Willoughby M L, Roberts P D, Bollum F J 1980 Detection of leukaemic lymphoblasts in CSF by immunofluorescence for terminal transferase. Lancet i: 1144
168 Janossy G, Bollum F J, Bradstock K F, Ashley J 1980 Cellular phenotypes of normal and leukaemic haemopoietic cells detected by selected antibody combinations. Blood 56: 430
169 Bradstock K F, Janossy G, Bollum F J, Milstein C 1980 Anomalous phenotype in human thymic acute lymphoblastic leukaemia Nature 284: 455
170 Janossy G, Prentice H G, Bradstock K F, Hoffbrand A V 1980 Recent advances in the diagnosis and treatment of thymic acute lymphoblastic leukaemia. In: Serrou B, Rosenfeld C (eds) New Trends in Human Immunology and Cancer Immunotherapy, Academic Press, Oxford
171 Rodt H, Netzel B, Kolb H J, Janka G, Haas R J, Rieder I, Belohradsky B, Thierfelder S 1980 Suppression of graft versus disease by incubation of bone marrow grafts with anti-T-cell globulin. Blut: in press

6

Chromosomes in Leukemia and Lymphoma with Special Emphasis on Methodology

Joseph R. Testa   Janet D. Rowley

INTRODUCTION

The renewed interest in the study of chromosomes in hematological malignancies is due to technical improvements that now permit the precise identification, not only of each human chromosome, but of portions of chromosomes as well. Use of chromosomal banding technics has revealed nonrandom chromosomal patterns in many of these diseases (e.g. the 9;22 translocation in chronic myelogenous leukemia [CML], the 15;17 translocation in acute promyelocytic leukemia [APL], and the presence of 14q+ chromosomes in malignant lymphomas). Correlations between karyotype and clinical findings have been found in several hematologic disorders. More data are available for the leukemias than for the lymphomas because of the relative ease of obtaining bone marrow and peripheral blood specimens from leukemia patients. Lymph nodes, effusions, the spleen and other infiltrated solid tissues are usually the most useful sources for chromosomal studies on lymphoma patients. Initial biopsies of lymphoma patients are often done prior to referral, and repeat samples usually cannot be obtained after treatment. In contrast, serial samples from leukemia patients permit the study of cytogenetic patterns during the various stages of the patients' clinical course.

Several extensive reviews of the types and frequency of chromosomal abnormalities in leukemia and lymphoma have recently been published.[1-4] Therefore, only a brief account of chromosomal findings in these diseases will be presented here. This chapter will be confined primarily to a discussion of the methods for obtaining successful cytogenetic analyses of patients with hematologic malignancies.

METHODOLOGY

Successful cytogenetic analysis of patients with hematologic malignances depends on a number of factors. Of utmost importance is the attention paid to the details of cell culture, staining and karyotypic analysis. Thus, we have been very specific in our description of the procedures that work well in our laboratory; some methods, however, particularly chromosome banding technics, may have to be modified to give optimal results in other laboratories. Wherever applicable, alternative methods have been presented because, in a particular patient, some may be successful whereas others are not.

The success rate varies with the specific type of disease. For example, about 90 per cent of the samples from our myeloid-leukemia patients are successful (at least five analyzable banded metaphases); since we obtain multiple samples from many of these patients, the percentage of patients with at least one successful sample is even higher than 90 per cent. We request an additional sample if the original one appears inadequate. Our success rate is about 60 to 70 per cent for samples from non-Hodgkin lymphoma patients.

CULTURE PROCEDURES

Bone marrow aspirate

Procedure

1. Using sterile technic, collect 1 to 2 ml of bone marrow aspirate in a heparinized syringe *or* use a dry syringe and transfer the marrow to a conical graduated centrifuge tube containing 0.1 ml of sodium heparin (stock solution = 1000 units/ml) and 5 ml of RPMI medium 1640 or Hanks' balanced salt solution. Note: if a previous aspirate has been obtained for cytological preparations, the needle should be rotated 180° before a second sample is aspirated for chromosome study. This procedure increases the likelihood of obtaining marrow spicules in the second aspirate.

2. Distribute approximately 0.5 to 1 ml of this suspension to each of several tissue culture flasks (25 cm² growth area) containing 5 ml of RPMI medium 1640 supplemented with 1 ml of fetal calf serum and 0.05 ml of antibiotic mixture (10 000 units/ml of penicillin and 10 000 μg/ml of streptomycin).

3. Incubate cultures at 37°C for 24 h and process the remaining 3 to 5 ml of the original medium plus marrow cell suspension directly. Note: we incubate marrow and blood without supplemental CO_2 and humidity. The caps of the flasks are tightened. We place the flasks with the cap end up into the incubator.

4. Cells in mitosis are harvested from both direct and 24 h cultured samples by addition of 0.1 ml of vincaleucoblastine (Velban) (stock solution = 0.5 μg/ml) or 0.1 ml of N-desacetyl-N-methylocolchicine (Colcemid) (stock solution = 10 μg/ml) and incubated at 37°C for 30 min. The centrifuge tube containing the direct marrow sample is placed in a beaker of pre-warmed water (37°C) for more rapid heating. Sterile technic can be abandoned once harvesting begins.

5. Centrifuge samples at 800 to 1000 r/min for 10 min and remove supernatant with a Pasteur pipette. If the sample is very cellular (i.e. with a cell pellet of about 1 ml or more), divide it among two or more tubes. If the sample is considerably diluted with blood, remove the leukocyte-rich plasma and buffy coat to another tube and discard the red cells. Add hypotonic KCl (0.075 mol/l or 5.6 g/l) in small amounts while gently resuspending the cells. The hypotonic KCl is pre-warmed to 37°C by storage in an incubator. A total of about 10 to 12 ml of hypotonic KCl is added for approximately 0.5 ml of cell sediment. Incubate the tubes for 20 min in a water-filled beaker at 37°C.

6. Centrifuge at 600 to 800 r/min for 10 min. Pipette off all but about 0.5 ml of the supernatant and resuspend the cells. Gradually add 8 to 10 ml of freshly made 1:3 fixative (1 part glacial acetic acid plus 3 parts absolute ethanol or methanol) while continually resuspending the cells and breaking up small clumps. Alternatively, some investigators add the unfixed resuspended cells to a new tube containing 8 to 10 ml of fixative. This may minimize clumping of the cells during fixation. Let stand for at least 1 h in the freezer ($-4°C$ to $-25°C$); samples left in the freezer overnight may give better results.

7. Centrifuge at 800 to 1000 r/min for 10 min. Discard the supernatant. We resuspend cells in 8 to 10 ml of freshly made fixative of 45 per cent glacial acetic acid and 55 per cent absolute ethanol; this fixative is used for all subsequent changes until the packed cells appear white and the supernatant is nearly colorless (usually 3 or 4 changes of fixative). Many investigators use 1:3 fixative at all times.

8. Samples can be stored in the freezer at any point after the addition of 1:3 fixative. The quality of the material will be nearly unchanged for several years when it is stored in a freezer. Slides should not be prepared until they are ready to be scanned, since it usually becomes increasingly difficult to band metaphases as slides become older.

9. To make slide preparations, first discard the supernatant. Then add enough fresh fixative (45 per cent glacial acetic acid, 55 per cent ethanol) to produce a slightly milky cell suspension (the amount of fresh fixative needed is approximately equal to five times the volume of the packed cells).

10. Drop 3 to 5 drops of cell suspension on to a clean, water-filled slide (flood slide with tap water or, preferably, distilled water prior to dropping on cells). Shake off the water drops, and blow on the slide to distribute the cells. Wipe the bottom of the slide with absorbent paper and then dry with a hair dryer or over the flame of an alcohol burner, *avoiding over-exposure to heat*. Check the cell density and the spreading of chromosomes in metaphase cells under a microscope with phase contrast optics. Adjust the density of the suspension, if necessary. Another change of fixative may improve the spreading of chromosomes.

Bone core biopsy

If an aspirate cannot be obtained because the marrow is highly fibrotic or because it is tightly 'packed' with cells, a bone core biopsy can give good results in most cases.

Procedure

1. After obtaining a core sample for cytological preparations, reposition the needle before obtaining a second core sample for chromosome analysis.
2. Place the biopsy specimen in a sterile tube containing 0.1 ml sodium heparin plus 5 ml RPMI medium 1640.
3. Using sterile procedure, place the contents of the tube into a Petri dish. Hold the core sample with a forceps and use a scalpel to slice sections as thin as possible.

4. The rest of the procedure is identical to that used for aspirates (beginning with Step 2).

Peripheral blood

For patients who have a high WBC count ($>15\,000/mm^3$) or more than about 10 per cent circulating immature myeloid cells (myelocytes or younger), peripheral blood cultured without the addition of phytohemagglutinin (PHA) can be used instead of, or in addition to, marrow. Although the proportion of normal and abnormal cells may be different, the chromosomal pattern of these dividing myeloid cells is identical to that seen in marrow cells. This procedure can also be useful in patients from whom it is not possible or convenient to obtain a marrow sample. In addition, metaphases from unstimulated blood may often show better banding than those from marrow.

A portion of the peripheral blood sample can be cultured with PHA for 72 h, so that lymphocytes are stimulated to divide; the karyotype of such cells is generally representative of the patient's constitutional chromosomal pattern.

Procedure

1. Using sterile procedure, wet the inside of a syringe with sodium heparin (0.1 ml), or use a dry syringe and transfer the blood to a centrifuge tube containing 0.1 ml of sodium heparin. Withdraw 10 ml of blood from the patient and put into a sterile centrifuge tube with screw cap (avoid flaming). Invert the tube gently several times to mix; avoid forming bubbles, as they tend to damage leukocytes.
2. Centrifuge at 600 to 800 r/min for 10 min. This should yield 4 to 6 ml of supernatant plasma and buffy coat; if not, repeat centrifugation.
3. Transfer the leukocyte-rich plasma and buffy coat to a second sterile centrifuge tube by using a sterile Pasteur pipette, minimizing the number of red cells. Resuspend the buffy coat in the plasma.
4. Distribute approximately 1 ml of the plasma-leukocyte suspension to each of several 25 cm² tissue culture flasks containing about 5 ml of medium such as McCoy's 5a or RPMI 1640 supplemented with 0.05 ml of antibiotic mixture (10 000 units/ml penicillin; 10 000 μg/ml streptomycin). One ml of fetal calf serum can also be added, but this is not necessary. If the patient's WBC count is greater than 10 000/mm³, add less than 1 ml of suspension.
5. Add 0.1 ml of PHA to each 72 h culture flask and incubate all cultures at 37°C for 24, 48 or 72 h.
6. To harvest mitoses, add 0.1 ml Velban (0.5 μg/ml) or 0.1 ml Colcemid (10 μg/ml) to the flasks at approximately 23, 47 or 71 h and allow to incubate further for 1 h or less. Sterile procedure may be abandoned at this point.
7. Transfer each culture to a centrifuge tube and continue to process as in the bone marrow aspirate procedure (starting with Step 5). However, incubate in hypotonic KCl for 17 min instead of 20 min.

Additional note: if the WBC count is more than about 50 000/mm³, of if there are more than about 50 per cent circulating immature myeloid cells, there may be substantial cell degeneration in 48-h cultures. Direct preparations of 24-h cultures may yield better results.

Lymph nodes

Procedure

1. Using sterile procedure, transfer the lymph node sample to a centrifuge tube containing 5 ml of RPMI medium 1640, 1 ml of fetal calf serum, and 0.05 ml of antibiotic-antimycotic (10 000 units/ml penicillin, 10 000 μg/ml strepto-mycin, and 25 μg/ml amphotericin B). The sample should be pea-sized or larger; smaller samples often yield unsatisfactory results.
2. Transfer the contents of the tube into a Petri dish.
3. Hold the tissue with a forceps; cut into very small pieces with scissors, or cut tissue with two scalpels in a cross-cutting style. If cutting is difficult, pipette off 2 to 3 ml of the liquid.
4. Break up the tissue further by gently forcing it up and down inside a Pasteur pipette several times.
5. Suspend the cells and distribute approximately equal amounts (1 to 2 ml) of the suspension to each of three 25 cm^2 culture flasks containing 5 ml RPMI medium 1640, 1 ml fetal calf serum, and 0.05 ml antibiotic-antimycotic mixture.
6. We usually put flasks in a humidified incubator (37°C) with 95 per cent air and 5 per cent CO_2. Lay flasks flat with caps loose. Other investigators have also obtained satisfactory results by incubating without supplemental CO_2 and humidity, and with flask caps tightened.
7. At 3 to 5 h or at about 23 h, harvest metaphases by adding 0.1 ml Velban (0.5 μg/ml) or 0.1 ml Colcemid (10 μg/ml) and return to the humidified CO_2 incubator for an additional 45 min. Note: if the sample is obtained in the morning, we culture some cells for 4 to 6 h and others for 24 h; if the sample is obtained in the late afternoon, the cells are usually cultured for 24 h only, although it may be advisable to process some cells directly (without culture) as well.
8. Continue to process as in the bone marrow aspirate procedure (starting with Step 5).

Spleen
Spleen biopsies are occasionally studied cytogenetically. The procedure used is basically the same as that for lymph node samples.

Effusions
Effusion samples are transferred to a centrifuge tube and centrifuged at 800 to 1000 r/min for 10 min. The supernatant is discarded, and the cells are resuspended in 5 ml RPMI medium 1640. The rest of the procedure is identical to that for bone marrow aspirates (beginning with Step 2).

STAINING TECHNICS

Chromosomes from malignant cells generally have poor morphology and do not band nearly as well as do chromosomes from cells such as PHA-stimulated lymphocytes. Since metaphases may be scarce in the bone marrow and often show poor banding patterns, several culture procedures and various staining technics should be tried. Frequently, the metaphases obtained from the 24-h bone marrow culture have chromosomes with clearer banding patterns than those from direct marrow preparations. However, it is recommended that material from more than one source be analyzed to determine which one will provide the most suitable metaphase cells. Good metaphases give good results with any banding technic; however, it is our experience that, with metaphases of poor quality, quinacrine-banding may give useful results when other technics fail. For complex rearrangements, several different staining technics are useful in defining breakpoints and identifying markers.

Conventional staining technic

Procedure

1. Let slides dry overnight before staining.
2. Mix 1 part stock Leishman-Giemsa staining solution plus 9 parts distilled water just before using. The stock solution is 1 part Leishman stain plus 3 parts Giemsa stain. Leishman stain can be made by addition of 1.5 g of powder to 100 ml of absolute methanol, allowing it to dissolve, and filtering before use. Giemsa stain is made by addition of 0.5 g of powder to 33 ml of glycerine at 55 to 60°C for 1.5 to 2 h, and then adding 33 ml of methanol.
3. Place slides on a staining rack and flood with stain. Allow to stand for 5 to 10 min.
4. Rinse slides with distilled water.
5. Place slides on end and allow to dry thoroughly. Note: we do not mount slides with coverslips because such slides cannot be reused for other staining procedures. However, care must be taken to avoid damaging the cells on these slides.
6. Slides are scanned, and the stage coordinates of suitably spread, intact metaphases are recorded. The chromosome number is counted for each of these cells. Whenever possible, 30 to 50 metaphases are counted. Metaphases are photographed at a DIN setting of 23 to 24 with Kodak Panatomic-X film. This is a fine-grained film with an ASA of 32 (DIN 16), which can be 'pushed' to ASA 160 (DIN 23) by development in Diafine (Acufine, Inc.). By 'pushing' the film, we have been able to shorten exposure times without appreciably increasing the film graininess. We use the same procedure to develop films of quinacrine-banded metaphases (see below); for these metaphases, however, a camera DIN setting of 26 is most satisfactory (shorter exposure times and increased contrast). Printing is done in our laboratory with a Rapidoprint LD14 (Agfa-Gevaert) automatic print processor. We employ Ilfoprint YR3.24P contrast 3, semi-matte paper (which can be written on with pencil) for routine use, and Rapidoprint FPI, contrast 4,

glossy paper for use in publications. Additional note: in samples in which more than one clone is observed, chromosomes from cells of the malignant clone may have poorer morphology. Thus, it is important to photograph and analyze metaphases of varying quality to minimize this bias. We also analyze all hyperdiploid and most hypodiploid metaphases.

7. The slides are destained as follows:

   a. Clean slide thoroughly with xylol for 1 to 2 min.
   b. Rinse off xylol by immersing slide in 100 per cent ethanol for 5 s.
   c. Immerse in 95 per cent ethanol for 5 s.
   d. Immerse in 70 per cent ethanol for 5 s.
   e. Rinse gently under tap water for 5 s.
   f. Using a pipette, drop on fresh fixative (45 per cent glacial acetic acid, 55 per cent ethanol).
   g. Alternate steps 'e' and 'f' until slide is clear.

Note: steps a to d can be done by immersion of slides in Coplin jars containing the specified liquids. Alternatively, the liquids may be squirted on to the slides with polyethylene wash bottles, provided that this action is done very gently, without application directly to the cell area, and without creation of aerosol.

Quinacrine (Q)-banding technic (modified from Caspersson et al[5])

Procedure

1. Store slides in a Coplin jar in 95 per cent ethanol, preferably overnight.
2. Slides are stained by immersion in a Coplin jar containing a solution of quinacrine mustard (0.05 per cent quinacrine mustard dissolved in MacIlvaine's buffer at pH 5.5) for 30 to 60 min. To make the staining solution, dissolve 25 mg of quinacrine mustard in 50 ml of buffer for 24 h, then filter before storing the solution in a refrigerator. To prevent deterioration, the solution is kept in the dark by wrapping the container with aluminum foil. The buffer is made by mixing 66.38 ml of 0.1 mol/l citric acid (anhydrous, 19.212 g/l), stored in a refrigerator, with 83.63 ml of 0.2 mol/l disodium phosphate (anhydrous, 28.396 g/l) just before using. The staining solution can be used repeatedly for 6 months or longer, provided it is filtered occasionally.
3. Drain excess stain off slide.
4. Rinse in two changes of MacIlvaine's buffer (pH 5.5).
5. Place several drops of MacIlvaine's buffer (pH 5.5) on the slide and mount with a coverslip. Remove excess buffer by covering mounted slide with absorbent paper and pressing gently. For sharp bands, it is important to have only a thin layer of buffer. The edge of the coverslip can be sealed with rubber cement or nail polish to prevent evaporation of the buffer during examination of the slide.
6. We photograph Q-banded metaphases on Kodak Panatomic-X film with a DIN setting of 26, using a Zeiss photomicroscope with epi-illumination; the microscope is equipped with an HBO 50 W mercury bulb (Osram), KP440 nm and KP490 nm exciter filters, an LP460 nm reflector, and an

LP470 nm barrier filter. The film is automatically exposed, with exposure times varying from about 15 to 45 s, depending on the state of the bulb and the degree of staining. We photograph with an Apo 100 × objective fitted with an iris diaphragm which is adjusted so that chromosomes fluoresce brightly, but with a minimum of background flare.

7. Remove coverslip under running water, or by flicking it off with a razor blade.
8. Store slides in 95 per cent ethanol for up to 1 week in case further fluorescence is required.
9. Q-banded metaphases are printed on Rapidoprint TP6 paper. Usually, 3 to 4 prints, with a gradation of exposure intensities, are made for each metaphase. If only one print is made, some chromosomes are too dull and some, too bright, for adequate examination of the banding pattern of each chromosome. Generally, the metaphases that are photographed with fluorescence technic are the same metaphases that were previously photographed with conventional Leishman-Giemsa staining (Fig. 6.1). From these duplicate photographs, metaphases are analyzed for any abnormalities of karyotype. The identity of chromosomes is recorded in pencil on the semi-matte print of the conventionally stained metaphase. Slides can be restained with Leishman-Giemsa, and metaphases can be analyzed directly with the microscope as well as on the photographs. Generally 15 metaphases are photographed and analyzed in detail. Ideally, however, 25 or more metaphases are analyzed

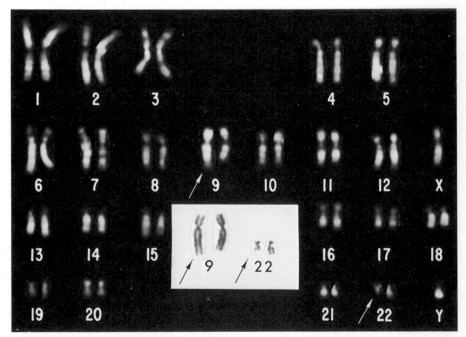

Fig. 6.1 Karyotype of a metaphase from the bone marrow of a patient with CML. The metaphase was stained with quinacrine mustard and examined with ultraviolet fluorescence. The arrows indicate the translocation between the long arm of No 9 and the long arm of No 22 [46,XY,t(9;22)(q34;q11)]. The inset depicts the same chromosomes 9 and 22 stained with Leishman-Giemsa. The partially deleted No 22 is the Ph[1] chromosome.

with banding technic to increase the likelihood of detecting mosaic patterns. Note: slides can be stained directly with quinacrine, without prior staining with Leishman-Giemsa.

Giemsa (G)-banding technic (modified from Sun et al[6])

G-banding gives basically the same pattern as Q-banding. Most investigators concentrate on one of these two technics and use the other only occasionally. G-banding may give less consistent results, but it requires no fluorescence equipment.

Procedure

1. Place fresh slides in an incubator at 60°C for 16 to 24 h.
2. Incubate slide in a Coplin jar containing 0.025 mol/l phosphate buffer (KH_2PO_4, 3.4 g/l, titrated to pH 6.8 with 50 per cent NaOH) at 56°C in a water bath for 10 min.
3. Blot gently and allow slide to dry.
4. Place slide on slide rack and flood with a Giemsa-trypsin mixture for 6 to 8 min. The mixture consists of 36.5 ml phosphate buffer (0.025 mol/l, pH 6.8), 12.5 ml ethanol, 1 to 2 ml of 0.1 per cent trypsin (1:250; Gibco) in pH 6.8 buffer, and 2 ml of filtered stock Giemsa stain. The mixture is prepared fresh every day. The trypsin is diluted in phosphate buffer (0.025 mol/l, pH 6.8), stored frozen in small quantities, and thawed before use.
5. Rinse thoroughly with tap water. Allow to air-dry.
6. Check staining and banding under the microscope.
7. If staining is too light, restain for 5 to 10 min in a solution containing 1 part Giemsa and 100 parts phosphate buffer (pH 6.8).
8. Photograph metaphases with Kodak High Contrast Copy film and print on Rapidoprint FP1, contrast 3 paper.

Additional note: some investigators obtain more consistent results with G-banding technics by controlling the humidity during slide preparation. After dropping several drops of cell suspension on the slide, the slide is held over steam (e.g. steam from a pot of simmering water with the lid removed) for 5 to 10 s and is then air-dried.

Reverse (R)-banding technic[7]

The R-banding technic gives patterns which are basically the opposite of those obtained with Q- or G-banding technics. Bands which appear unstained, or pale, with Q- or G-banding generally stain darkly with R-banding (Fig. 6.2). The R-banding technic is particularly useful for detection of small deletions, since the telomeres stain darkly with this procedure.

Procedure

1. Slides 15 to 21 days old generally give optimal results.
2. Two slides are placed in a 50 ml porcelain Coplin jar containing fresh phosphate buffer (32 ml of 0.07 mol/l $Na_2HPO_4 \cdot 12H_2O$ and 68 ml of 0.07 mol/l KH_2PO_4 adjusted to pH 6.5 by addition of 0.07 mol/l $Na_2HPO_4 \cdot 12H_2O$

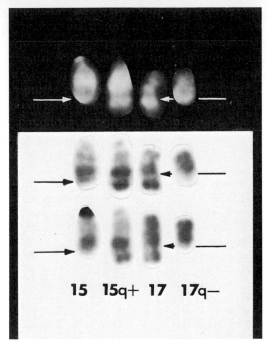

15 15q+ 17 17q−

Fig. 6.2 Partial karyotypes of chromosome pairs No 15 and No 17 from three different metaphases obtained from unstimulated peripheral blood of an APL patient. The partial karyotype shown in the top row is from a Q-banded metaphase; the partial karyotypes shown in the middle and bottom rows are from reverse (R)-banded metaphases. The long arm is short in the abnormal No 17 (17q−) and long in the abnormal No 15 (15q+) due to a reciprocal translocation between these chromosomes. Probable breakpoints are identified with arrows. R-banding appeared to be more informative in the analysis of this rearrangement, since the band proximal to the arrow in No 15, q24, stains darkly when this technic is used. The apparent presence of q24 in both the normal 15 and in the 15q+ suggests a translocation breakpoint distal to q24 [t(15;17)(q25?;q22)]. (Reprinted from *Virchows Archiv B Cell Pathology.*)

to the solution) and incubated in a water bath kept at exactly 85°C for 20 to 25 min. The lid should be kept on the Coplin jar during the incubation period. The level of the water in the water bath should be even with the level of the buffer in the Coplin jar for uniform heating of the slides. The buffer is preheated for 5 min to reach 85°C and is changed after heating of every two slides.

Move slides up and down at 3 to 5 min intervals during the incubation period. This procedure removes air bubbles that form on the surface of the slides while the temperature is at 85°C. If these bubbles are not removed, patchy banding may result.

Glass Coplin jars may break at 85°C. Pyrex or metal containers may be used instead of the porcelain jar.

Slides should be placed in the Coplin jar as soon as the buffer reaches 85°C (approximately 5 min after the buffer-filled Coplin jar is placed in the pre-heated water bath), since the pH (6.5) of the buffer may change within a short time. When the pH becomes higher, the fluorescence of the chromosomes becomes more green.

3. Slides are stained for 4 to 6 min with 0.01 per cent acridine orange, prepared in phosphate buffer (pH 6.5).
4. Rinse slides in phosphate buffer (pH 6.5) for 1.5 to 2 min and mount in the same buffer without sealing the coverslip. Remove excess buffer by covering the mounted slide with absorbent paper and pressing gently. Optimum results are obtained when the layer of buffer between the coverslip and slide is as thin as possible. A thick layer of buffer results in rapid fading under ultraviolet light.
5. Slides are examined with ultraviolet-lightmicroscopy. Chromosomes should show orange and green bands with green telomeres. Metaphases are usually photographed with color transparency film (Kodachrome 64). We use a Zeiss photomicroscope with epi-illumination; the microscope is equipped with a 50 W mercury bulb, a BG12 and an LP420 nm exciter filters, an LP510 nm dichroic reflector, and an LP520 nm barrier filter. The DIN setting is 27. With a 100 W halogen light source, a KP490 nm exciter filter replaces the BG12; also, a KP560 nm barrier filter is used in addition to the LP520 nm barrier filter.
6. Black-and-white prints (Rapidoprint, FP1, contrast Nos 2 or 3) are made from the color transparency film. Green bands on this film appear dark in the black-and-white prints; these bands correspond to lightly stained Q- or G-bands. Orange bands on the transparency film appear light, or unstained, in black-and-white prints; these bands generally correspond to the brightly stained Q-bands or dark G-bands.

Additional comments: if the incubation time is too long, the chromosomes appear fuzzy and only show orange-red fluorescence. Overstaining also results in this type of fluorescence. When overstaining is the cause of such fluorescence, it can be corrected by additional rinsing. Understaining results in green fluorescence and no banding; this can be corrected with an additional short time in stain, followed by rinsing and remounting. When it is necessary to do additional rinsing or staining, coverslips should be removed with a razor blade. Unsatisfactory color differentiation will result when the coverslip is removed by flooding with water.

In general, shorter incubation times are required for older slides. For example, slides 1.5 to 2 months old require an incubation time of 14 to 18 min. Slides older than 2 months do not typically yield good results. However, older slides retreated for 2 to 3 days in fixative may show improved color differentiation. Slides less than a week old tend to fade quickly under ultraviolet light.

When sequential staining of a metaphase is performed, Q-banding followed by R-banding yields excellent results. Frequently, the R-banding obtained after Q-banding is superior to that with R-banding alone. R-banding of metaphases that have already been sequentially stained with conventional Leishman-Giemsa and quinacrine may be less satisfactory. It is also possible to obtain C-bands after R-bands (see below).

C-banding technic (modified from Stefos and Arrighi[8])
Unlike Q-, G- and R-banding technics, constitutive heterochromatin (C)-banding cannot be used for differentiation of all of the chromosomes. Instead, it is

used to identify areas of constitutive heterochromatin on the long arm of chromosomes 1, 9, 16 and Y. The technic also reveals centromeric positions, which are valuable in providing information on the nature of certain rearrangements.

Procedure

1. Immerse the slide for 30 to 45 s in $2 \times SSC$ (0.03 mol/l trisodium citrate [8.82 g/l] and 0.3 mol/l NaCl [17.53 g/l]) which has been adjusted to pH 12 with 1 mol/l NaOH.
2. Rinse three times in $2 \times SSC$ adjusted to pH 7.0 (5 min in each bath).
3. Incubate slide for 1 h in a Coplin jar containing $2 \times SSC$ (pH 7.0) which is maintained at 65°C in a water bath.
4. Rinse for 10 s in 0.2N HCl. This step is optional, but may make the C-bands clearer.
5. Rinse briefly in $2 \times SSC$ (pH 7.0).
6. Rinse twice in 70 per cent ethanol (5 min in each bath).
7. Rinse twice in 95 per cent ethanol (5 min in each bath).
8. Air-dry slide.
9. Stain in Giemsa solution (1 part Giemsa stain plus 9 parts buffer, pH 6.8) for 10 min. The buffer is made by dissolving one buffer tablet (Gurr) in 100 ml of distilled water. Alternatively, Sörensen's buffer (pH 6.8) may be used (50.8 ml of KH_2PO_4 solution [9.078 g/l] and 49.2 ml $Na_2HPO_42H_2O$ solution [11.876 g/l]).
10. Wash 1 min in running tap water.
11. Air-dry slide.
12. Examine metaphases with both bright-field and with phase optics. Often phase optics shows more distinct C-banding. If the C-bands are not dark enough, slides can be stained for an additional time and re-examined.
13. Photograph with Panatomic-X film and print on Rapidoprint FP1, contrast 2 paper.

Additional comments: it is usually possible to C-band metaphases that have been examined previously with both conventional Leishman-Giemsa stain and with fluorescence. However, prolonged exposure to ultraviolet light may be detrimental to subsequent C-banding; therefore exposure should be as brief as possible.

Rubenstein et al[9] recently reported that it is possible to obtain C-bands after sequential Q- and R-banding. For this sequence, C-bands are obtained by treatment of slides with 0.9 per cent NaCl for 1 to 2 min. The slides are then immersed in a freshly prepared 6 per cent aqueous solution of barium hydroxide at room temperature for 17 min. Slides are then rinsed thoroughly with 70 per cent ethanol and saline and incubated at 60°C in $2 \times SSC$ (pH 7.0) for at least 3 to 4 h. Slides are then rinsed with tap water, stained with 5 per cent Giemsa for 5 min, rinsed again with tap water, and allowed to air-dry. If C-bands are to be obtained after R-bands, it is necessary to limit the treatment time with phosphate buffer at 85°C during the R-banding procedure; C-bands cannot be obtained if slides are treated for more than 15 min.

CHROMOSOMAL NOMENCLATURE

The chromosomes are identified according to the Paris Conference nomenclature,[10] and the karyotypes are expressed as recommended under this system. The total chromosome number is indicated first, followed by the sex chromosomes, and then by the gains, losses, or rearrangements of the autosomes. A plus or minus sign before a number indicates a gain or loss, respectively, of a whole chromosome; plus or minus after a number indicates a gain or loss of part of a chromosome. The letters 'p' and 'q' refer to the short and long arms of the chromosome, respectively; 'i' and 'r' stand for isochromosome and ring chromosome. *Mar* is marker, *del* is deletion, *ins* is insertion, and *inv* is inversion. Translocations are identified by 't' followed by the chromosomes involved in a first set of parentheses; the chromosome bands in which the breaks occurred are indicated in a second pair of parentheses. Uncertainty in the chromosome or band involved is signified by a question mark.

CHROMOSOME ABNORMALITIES IN LEUKEMIA

CHRONIC MYELOID LEUKEMIA (CML)

Chronic phase

The Philadelphia (Ph[1]) chromosome is seen in bone marrow cells from approximately 85 per cent of patients with CML.[11] This abnormality was first described in 1960 by Nowell and Hungerford[12] as a deletion of part of the long arm of a G-group chromosome. With the use of banding technics, the Ph[1] chromosome was identified as a 22q−,[13,14] and it was shown, in 1973, to result from a previously undetected translocation involving No 9[15] (Fig. 6.1). Cells from 802 patients with Ph[1]-positive (Ph[1]+) CML have been studied with banding; 739 (92 per cent) of these patients had the usual 9;22 translocation [t(9;22)(q34;q11)] (reviewed by Rowley[16]). Of the remaining 63 patients, 60 had a variant translocation; three had a 22q−, but no translocation was apparent. Of the patients with variant rearrangements, in 29 the translocation involved No 22 and one of several chromosomes other than 9, whereas 31 had a complex, three-way translocation. All but two of the three-way rearrangements involved Nos 9 and 22 and a third chromosome, with the breakpoints in 9 and 22 occurring in the same bands that are involved in the typical t(9;22).

Ph[1]+ patients tend to have a better prognosis than Ph[1]− patients. The median survival of Ph[1]+ patients is about 30 to 40 months, compared to only 12 to 15 months for Ph[1]− patients.[11]

Acute phase

Leukemic cells from 242 patients in the acute phase of Ph[1]+ CML have undergone a karyotypic analysis with banding.[16] The 46,Ph[1]+ cell line remained unchanged in 40 patients (17 per cent), whereas other chromosomal abnormalities were superimposed on this cell line in 202 (83 per cent). The four most frequent changes were a +8 (95 patients), the addition of a second Ph[1] (22q−) chromosome (73 patients), an isochromosome of the long arm of No 17 (56 patients), and a $+19$ (38 patients). These changes often occur in combination in a given patient. A $+19$ seems to have lesser importance because, unlike the other three abnormalities, it was never observed as the only new change in the acute phase.

A change in the karyotype is usually considered to be a grave prognostic sign. The median survival from the time of change until death was found by Whang-Peng et al[11] to be 2 to 5 months; more recently, the same group reported similar results in a new series of patients.[17] In some patients, karyotypic change precedes the clinical signs of blast crisis by 2 to 4 months.[3]

Ph[1]-negative CML

Soon after the translocation had been described in Ph[1]$+$ CML, a number of investigators reported that Ph[1]$-$ patients had a normal karyotype.[18] Since then, there have been a few reports of abnormalities in Ph[1]$-$ patients, including loss of the Y,[18–20] gain of a C-group chromosome,[21] a 6;14 translocation in one case[22] and, in one child, a 9;11 translocation.[23] Two Ph[1]$-$ patients reported by Mintz et al[22] acquired a $+8$ in the blastic phase. Additional patients with Ph[1]$-$ CML will need to be studied before the pattern of aberrations can be determined.

ACUTE LEUKEMIA

Acute non-lymphocytic leukemia (ANLL)

Since we recently reviewed the cytogenetics of ANLL,[24, 25] only a brief summary will be presented here, together with some recent developments.

Approximately 50 per cent of ANLL patients studied with banding technics have detectable karyotypic abnormalities. These abnormalities usually are not seen when the patient is in remission. They reappear in relapse, however, and sometimes there is evidence of additional karyotypic change superimposed on the original aberration.

ANLL patients who have karyotypic abnormalities have modal chromosome numbers that cluster in the diploid range; 80 to 85 per cent of these patients have 45 to 47 chromosomes in cells from abnormal clones. Although there is substantial variability, certain nonrandom abnormalities occur in ANLL. Of 110 patients whom we reviewed,[25] 27 (25 per cent) had a $+8$, which was the most frequent aberration reported; -7, the next most frequent change, was seen in 14 patients.

Two rearrangements observed in ANLL patients have special significance. The first is an 8;21 translocation [t(8;21)(q22;q22)], which was first identified with banding by Rowley.[26] This abnormality was observed in 9 of the 110 chromosomally abnormal patients whom we reviewed.[25] The t(8;21) is unique because its presence is often accompanied by the loss of a sex chromosome, an X in females (33 per cent) and the Y in males (59 per cent), which is otherwise a rare occurrence in ANLL.[24] Chromosomes 8 and 21 can also participate in translocations involving three chromosomes, with breaks in 8 and 21 in the same bands as in the typical t(8;21).[27] Thus, variant 8;21 translocations follow a pattern analogous to that in variant three-way 9;22 translocations in CML.

The second significant rearrangement involves chromosomes 15 and 17 in

APL. We studied this rearrangement in an APL patient by using multiple banding technics; R-banding appeared to be the most informative, indicating a reciprocal translocation with breakpoints distal to q24 in No 15, and in q22 in No 17 [t(15;17)(q25?;q22)][28] (Fig. 6.2). The same abnormality has also been seen in APL patients reported from other laboratories.[29-32] The possibility that there is an unusual geographic distribution of this association was raised by Teerenhovi et al,[33] who reported on 12 APL patients in Finland and Sweden without observing a single case of a t(15;17). In contrast, we have seen a t(15;17) in all six of our APL patients for whom a sufficient number of metaphases could be analyzed,[34] and Van Den Berghe et al[32] of Belgium reported a t(15;17)(q26;q22) in 11 of 16 APL patients. Whether this geographical difference is related to an etiologic difference, a difference in genetic susceptibility, or some other factor is presently unknown.

Although early studies indicated that clonal karyotypic evolution rarely occurred in ANLL, we have recently found evolution of the karyotype in 17 of 60 (28 per cent) ANLL patients for whom serial cytogenetic analyses were obtained.[35] The pattern of chromosomal evolution was nonrandom; the most frequent evolutionary change was a +8, found in 10 of 17 (59 per cent) patients who evolved. The incidence of evolution and the type and frequency of particular evolutionary changes were similar in patients who initially had normal and in those who initially had abnormal karyotypes.

Acute lymphoblastic leukemia (ALL)

A review of ALL patients studied by a number of investigators showed that very few abnormal cases were hypodiploid, but that most were pseudodiploid or hyperdiploid; about 40 per cent of the abnormal cases had modal numbers above 50.[24] Approximately 50 per cent of the ALL patients reviewed had an abnormal karyotype.

Metaphase chromosomes from ALL patients have particularly poor morphology with indistinct bands, making an accurate karyotypic analysis difficult. Cimino et al[36] recently summarized the cytogenetic data on ALL patients reported by a number of laboratories, including their own. Preliminary data on 57 patients with abnormal karyotypes who were studied with banding indicate that the chromosomal pattern is quite variable; however, some nonrandom abnormalities have emerged. The chromosome pattern in ALL differs from that observed in ANLL. The most frequent abnormality, seen in 12 of the 57 patients, is the presence of a Ph[1] chromosome. This probably reflects a bias in the reporting of these interesting cases. It is too early to determine accurately the incidence of the Ph[1] chromosome in ALL. However, a Ph[1] chromosome may occur in up to 25 per cent of adult ALL patients[37] and in about 4 per cent of children with ALL.[38] The identification, by Whang-Peng et al,[39] of 'Ph[1]' as a 21q− in two of four Ph[1]+ ALL patients shows that the use of banding is essential. Most of the Ph[1] chromosomes identified with banding by a number of investigators involve a 9;22 translocation which appears to be identical to that seen in most patients with CML; however, in contrast to CML, in ALL patients the Ph[1]+ cell line disappears during remission.[24]

A gain of No 21 was found in 10 of the 57 abnormal ALL patients reviewed by Cimino et al.[36] A gain of No 14 was seen in 7 cases and a deletion of 6q in 6 cases. The only two patients with B-cell ALL reported had additional material on the end of one No 14 (14q +) (Oshimura et al,[40] Cimino et al[36]); a 14q + is also found in various other lymphoproliferative disorders of B-cell origin, as will be discussed below.

MALIGNANT LYMPHOMA (ML)

Although much fewer chromosomal data are available for ML than for leukemia, certain patterns have already been observed. Affected cells from patients with non-Hodgkin lymphomas, both histiocytic and lymphocytic, generally have modal numbers in the diploid range, whereas about 70 per cent of patients with Hodgkin disease have numbers in the triploid, tetraploid, or higher, range (reviewed in Mark[1]). The incidence of karyotypic abnormalities is quite high in lymphoma patients; for example, in a study of 27 patients with ML of various histologic types, Fukuhara and Rowley[41] found only one case with a normal karyotype. The karyotype in lymphoma cells may be very complex; however, the abnormalities tend to be consistent in cells from an individual patient.

The most frequent abnormality seen in ML is the 14q + anomaly. In 1972, Manolov and Manolova[42] reported a 14q + in 10 of 12 patients with African Burkitt lymphoma (BL). Subsequent studies of African BL tumors[43] and African and American BL cell lines[43,44] showed that the 14q + resulted from a consistent 8;14 translocation [t(8;14) (q24;q32)]. This translocation has also been reported in one case each of chronic lymphocytic leukemia,[45] lymphosarcoma[43] and poorly differentiated lymphocytic lymphoma[41] and in two cases of histiocytic lymphoma.[41,46] However, non-BL differs from BL in that the origin of the translocated segment of the 14q + is inconsistent in non-BL; translocations between 14q and other chromosomes, especially Nos 1, 11 and 18, have been observed in various non-BLs (reviewed in Fukuhara and Rowley[41]). A 14q + is found in about 50 per cent of non-BL patients, being seen in 17 of 27 lymphomas studied by Fukuhara and Rowley[41] and in 17 of 45 non-Hodgkin lymphoma patients reviewed by Mark et al,[46] including 13 of their own cases.

Structural rearrangements other than those involving No 14 are also frequently observed in non-Hodgkin and non-BL; these often involve Nos 1, 3, 9 and 11 (Mark et al[46]). Gains of Nos 3 and 7 and gain or loss of No 8 are also frequent in these diseases.[46]

MULTIPLE MYELOMA (MM)

Chromosome studies in patients with MM and plasma cell leukemia have recently been reviewed by Wurster-Hill et al.[47] Chromosome abnormalities can be found in at least 50 per cent of these patients; however, there is some question as to how many of these patients show clonal chromosomal abnormalities. Liang and Rowley[48] saw clonal changes in less than half of their MM patients, and these were seen mainly in patients who had accelerated disease. The modal chromosome number is usually in the diploid or hyperdiploid range; however, Wurster-Hill et al[47] reported hypodiploid modes in 4 of 19 (21 per cent) of their own patients. Chromosomal abnormalities in MM patients appear to be highly variable; but the number of patients studied thus far with banding is small.

A 14q + marker has been observed in 3 of the 19 patients with MM or plasma cell leukemia studied by Wurster-Hill et al[47] and in 4 of the 22 studied by Liang and Rowley.[48] All of the 14q + clones reported in these patients were found in bone marrow or in unstimulated peripheral blood and thus appear to be representative of plasma cells of the B-cell population, although other abnormalities may also be found in PHA-stimulated blood of these patients (Wurster-Hill et al[47]). Thus, the consistent involvement of 14q in various rearrangements may be the abnormality common to a number of lymphoproliferative disorders, particularly those of B-cell origin.

CONCLUSION

The use of banding technics has resulted in a number of significant observations regarding chromosomal patterns in hematologic diseases. In the future, the application of newer technics, including methods for producing more elongated chromosomes and in situ hybridization, should allow even more precision in the delineation of subtle chromosome rearrangements that are undetectable at the present time.

Acknowledgment

Studies carried out in our laboratory which are referred to here were supported in part by Grant CA-16910 awarded by the National Institutes of Health, by The University of Chicago Cancer Research Foundation, and by an Otho S. A. Spraque institutional grant. The Franklin McLean Memorial Research Institute is operated by The University of Chicago for the United States Department of Energy under Contract EY-76-C-02-0069.

REFERENCES

1 Mark J 1977 Chromosomal abnormalities and their specificity in human neoplasms: An assessment of recent observations by banding techniques. In: Advances in Cancer Research vol 24. Academic Press, New York pp 165–122
2 Mitelman F, Levan G 1978 Clustering of aberrations to specific chromosomes in human neoplasms. III. Incidence and geographic distribution of chromosome aberrations in 856 cases. Hereditas 89: 207–232
3 Rowley J D 1978 Chromosomes in leukemia and lymphoma. Seminars in Hematology 15: 301–319
4 Sandberg A A 1980 The chromosomes in human cancer and leukemia. Elsevier/North-Holland, New York
5 Caspersson T, Zech L, Johansson C, Modest E J 1970 Identification of human chromosomes by DNA-binding fluorescent agents. Chromosoma 30: 215–227
6 Sun N C, Chu E H Y, Chang C C 1974 Staining method for the banding patterns of human mitotic chromosomes. Caryologia 27: 315–324
7 Verma R S, Lubs H A 1976 Additional observations on the preparation of R banded human chromosomes with acridine orange. Canadian Journal of Genetics and Cytology 18: 45–50
8 Stefos K, Arrighi F E 1971 Heterochromatic nature of W chromosome in birds. Experimental Cell Research 68: 228–231
9 Rubenstein C T, Verma R S, Dosik H 1978 Centromeric banding (C) of sequentially Q- and R-banded human chromosomes. Human Genetics 40: 279–283

10 Paris Conference 1971 Standardization in human cytogenetics. In: Birth Defects: Original Article Series vol 8 no 7 1972. The National Foundation, New York

11 Whang-Peng J, Canellos G P, Carbone P P, Tjio J H 1968 Clinical implications of cytogenetic variants in chronic myelocytic leukemia (CML). Blood 32: 755–766

12 Nowell P C, Hungerford D A 1960 A minute chromosome in human chronic granulocytic leukemia. Science 132: 1497

13 Caspersson T, Gahrton G, Lindsten J, Zech L 1970 Identification of the Philadelphia chromosome as a number 22 by quinacrine mustard fluorescence analysis. Experimental Cell Research 63: 238–244

14 O'Riordan M L, Robinson J A, Buckton K E, Evans H J 1971 Distinguishing between the chromosomes involved in Down's syndrome (trisomy 21) and chronic myeloid leukemia (Ph[1]) by fluorescence. Nature 230: 167–168

15 Rowley J D 1973 A new consistent chromosomal abnormality in chronic myelogenous leukaemia identified by quinacrine fluorescence and Giemsa staining. Nature 243: 290–293

16 Rowley J D 1980 Ph[1]-positive leukaemia, including chronic myelogenous leukaemia. Clinics in Haematology 9: 55–86

17 Canellos G P, DeVita V T, Whang-Peng J, Chabner B A, Schein P S, Young R C 1976 Chemotherapy of the blastic phase of chronic granulocytic leukaemia: hypodiploidy and response to therapy. Blood 47: 1003–1009

18 Rowley J D 1977 Population cytogenetics in leukemia. In: Hook E B, Porter I H (eds) Population cytogenetics. Academic Press, New York pp 189–216

19 Hossfeld D K, Wendehorst E 1974 Ph[1]-negative chronic myelocytic leukemia with a missing Y chromosome. Acta Haematologica 52: 232–237

20 Singh I P, Ghosh P J 1977 Giemsa banding analysis in myeloproliferative and lymphoproliferative disorders (Abstract). Fifth International Congress on Human Genetics, Amsterdam. Excerpta Medica p 153

21 Canellos G P, Whang-Peng J, DeVita V T 1976 Chronic granulocytic leukemia without the Philadelphia chromosome. American Journal of Clinical Pathology 65: 467–470

22 Mintz U, Vardiman J, Golomb H M, Rowley J D 1979 Evolution of karyotypes in Philadelphia (Ph[1]) chromosome-negative chronic myelogenous leukemia. Cancer 43: 411–416

23 Warburton D, Shah N 1976 A 9/11 translocation in a child with Ph[1]-negative chronic myelogenous leukemia. Journal of Pediatrics 88: 599–601

24 Rowley J D 1978 The cytogenetics of acute leukaemia. Clinics in Haematology 7: 385–406

25 Testa J R, Rowley J D 1978 Cytogenetic patterns in acute non-lymphocytic leukemia. Virchows Archiv B Cell Pathology 29: 65–72

26 Rowley J D 1973 Identification of a translocation with quinacrine fluorescence in a patient with acute leukaemia. Annales de Génétique 16: 109–112

27 Lindgren V, Rowley J D 1977 Comparable complex rearrangements involving 8;21 and 9;22 translocations in leukaemia. Nature 266: 744–745

28 Testa J R, Golomb H M, Rowley J D, Vardiman J W, Sweet D L 1978 Hypergranular promyelocytic leukaemia (APL): cytogenetic and ultrastructural specificity. Blood 52: 272–280

29 Kaneko Y, Sakurai M 1977 15/17 translocation in acute promyelocytic leukaemia. Lancet i: 961

30 Okada M, Miyazaki T, Kumota K 1977 15/17 translocation in acute promyelocytic leukaemia. Lancet i: 961

31 Scheres J M J C, Hustinx T W J, de Vaan G A M, Rutten F J 1978 15/17 translocation in acute promyelocytic leukaemia. Human Genetics 43: 115–117

32 Van Den Berghe H, Louwagie A, Broeckaert-Van Orshoven A, David G, Verwilghen R, Michaux J L, Sokal G 1979 Chromosome abnormalities in acute promyelocytic leukemia (APL). Cancer 43: 558–562

33 Teerenhovi L, Borgström G H, Mitelman F, Brandt L, Vuopio P, Timonen T, Almqvist A, de la Chapelle A 1978 Uneven geographical distribution of 15;17-translocation in acute promyelocytic leukaemia. Lancet ii: 797

34 Golomb H M, Testa J R, Vardiman J W, Butler A E, Rowley J D 1979 Cytogenetic and ultrastructural features of de novo acute promyelocytic leukemia; The University of Chicago experience (1973–1978). Cancer Genetics and Cytogenetics, 1: 69–78

35 Testa J R, Mintz U, Rowley J D, Vardiman J W, Golomb H M 1979 Evolution of karyotypes in acute nonlymphocytic leukemia. Cancer Research 39: 3619–3627

36 Cimino M C, Rowley J D, Kinnealey A, Variakojis D, Golomb H M 1979 Banding studies of chromosomal abnormalities in patients with acute lymphocytic leukemia. Cancer Research 39: 227–238

37 Bloomfield C D, Lindquist L L, Brunning R D, Yunis J J, Coccia P F 1978 The Philadelphia chromosome in acute leukemia. Virchows Archiv B Cell Pathology 29: 81–91

38 Chessells J M, Janossy G, Lawler S D, Secker Walker L M 1979 The Ph[1] chromosome in childhood leukemia. British Journal of Haematology 41: 25–41

39 Whang-Peng J, Knutsen T, Ziegler J, Leventhal B 1976 Cytogenetic studies in acute lymphocytic leukemia: Special emphasis in long-term survival. Medical and Pediatric Oncology 2: 333–351

40 Oshimura M, Freeman A I, Sandberg A A 1977 Chromosomes and causation of human cancer and leukemia. XXVI. Banding studies in acute lymphoblastic leukemia (ALL). Cancer 40: 1161–1172

41 Fukuhara S, Rowley J D 1978 Chromosome 14 translocations in non-Burkitt lymphomas. International Journal of Cancer 22: 14–21

42 Manolov G, Manolova Y 1972 Marker band in one chromosome 14 from Burkitt lymphomas. Nature 237: 33–34

43 Zech L, Haglund U, Nilsson K, Klein G 1976 Characteristic chromosomal abnormalities in biopsies and lymphoid-cell lines from patients with Burkitt and non-Burkitt lymphomas. International Journal of Cancer 17: 47–56

44 McCaw B K, Epstein A L, Kaplan H S, Hecht F 1977 Chromosome 14 translocation in African and North American Burkitt's lymphoma. International Journal of Cancer 19: 482–486

45 Fleischman E W, Prigogina E L 1977 Karyotype peculiarities of malignant lymphomas. Human Genetics 35: 269–279

46 Mark J, Ekedahl C, Dahlenfors R 1978 Characteristics of the banding patterns in non-Hodgkin and non-Burkitt lymphomas. Hereditas 88: 229–242

47 Wurster-Hill D H, McIntyre O R, Cornwell G G 1978 Chromosome studies in myelomatosis. Virchows Archiv B Cell Pathology 29: 93–97

48 Liang W, Rowley J D 1978 14q+ marker chromosomes in multiple myeloma and plasma-cell leukaemia. Lancet i: 96

7

Terminal Transferase

Mary Sue Coleman   John J. Hutton

INTRODUCTION

DISTRIBUTION AND BIOCHEMISTRY OF TERMINAL TRANSFERASE

Terminal deoxynucleotidyltransferase (terminal transferase) is an unusual deoxynucleotide polymerizing enzyme normally present at high levels only in thymus[1] and at low levels in the bone marrow.[2] It has not been detected in circulating or mitogen-stimulated lymphocytes.[2] Identification of transferase activity in circulating blast cells and cell lines from acute lymphoblastic leukemia and in some cases of chronic myelogenous leukemia in blastic crisis has raised the speculation that it may be localised in a primitive hematopoietic stem cell or lymphoid precursor.[2-6] *In vitro*, terminal transferase catalyzes and addition of deoxynucleoside triphosphates to the 3′-hydroxyl ends of oligo- and polydeoxynucleotide initiators without template instruction.[7] The enzyme has been purified to homogeneity from both calf[8] and human[9] cells.

CLINICAL CORRELATES

Assays of terminal transferase activity and antigen are of value in the classification of hematologic neoplasms. It is helpful to think of the measurement of terminal transferase as a 'positive test' for immature lymphoid cells. The assay is somewhat analogous to the determination of peroxidase in blast cells as a test for myeloid precursors. Interpretation of terminal transferase activity requires knowledge of the range of values obtained when assaying specific types of tissue in a particular laboratory. Terminal transferase activities in nucleated cells from the bone marrow and peripheral blood of patients without leukemia or lymphoma are used to define a normal range. The mean $\pm$ s.d. terminal transferase activities (1 unit = 1 nmol of dGTP polymerized per hour) in the bone marrow from 160 adults and 198 children were 2.7 ± 3.7 units/10^8 cells and 5.9 ± 19 units/10^8 cells, respectively, in our laboratory.[10] The distribution of individual (control) values is illustrated in Figure 7.1. The clustering of adult values in the range 0.1 to 0.3 units/10^8 cells and pediatric values in the range 2.0 to 4.0 accounts for the bimodal distribution. Activities of terminal transferase in the marrow of children and adults, when plotted separately, do not follow a normal distribution, but have a distinct tailing of activities greater than the mean. The five children with the highest values (over 20 units/10^8 cells) in marrow not involved with a hematologic neoplasm had diagnoses of idiopathic thrombocytopenic purpura, neuroblastoma and pulmonary actinomycosis. Terminal transferase activity in nucleated cells from the peripheral blood of adults and children is generally very low and may not be significantly different from zero.

Terminal transferase is present in large amounts in malignant cells from certain patients with leukemia and lymphoma. Tumor cells from any source (such as peripheral blood, bone marrow, pleural fluid, bulk tumor) are satisfactory for assay, provided they can be obtained in sufficient numbers. Our results of

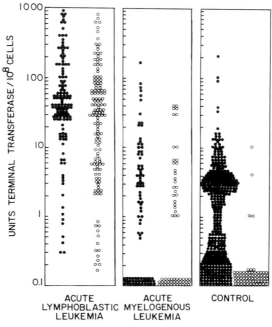

Fig. 7.1 Summary of terminal transferase activities in bone marrow (●) and peripheral blood (○) of children and adults with acute lymphoblastic leukemia or acute myelogenous leukemia. Control specimens were from patients without leukemia or lymphoma. Note that the activity scale is logarithmic. Each point represents a different patient.

the assay of nucleated cells from peripheral blood and bone marrow are summarized in Figure 7.1. Most patients with a diagnosis of acute lymphoblastic leukemia (ALL) have markedly elevated terminal transferase activities in their bone marrow and peripheral blood cells. A summary of studies of terminal transferase activity in ALL is presented in Table 7.1. Blasts from approximately 300 patients with ALL have been assayed and reported as having high levels of terminal transferase in 90 per cent of cases. Large numbers of patients have been studied by Kung et al[11] and Hutton et al[10] who report elevated terminal transferase activities in 87 per cent and 95 per cent of cases, respectively. There is a significant correlation (r=0.73) between terminal transferase activity in peripheral lymphoblasts and activity in the bone marrow.[12] The average terminal transferase activity is significantly lower in T marked lymphoblasts than

Table 7.1 Activity of terminal transferase in hematologic disease

Senior author and date	Number of patients studied	Fraction with 'high' transferase before treatment[a]				Lymphomas and lymphoma leukemias tested[b]
		Acute myelogenous leukemia	Acute lymphoblastic leukemia	Chronic myelogenous leukemia Stable	Blastic	
Catovsky (1978)[15]	5	—	—	—	1/5	no
Coleman (1976)[6]	27	—	7/7	—	—	no
Coleman (1978)[13]	26	0/3	20/23	—	—	no
Coleman (1974)[2]	6	1/5	—	—	—	no
Donlon (1977)[16]	57	—	2/2	0/1	1/1	yes
Gordon (1978)[17]	80	3/48	8/8	—	—	yes
Greenwood (1977)[12]	115	0/8	20/20	—	—	yes
Hoffbrand (1977)[18]	112	1/17	39/40	0/7	11/23	no
Hutton (1976)[5]	28	0/11	3/3	0/4	3/7	yes
Hutton (1979)[10]	1000	10/80	110/127	0/14	2/6	yes
Jaffe (1977)[19]	5	—	—	—	—	yes
Janossy (1979)[20]	34	—	—	—	10/34	no
Kung (1978)[11]	299	2/55	73/77	0/12	24/72	yes
Marks (1978)[21]	22	—	—	—	13/22	no
McCaffrey (1975)[22]	27	0/3	11/13	0/2	1/4	yes
McCaffrey (1973)[3]	3	0/1	1/1	—	—	yes
Mertelsmann (1978)[23]	89	—	11/11	—	—	yes
Oken (1978)[24]	1	—	—	—	1/1	no
Penit (1977)[25]	40	—	25/28	—	—	yes
Ross (1979)[26]	1	—	—	—	1/1	no
Saffhill (1976)[27]	1	—	—	1/1	—	no
Sarin (1977)[28]	142	1/22	18/18	0/30	12/30	no
Sarin (1976)[29]	22	0/3	2/2	0/9	4/4	no
Srivastava (1976)[30]	36	2/23	13/13	—	—	no
Srivastava (1977)[31]	26	—	—	—	6/26	no
Stass (1978)[32]	1	1/1	—	—	—	no
Vogler (1978)[14]	4	—	1/4	—	—	no
Wiernik (1979)[33]	40	3/30	10/10	—	—	no

[a] Terminal transferase was assayed by several different methods. Values were classified as 'high' by individual authors using a variety of criteria. The number of patients with specimens having high terminal transferase activity is recorded as the numerator with total patients as the denominator. Acute myelogenous leukemia = all variants of AML excluding CML in blast crisis; acute lymphoblastic leukemia = all variants of ALL, excluding lymphoid leukemia which occurs in patients with lymphoma. Patients were excluded unless malignant cells were studied before treatment of the leukemia.
[b] The histological classification of lymphomas is complex. The tissues assayed for terminal transferase varied from lymph nodes to pleural fluid. In the interests of clarity, whether investigators studied patients with lymphoma is noted, but original papers must be consulted for details and conclusions.

in null marked lymphoblasts.[13] There are at least two variants of ALL where terminal transferase activity in blasts may be very low (less than 3 units/10^8 cells, Fig. 7.1). Blasts from approximately 50 per cent of these patients who are diagnosed as ALL, but have low terminal transferase, bear immunoglobulin on their surface implying that the leukemia is of B-cell origin.[13] Cytologic features of the blasts in these cases are indistinguishable from Burkitt's leukemia. A second group of patients diagnosed as ALL with low terminal transferase have blasts with cytoplasmic IgM, but without surface immunoglobulin[14] and therefore are thought to have a 'pre-B' cell leukemia (see Ch. 5).

In patients with acute myeloblastic and myelomonocytic leukemia confirmed cytochemically, grouped as acute myelogenous leukemia (AML) in Table 7.1, terminal transferase activity in bone marrow and peripheral blood is generally within the 'control' range and is much lower than in ALL. In a study of adult leukemia from our laboratory, terminal transferase activity was considered to be elevated to the lymphoid range if it exceeded 10 units/10^8 nucleated cells from peripheral blood or 20 units/10^8 nucleated cells from bone marrow.[17] Using these criteria, 5 to 10 per cent of patients with AML had elevated terminal transferase activity in their blasts. Whether these patients will benefit from chemotherapy for lymphoid as well as myeloid leukemia is not known, but this is recommended for clinical trial.

At least 98 per cent of patients with chronic myelogenous leukemia (CML) in the stable (chronic) phase have low levels of terminal transferase in their blasts, whereas 35 per cent of patients in blast crisis have elevated levels of terminal transferase (Table 7.1). There are two large independent studies showing that patients with high levels of terminal transferase during blast crisis respond much more favorably to treatment with vincristine and prednisone than do patients with low levels of terminal transferase.[20–21] Patients in blast crisis with terminal transferase containing blasts should be identified prospectively and treated intensively with drugs effective in lymphoid leukemia.

High levels of terminal transferase can be present in malignant cells of patients with non-Hodgkin's lymphoma. This includes cells from diverse sites such as bone marrow, peripheral blood, pleural fluid, lymph nodes and testicle. Studies of terminal transferase in lymphoma are referred to in Table 7.1. It appears that terminal transferase is elevated in lymphoblastic lymphoma and the assay of terminal transferase may serve as a diagnostic tool. This group of patients is generally young, has a poor prognosis, and behaves clinically like patients with ALL.

Based upon information presently available, measurements of terminal transferase can be helpful in specimens from patients with:

1. Undifferentiated leukemias where blasts do not react with standard cytochemical stains. Cases of ALL may be identified
2. Blast crisis of CML initially and at relapse. High levels of terminal transferase in blasts are associated with 'lymphoid' crisis (see Ch. 5)
3. Leukemias with unusual morphological features, particularly where mixed proliferations of myeloid and lymphoid cells are suspected or the response to treatment is not as expected
4. Diffuse non-Hodgkin's lymphoma where lymphoblastic lymphoma is possible. Lymphoblastic lymphoma may respond best to treatment regimens appropriate for ALL.

It is critically important to emphasise that measurements of terminal transferase cannot diagnose malignancy. No data are available at present which demonstrate that measurements of terminal transferase can predict impending relapse in leukemias or lymphomas. Because the measurement is relatively expensive and difficult, it is not recommended in all cases of leukemia and lymphoma. This recommendation could change with advances in technology, particularly the commercial development of reliable assay kits or immunochemical reagents.

QUANTITATIVE BIOCHEMICAL ASSAY

PREPARATION OF SPECIMENS

At least 2×10^7 nucleated cells from marrow or peripheral blood are necessary to assay terminal transferase reliably. We have found that it is sufficient to use nucleated cells isolated from buffy coat for the assay of the enzyme in bone marrow. Mononuclear cells purified from buffy coat are generally prepared for assay of the enzyme in peripheral blood.

Reagents required:

Dextran, 6 per cent in saline—6 g dextran (Sigma-Clinical Grade, MW 234 000), 0.85 g NaCl in a total volume of 100 ml of distilled water. May be autoclaved to prolong storage.

Phosphate buffered saline 10 × —85 g NaCl, 2 g KCl, 11.5 g Na_2HPO_4. Dilute to 1 liter with distilled H_2O. Dilute 1:10 with distilled H_2O before use. Final pH should be 7.

4 per cent EDTA—4 g disodium ethylenediaminetetraacetate in 100 ml of distilled H_2O.

Hypaque-Ficoll (34 per cent—9 per cent). Ficoll (9 per cent mass/vol solution)—9 g Ficoll (Sigma, type 400, MW 400 000) in a total volume of 100 ml of distilled H_2O. Hypaque (sodium diatrizoate 34 per cent mass/vol solution)—add 14.1 ml distilled H_2O to 30 ml 50 per cent Hypaque (Winthrop Laboratories). Mix 100 ml 9 per cent Ficoll with 41.7 ml 34 per cent Hypaque. May be autoclaved to prolong storage. Store in the refrigerator protected from light.

1. Separation of nucleated cells

The sample of marrow or peripheral blood should be collected in a syringe containing a small amount (1/10 volume) of 4 per cent EDTA, since even small amounts of heparin inhibit terminal transferase. The sample is placed in a plastic tube with 1/10 volume of 6 per cent dextran in saline. The tube is mixed and allowed to stand at room temperature until erythrocytes sediment (about 30 min). Taking care to avoid contamination of nucleated cells with mature erythrocytes, the leukocyte-rich supernatant is withdrawn, diluted twofold with phosphate buffered saline and placed in a plastic conical centrifuge tube. With bone marrow, this type of cell separation is usually adequate. The sample is centrifuged at 300 × g for 10 min. The supernatant solution is discarded and the pellet is resuspended in 10 ml of phosphate buffered saline. The total number of cells in the 10 ml volume is determined. This should be done with an electronic cell counter. The suspension is then centrifuged at 300 × g for 10 min, the supernatant solution is discarded and the pellet is frozen at $-20°C$ until used for assay. Sample identification and total number of nucleated cells must be carefully recorded. The pellet should be pink, indicating minimal contamination by red cells.

2. Separation of mononuclear cells from peripheral blood or bone marrow

The supernatant solution containing nucleated cells (from preceding dextran sedimentation) is carefully removed and layered over an equal volume of Hypaque-Ficoll solution in a graduated 40 ml conical centrifuge tube. The tubes are centrifuged at $300 \times g$ in a swinging bucket rotor for 30 min at room temperature. The lymphocytes and leukemic blasts layer as a white band between the plasma and Hypaque-Ficoll. Granulocytes and erythrocytes sediment to the bottom of the tube. Using a disposable pipette, the lymphocytes and blasts are removed from the interface and placed in a 15 ml conical centrifuge tube. An aliquot of cells should be stained with Wright-Giemsa and examined morphologically. Phosphate buffered saline is added to cells to a volume of about 14 ml, mixed thoroughly and centrifuged at $300 \times g$ for 20 min. All but 1 ml of the supernatant is drawn off and discarded. The pellet is resuspended in 1 ml of the supernatant and then diluted to 10 ml with phosphate buffered saline. Nucleated cells are counted and total volume is recorded. The total number of cells in the tube is then calculated and recorded. After centrifugation of the cell suspension at $300 \times g$ the cell pellet is frozen at $-20°C$.

3. Other tissues

A variety of other tissues (pleural fluid, spinal fluid, lymph nodes, testicular tissue) are of interest in disease states and can be used in the assay of terminal transferase. Fluid samples are centrifuged at $300 \times g$ for 10 min to collect cells. Pelleted cells are resuspended in 10 ml phosphate buffered saline, mixed thoroughly and counted. The total number of cells is recorded. Smears of the cells should be stained with Wright-Giemsa and examined morphologically to determine the types of cells recovered. After centrifugation at $300 \times g$ for 10 min, pelleted cells are stored frozen. Solid tissue specimens (testis, lymph nodes) are minced with scissors in phosphate buffered saline. The tissue pieces are gently forced through a No 40 wire mesh screen. A suspension of single cells is made up to 10 ml in volume with phosphate buffered saline and the cells are counted. Total cell number is recorded and morphology confirmed by Wright-Giemsa stain of smears.

Potential problems. The most common problem encountered is the lack of a sufficient number of cells for an accurate assay. If heparin, an inhibitor of terminal transferase, has been used inadvertently, then cells must be washed several times with phosphate buffered saline following separation procedures. In order to calculate terminal transferase activity, the total number of nucleated cells in a specimen must be known. If errors in cell counts are suspected, then DNA determination can be helpful to confirm cell number (10 μg DNA per 10^6 cells).

METHOD OF EXTRACTION

The method of extraction of terminal transferase from fresh or frozen cells has a major effect on the yield of enzyme obtained in the extract.[34] A reasonably high salt concentration is necessary for optimal enzyme extraction, but dialysis of small samples and column fractionation procedures as used by others[21-31] are detrimental to recovery of activity.[34] Terminal transferase is best extracted from cells with phosphate buffer.

Reagents required:

0.25 mol/l potassium phosphate buffer, pH 7.5 containing 1 mmol/l 2-mercaptoethanol. (18.85 ml 1 mol/l K_2HPO_4, 6.15 ml 1 mol/l KH_2PO_4, 0.1 ml 1 mol/l 2-mercaptoethanol.) Bring volume to 100 ml, check and adjust pH. This is the 'extraction buffer'.

Extraction buffer is added to the cell pellet collected from human tissue. The volume of buffer is dictated by the total number of cells in the pellet. A final concentration of at least 1×10^8 cells/ml should be obtained. Therefore, for 1×10^7 cells, 0.1 ml extraction buffer is used; for 1×10^8 cells, 1 ml extraction buffer is used. The cell pellet and buffer are thoroughly mixed. Cell breakage (>95 per cent) is achieved by sonication or by homogenization in a glass–Teflon homogenizer. Since leukemic patients may be infected with hepatitis, it is advisable to perform these operations in a biohazard hood to protect personnel from aerosols. The total volume is recorded and the suspension of broken cells is centrifuged for 1 h at $100\,000 \times g$. The supernatant solution is removed and placed in a small tube. It can be stored at $-70°C$ for several months or years before assay.

METHOD OF ASSAY

Two methods of assay of terminal transferase will be described. They are the same in principle, but employ different initiators and different methods of processing of reaction product. Each depends upon the addition of ^{3}H-dGTP monomer to oligo d(pA) initiator. The initiators differ in chain length and availability from commercial suppliers.

1. Preparation of substrates

a. oligo d(pA)$_{12-18}$.

This substrate has been widely used as an initiator for the terminal transferase assay. It is quite satisfactory for assay of crude tissue extracts if the product is detected by ion exchange adsorption (see below). When this short initiator is used, the products of the assay are acid soluble and cannot be reliably precipitated on to glass fiber disks by TCA.[35] Oligo p(dA)$_{12-18}$ is available from P-L Biochemicals (Milwaukee, WI, USA), Collaborative Research (Waltham, MA, USA) or Miles Laboratories (Elkhart, IN, USA). In order to prepare a solution that is 0.12 mmolar in 3′OH groups from 100 units of oligo d(pA)$_{12-18}$, the following procedure is used. (1) 100 units of oligo d(pA)$_{12-18}$ is dissolved in 6.9 ml of distilled water. (2) 10 μl of the solution is diluted to 1 ml in water and the absorbance at 260 nm is determined. This value should be approximately 0.14 absorbance units if 100 units of the oligomer are present. (3) The millimolar extinction coefficient at 260 nm of oligo d(pA)$_{12-18}$[36] is approximately 10. Therefore, the concentration of the solution is:

$$\frac{14.4\ A_{260}\ \text{units/ml} \div 10\ A_{260}\ \text{units/1 mmolar soln}}{\text{average chain length of 12}} =$$

0.12 mmol/l 3′OH groups in the 6.9 ml volume of oligo d(pA)$_{12-18}$.

b. *Oligo d(pA)$_{\overline{50}}$*

The use of an initiator of longer chain length, such as oligo d)pA)$_{\overline{50}}$, is advantageous in assays of crude tissue extracts.[2] This initiator is sufficiently long so that several endonucleolytic cleavages will not affect the acid insolubility of the product. At the same time, it is short enough to obtain a high concentration of 3'OH groups. Oligo d(pA)$_{\overline{50}}$ is not commercially available at the present time and must be synthesized in the laboratory according to procedures developed by Bollum.[37] A kit containing d(pA)$_{\overline{50}}$ has recently been offered commercially for assay of terminal transferase (Bethesda Research Laboratories, Inc., Rockville, MD, USA).

Reagents required:
   200 units d(pA)$_4$ (Collaborative Research) in 10 ml distilled H$_2$O.
   10 000 units of terminal transferase from calf thymus (Bethesda Research Laboratories).
   250 μmol unlabeled dATP in approximately 4 ml distilled H$_2$O.
   80 mmol/l MgCl$_2$.
   1 mol/l potassium cacodylate, pH 7.5 5 mol/l cacodylic acid should be run through an ion exchange column (3 × 10 cm) made from Chelex-100 (Bio-Rad 100–200 mesh, sodium form) to remove heavy metals. Dilute the purified 5 mol/l stock to 1 mol/l and adjust pH to 7.5 with 10 mol/l KOH.
   10 mmol/l 2-mercaptoethanol.
   20 mg/ml bovine serum albumin.
   100 units inorganic pyrophosphatase.
   5 mol/l NaCl.
   95 per cent ethanol.

Two hundred units of d(pA)$_4$ are dissolved in a total volume of 10 ml of distilled water. A 10 μl aliquot is diluted to 1 ml in water for measurement of absorbance at 260 nm. If the concentration of d(pA) monomer is 2.0 mmolar, then using the calculation described previously the actual concentration of 3'OH groups is 0.5 mmolar. The amount of dATP added to the reaction is adjusted to give a ratio of 1 to 50 of d(pA)$_4$ to dATP. Therefore with 5 μmol of d(pA)$_4$ (10 ml of a 0.5 mmolar solution) 250 μmol of dATP is required. To the reaction is added in final concentration, 8 mmol/l MgCl$_2$, 0.2 mol/l potassium cacodylate, pH 7.5, 10 mmol/l 2-mercaptoethanol, 1 mg/ml bovine serum albumin, 100 units inorganic pyrophosphatase and 10 000 units of terminal transferase. The total reaction volume will be about 25 ml. The reaction mixture is incubated in a 40 ml glass centrifuge tube at 35°C for at least 25 h. In order to monitor the polymerization of dATP, spectrophotometric readings at 260 nm are taken of a 1/300 dilution of a small aliquot from the reaction at several intervals during the incubation period. When the optical absorbance at 260 nm stabilizes at approximately 0.4 (after 25 to 30 h), 3 ml of 5 mol/l NaCl is added to the reaction (final volume should be about 30 ml). To the reaction mixture is then added 2 volumes (60 ml) of 95 per cent ethanol. The solution is stored at 4°C for 1 day to allow product precipitation and is then centrifuged at 1000 × g for 20 min and without pause at 6000 × g for an additional 16 min. The pellet is dissolved in 30 ml of H$_2$O. Precipitation is repeated by adding 3 ml of 5 mol/l NaCl, 2 volumes of 95 per cent ethanol and then storing the solution overnight at 4°C. The solution is centrifuged as before and the pellet is dissolved in phosphate buffered saline. This solution is dialyzed first against 4 l of phosphate buffered saline and then against 4 l of distilled H_2O. Absorbance units/ml at 260 nm are measured for the final solution and the concentration is adjusted to about 0.13 mmolar (3'OH) groups.

Sample calculation
Final volume is 32 ml. The absorbance at 260 nm of a 1/300 dilution of a small aliquot is 0.21. Therefore, the total absorbance units are $0.21 \times 300 = 63$ A_{260} units/ml. The millimolar extinction coefficient of $d(pA)_{50}$ at 260 nm[36] is about 9.65. The concentration of 3'OH groups is:

$$\frac{63 \text{ total } A_{260} \text{ units} \div 9.65 \text{ } A_{260} \text{ units}/1 \text{ mmolar soln}}{50 \text{ (average chain length)}} = 0.13 \text{ mmolar}$$

From this synthesis about 40 ml of $d(pA)_{\overline{50}}$ is obtained at a concentration of 0.13 mmolar. This amount of the initiator is sufficient for about 3500 terminal transferase assays.

c. dGTP
When assaying terminal transferase in crude tissue extracts, the polymerization of dGTP on to an oligo dA initiator is the preferred reaction. As dGTP polymerises, it aggregates and produces a product which is inaccessible to exonuclease activities.[8] Therefore, it is the nucleotide substrate of choice. The unlabeled compound can be used directly from the manufacturer at a purity of 90 to 95 per cent. If greater purity is desired, the following procedure can be used with 1 g of dGTP.[38]

Reagents required:
    1 g dGTP (Sigma, St. Louis, MO, USA or P.L. Biochemicals, Milwaukee, WI, USA).
    1 l 0.05 mol/l NaCl.
    2 l 0.05 mol/l NaCl in 0.02 mol/l sodium acetate, pH 4.7.
    2 l 0.5 mol/l NaCl in 0.02 mol/l sodium acetate, pH 4.7.
    500 ml 0.01 mol/l sodium carbonate.
    1 l 0.1 mol/l NaOH.
    1 l 0.1 mol/l HCl.
    25 g QAE Sephadex A25 (Pharmacia, Uppsala).
    10 mCi ^3H . dGTP (5–15 Ci/mmol).

Preparation of QAE Sephadex A25 column. Suspend 25 g of QAE Sephadex A25 in water and allow to swell for 3 h. Pour a 3×38 cm column and wash with 1 l of 0.1 mol/l NaOH, then with water until neutral. Repeat the procedure with 1 l 0.1 mol/l HCl and rinse with distilled water until neutral. Equilibrate with 0.05 mol/l NaCl, 0.02 mol/l sodium acetate, pH 4.7.

Purification of dGTP. Unlabeled dGTP (1 g) is dissolved in 10 ml of water and loaded on to the QAE-Sephadex A25 column. Approximately 10 ml of 0.05 mol/l NaCl is layered and washed into the column to allow binding of dGTP. A linear gradient for the column is prepared consisting of 21 of 0.05 mol/l NaCl, 0.02 mol/l sodium acetate, pH 4.7 and 21 of 0.5 mol/l NaCl, 0.02 mol/l sodium acetate and allowed to run through the column for 17 h (4 ml/min). Absorbance at 260 nm can be monitored with a spectrophotometer equipped with a flow cell or by manual reading of the fractions. The fractions comprising the broad peak of dGTP are pooled (approximately 500 ml) and diluted five-fold with distilled water and titrated to pH 8 with NH_4OH. At this stage of the preparation, the volume will be approximately 2500 ml. A new column of QAE-Sephadex A25 (3×8 cm) equilibrated with 0.05 mol/l NaCl is used to absorb dGTP from the solution. The column is then washed with 0.01 mol/l sodium carbonate (350 ml) followed by distilled H_2O (200 ml). The bound dGTP is eluted with 250 ml of 1 mol/l ammonium bicarbonate collected in 50 ml fractions. The fractions having a significant absorbance (>2) at 260 nm are pooled and dried by rotary evaporation, lyophilization or in a water bath with the aid of an air stream. The dry powder is dissolved in 30 ml of distilled H_2O and re-dried. The powder is finally dissolved in 30 ml of distilled water. From this solution 10 μl is diluted to 10 ml and absorbance is measured at 260 nm. The final concentration is calculated by use of a millimolar extinction coefficient for dGTP at 260 nm of 11.4. Therefore, if the absorbance reading at 260 nm is 0.4 at a 1 to 1000 dilution the concentration is

$$\frac{0.4 \times 1000}{11.4} = 35 \text{ mmol/l}$$

The dGTP stock solution should be divided into 2 ml portions and stored in small tubes at $-20°C$.

Preparation of $^3H.dGTP$ solutions. In order to assay quantitatively for terminal transferase, the concentration of nucleotide must be maintained at 1 mmolar in the reaction mixture.[34] Therefore, the $^3H.dGTP$ is diluted with unlabeled dGTP. Ethanol, in which most radioactive compounds are supplied, must be removed since it inhibits terminal transferase activity. In order to prepare a 10 mmolar $^3H.dGTP$ stock solution sufficient for approx. 160 terminal transferase assays, the following procedure is used. To 10 mCi of $^3H.dGTP$ is added 50 μmol of unlabeled dGTP (either powder or stock solution). This solution is lyophilized or evaporated to dryness by rotary evaporation. The dry powder is redissolved in 4.0 ml of distilled water. A 10 μl aliquot is diluted to 4.0 ml and the absorbance is recorded at 260 nm. Using a millimolar extinction coefficient of 11.9 for dGTP, the concentration of the $^3H.dGTP$ solution is calculated. The stock solution is diluted to 10 mmolar and stored at $-20°C$ in 1 ml aliquots, to avoid excessive freeze-thaw cycles.

Estimation of specific activity. A 10 μl aliquot of the 10 mmolar stock solution of $^3H.dGTP$ is diluted to 4.0 ml and 10 μl is spotted (in duplicate) on 1×1 cm squares of Whatman DE-81 paper or GF/C paper (depending on assay) and dried thoroughly. The DE-81 squares are placed in scintillation vials to each of which is added 1 ml of a tissue solubilizer (e.g. Soluene 350, Packard Instruments, Downer's Grove, Ill. The vials are placed at 50°C 1 h for digestion. Scintillation fluid is then added. GF/C squares can be placed directly in scintillation fluid without prior solubilization. These samples are counted in a liquid scintillation counter. If the stock solution is 10 mmolar and 10 μl of a 1/400 dilution is spotted, then 250 pmol of ^{3}H. dGTP is on the DE-81 square. For a value of 25 000 counts per minute, the specific activity of the ^{3}H . dGTP is 100 cpm/pmol (25 000 cpm ÷ 250 pmol).

2. Assay procedures

a. *Measurement of terminal transferase using oligo* $d(pA)_{12-18}$ *and ion exchange chromatography*[35]

Reagents required:
  10 mmol/l ^{3}H . dGTP (approximately 100 cpm/pmol).
  10 mmol/l 2-mercaptoethanol.
  8 mmol/l $MgCl_2$.
  1 mol/l potassium cacodylate, pHn 7.5.
  0.12 mmol/l $d(pA)_{12-18}$.
  DE-81 paper (Whatman) 23 cm × 10 cm.
  5 per cent potassium dibasic phosphate.
  Soluene-350 (Packard Instrument Co.) or any tissue solubilizer.
  Dimilume-30 (Packard Instrument Co.) or any scintillation fluid that is compatible with the solubilizer.

The enzyme assay is carried out in a total volume of 125 μl in 10 × 75 mm tubes. Reaction mixtures are prepared by mixing to a total volume of 100 μl per reaction, one part 10 mmolar H . dGTP, one part 0.12 mmolar $d(pA)_{12-18}$, one part 10 mmolar 2-mercaptoethanol, one part 80 mmolar $MgCl_2$, two parts 1 mol/l potassium cacodylate, pH 7.5, and two parts of H_2O. If 10 samples are to be assayed, the reaction mixture is made as a stock solution in a total volume of 1.1 ml and a 100 μl aliquot is placed into each tube. The reaction tubes are incubated at 35°C. To start the reaction, 25 μl of the 100 000 × g supernatant solution from the cell extract is added. At timed intervals (for example, 4, 8, 12 and 16 min) 25 μl aliquots are removed from the reaction system and spotted at the origin of a strip of DE-81 chromatography paper. The chromatography paper is cut to the dimensions of 23 cm wide and 10 cm long. Each sheet has 12 penciled channels (2 cm wide) for product application. Sheets are developed in 5 per cent potassium dibasic phosphate by descending chromatography for 2 h. The DE-81 paper is dried and the oligomer product is cut out at the origin (1 cm square) of each channel. In this system, the ^{3}H . dGTP migrates at the solvent front and the labeled product is immobile at the origin. The DE-81 squares are placed in glass scintillation vials with 1 ml of Soluene-350 and digested at 50°C (1 h). Following digestion, 10 ml volumes of Dimilume-30 scintillation cocktail are added to each vial for counting in a liquid scintillation counter. In order to calculate the specific activity of terminal transferase in the crude extract, the radioactive counts are converted to nmoles ^{3}H . dGTP incorporated into product/10^8 cells/hour. Given representative data, a sample calculation is as follows: (1) extract concentration: 1 × 10^8 cells/ml; (2) specific activity ^{3}H . dGTP: 108 cpm/pmol.

[4 min time point] 4050 cpm ÷ 108 cpm/pmol ÷ 1 × 10^8 cells/ml ÷ 0.005 ml
extract × 15 intervals/h = 112 500 pmol/10^8 cells/h or
113 nmol/10^8 cells/h

[8 min time point] 8200 cpm ÷ 108 cpm/pmol ÷ 1 × 10^8 cells/ml ÷ 0.005 ml
extract × 7.5 = 114 000 pmol/10^8 cells/h or 114 nmol/10^8
cells/h

Average value = 114 nmol/10^8 cells/h

Values are obtained at four time points and averaged to obtain the specific activity. A linear incorporation of radioactivity with increasing time should be observed and the specific activity calculated at the four time points should be nearly identical. If product incorporation does not increase with time despite the use of an adequate number of cells, then the enzyme activity should be considered 'not detected'.

Potential problems. Since the K_m for the nucleotide substrate (dGTP) in the assay of terminal transferase is relatively high (0.1 mmolar), it is critical that the concentration of dGTP be maintained at 1 mmolar final concentration in the

Table 7.2 Terminal transferase activity in mammalian hematopoietic tissue

Cell type	Species	Specific activity (nmol ^{3}H . dGTP/10^8 cells/h)
Thymus	Rat or human	10–25
Bone marrow lymphocytes	Human	1–5
Blasts in acute lymphoblastic leukemia	Human	10–1000
Peripheral lymphocytes	Human	0

assay.[34] When low activity is regularly observed in a laboratory, it can most often be attributed to less than optimal concentration of dGTP. For every assay, a background or control sample should be included to determine the non-specific binding of ^{3}H . dGTP to DE-81 paper. This is usually accomplished by preparing one reaction tube without cell extract, spotting 25 μl on the chromatogram and developing along with the complete assay. If the background radioactivity is inordinately high (greater than 500 cpm), then the purity of the ^{3}H . dGTP should be checked by paper chromatography.[39] If significant contamination of dGTP is present (greater than 10 per cent), purification procedures or change in supplier are warranted. When using a short oligonucleotide initiator, like d(pA)$_{12-18}$, it is very important that ion exchange chromatography be used instead of acid precipitation of product, since the product is not always long enough to be 'acid precipitable'.[35]

Table 7.2 lists representative ranges of terminal transferase activity obtained in our laboratory. If laboratory values are significantly different, a careful examination of assay procedures is in order.

b. *Terminal transferase assay using oligo d(pA)*$_{\overline{50}}$ *and acid precipitation*[8, 35]

Reagents required:
0.13 mmol/l d(pA)$_{\overline{50}}$.
10 mmol/l ^{3}H . dGTP (100 cpm/pmol).

10 mmol/l 2-mercaptoethanol.

80 mmol/l $MgCl_2$.

1 mol/l potassium cacodylate, pH 7.5.

Glass fiber paper (Whatman GF/C) cut into 2×2 cm squares.

5 per cent TCA in 1 per cent sodium pyrophosphate.

5 per cent TCA.

95 per cent ethanol.

Anhydrous diethyl ether.

Toluene based scintillation fluid.

The enzyme assay is carried out in a total volume of 125 μl as described earlier except that one part of 0.13 mmolar $(d(pA)_{50}$ is substituted for $d(pA)_{12-18}$. The reaction is initiated by the addition of 25 μl of the 100 000 $\times g$ supernatant of the cell extract. At timed intervals, 25 μl aliquots are removed from the reaction tube and spotted on to 2×2 cm GF/C squares which have been numbered with India ink. The square is then dropped into a beaker containing cold 5 per cent TCA containing 1 per cent sodium pyrophosphate (10 ml for each square) for batch processing.[40] When all squares have been collected, they are washed by swirling the beaker gently for 2 min. The TCA is poured off and fresh 5 per cent TCA (10 ml per square) is added, and squares are washed for 2 min with constant swirling. This process is repeated twice. After the final wash, TCA is poured off and 95 per cent ethanol (10 ml per square) is added. The washing process is repeated twice. For final drying of the GF/C squares, anhydrous ether (use fume hood) is added twice for 10 min. The squares are carefully removed, arranged in numerical order and allowed to dry in a hood for 10 min. The squares are then placed in scintillation vials with a toluene based scintillation fluid for counting. Calculations for specific activity are identical to those explained earlier.

Potential problems. Use of the oligo $d(pA)_{\overline{50}}$ initiator with acid precipitation of the product is the best and most convenient method of assay for terminal transferase in crude tissue extracts.[35] However, it can involve a considerable investment of time, since the oligo $d(pA)_{\overline{50}}$ is not commercially available and must be synthesized in the laboratory. A kit (with $d(pA)_{\overline{50}}$ included) for assay of clinical samples has recently become commercially available (Bethesda Research Laboratories, Rockville, MD, USA). While we have not tested this product extensively, it has been offered at a reasonable cost and should be very useful for clinical laboratories. In lieu of the assay kit, the easiest method for clinical samples uses the oligo $d(pA)_{12-18}$ initiator and ion exchange separation of product.

IMMUNOLOGIC METHODS FOR DETECTION OF TERMINAL TRANSFERASE

Because the quantitative assay of enzyme activity is reasonably complex and requires a substantial number of cells, it is of great importance to develop immunocytochemical procedures for detection of terminal transferase. While the immunocytochemical procedure is much simpler than the quantitative assay, development of and access to the appropriate immunologic reagents is currently difficult. However, antibody to calf thymus terminal transferase has been raised in rabbits[41] and mice.[42] Results using radioimmune[42] and immunofluorescence[43–47] tests are available. The antiserum to the calf enzyme does cross react with human terminal transferase[41] although the two enzymes differ significantly in structure.[9,48] In a comparative study of the quantitative assay and the immunofluorescence test on dried smear preparations of bone marrow and peripheral blood we have found that there is substantial, but not complete, agreement between the two[10] (Fig. 7.2).

It is generally true that low levels of terminal transferase activity are associated with a lack of reactivity with specific antiserum to terminal transferase. However, a high level of terminal transferase activity in a specimen is not always

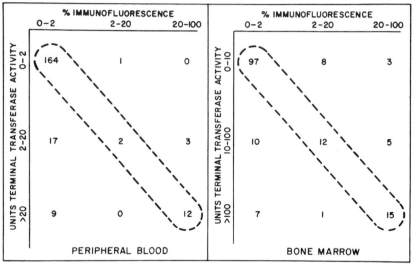

Fig. 7.2 The samples depicted (given in numbers) were collected from patients with many types of diseases. The activity of terminal transferase was quantitatively measured in nucleated cells. Immunocytochemical studies of nucleated cells were done in collaboration with Dr F. J. Bollum utilizing antibody to calf terminal transferase which he raised in rabbits.[41,43–45] The percentage of nucleated cells that react with antiserum is recorded. No attempts were made to quantitate the level of immunofluorescence in individual cells.

associated with a high percentage of cells reacting with antiserum to calf transferase. Discrepancies between the percentage of immunofluorescent cells and quantitative enzymatic activity suggests heterogeneity among cells in content of terminal transferase, as well as the possibilities of enzymatically active enzyme that is not antigenically reactive and vice versa. Specimens for immunocytochemical and enzymatic assay are prepared in different ways. Some of the disagreement between the two types of procedures may be associated with technical difficulties in cell isolation. It is also possible that antiserum to human transferase, when available, will react more strongly with human cells than does antiserum to the calf enzyme. As with all new technics, it is essential that investigators check the results of immunocytochemical assay with the quantitative assay. Within the near future, at least one biochemical supply house, Bethesda

Research Laboratories, Rockville, MD, USA, will have $F(ab')_2$ fragments of rabbit anti-calf transferase available for commercial distribution. Human terminal transferase has been purified to homogeneity in our laboratory,[9] and antiserum to it should also be available in the near future.

Measurements of terminal transferase activity and antigen are useful objective markers of certain types of malignant lymphoid cells and can be of value in the classification of hematologic neoplasms. More detailed studies of this enzyme in human cells will be required before all of the changes in terminal transferase activity and distribution in disease can be interpreted.

REFERENCES

1 Chang L M S 1971 Development of terminal deoxynucleotidyl transferase activity in embryonic calf thymus gland. Biochemical Biophysical Research Communication 44: 124–131
2 Coleman M S, Hutton J J, De Simone P, Bollum F J 1974 Terminal deoxyribonucleotidyl transferase in human leukemia. Proceedings of the National Academy of Sciences of the USA, 71: 4404–4408
3 McCaffrey R, Smoler D F, Baltimore D 1973 Terminal deoxynucleotidyl transferase in a case of childhood acute lymphoblastic leukemia. Proceedings of the National Academy of Sciences of the USA, 521–525
4 Sarin P S, Gallo R C 1976 Terminal deoxynucleotidyl transferase as a biological marker for human leukemia. In: Neth R, Gallo R, Mannweiler R, Maloney R, Maloney W (eds) Modern trends in human leukemia vol II. J F Lehmanns, Munich, pp 491–502
5 Hutton J J, Coleman M S 1976 Terminal deoxynucleotidyl transferase measurements in the differential diagnosis of adult leukemias. British Journal of Haematology 34: 447–456
6 Coleman M S, Greenwood M F, Hutton J J, Bollum F J, Lampkin B, Holland P 1976 Serial observations on terminal deoxynucleotidyl transferase activity and lymphoblast surface markers in acute lymphoblastic leukemia. Cancer Research 36: 120–127
7 Bollum F J 1966 Preparation of oligodeoxynucleotides. In: Cantoni G L, Davies D R (eds) Procedures in nucleic acid research vol I. Harper and Row, New York, pp 592–599
8 Chang L M S, Bollum F J 1971 Deoxynucleotide-polymerizing enzymes of calf thymus gland. V. Homogeneous terminal deoxynucleotidyl transferase. Journal of Biological Chemistry 246: 909–916.
9 Deibel M R, Coleman M S 1979 Purification of a high molecular weight human terminal deoxynucleotidyl transferase. Journal of Biological Chemistry 254: 8634–8640
10 Hutton J J, Coleman M S, Keneklis T P, Bollum F J 1979 Terminal deoxynucleotidyl transferase as a tumor cell marker in leukemia and lymphoma: results from 1000 patients. In: Fox M (ed) Advances in medical oncology research and education vol 4 Biological basis for cancer diagnosis. Pergamon Press, Oxford, pp 165–175
11 Kung P C, Long J C, McCaffrey R P, Ratliff R, Harrison T A, Baltimore D 1978 Terminal deoxynucleotidyl transferase in the diagnosis of leukemia and malignant lymphoma. American Journal of Medicine 64: 788–794
12 Greenwood M F, Coleman M S, Hutton J J, Lampkin B, Krill C, Bollum F J, Holland P 1977 Terminal deoxynucleotidyl transferase distribution in neoplastic and hematopoietic cells. Journal of Clinical Investigation 59: 889–899
13 Coleman M S, Greenwood M F, Hutton J J, Holland P, Lampkin B, Krill C, Kastelic J E 1978 Adenosine deaminase, terminal deoxynucleotidyl transferase (TdT), and cell surface markers in childhood acute leukemia. Blood 52: 1125–1131
14 Vogler L B, Crist W M, Bockman D E, Pearl E R, Lawton A R, Cooper M D 1978 Pre-B-cell leukemia. A new phenotype of childhood lymphoblastic leukemia. New England Journal of Medicine 298: 872–878
15 Catovsky D, O'Brian M, Cherchi M, Benavides I 1978 Ultrastructural, cytochemical and surface marker analysis of cells during blast crisis of chronic granulocytic leukaemia. Bolletino dell' Istituto Sieroterapico Milanese 57: 344–354
16 Donlon J A, Jaffe E S, Braylan R C 1977 Terminal deoxynucleotidyl transferase activity in malignant lymphomas. New England Journal of Medicine 297: 461–464

17 Gordon D S, Hutton J J, Smalley R V, Meyer L M, Vogler W R 1978 Terminal deoxynucleotidyl transferase (TdT), cytochemistry, and membrane receptors in adult acute leukemia. Blood 52: 1079–1088.

18 Hoffbrand A V, Ganeshaguru K, Janossy G, Greaves M F, Catovsky D, Woodruff R K 1977 Terminal deoxynucleotidyl transferase levels and membrane phenotypes in diagnosis of acute leukemia. Lancet ii: 520–523

19 Jaffe E S, Braylan R C, Nauba K, Frank M, Berard C W 1977 Functional markers: a new perspective on malignant lymphomas. Cancer Treatment Reports 61: 953–962

20 Janossy G, Woodruff R K, Pippard M J, Prentice G, Hoffbrand A V, Paxton A, Lister T A, Bunch C, Greaves M F 1979 Relation of 'lymphoid' phenotype and response to chemotherapy incorporating vincristine-prednisolone in the acute phase of Ph′ positive leukemia. Cancer 43: 426–434

21 Marks S M, Baltimore D, McCaffrey R 1978 Terminal transferase as a predictor of initial responsiveness to vincristine and prednisone in blastic chronic myelogenous leukemia. New England Journal of Medicine 298: 812–814

22 McCaffrey R, Harrison T A, Parkman R, Baltimore D 1975 Terminal deoxynucleotidyl transferase activity in human leukemic cells and in normal human thymocytes. New England Journal of Medicine 292: 775–780

23 Mertelsmann R, Mertelsmann I, Koziner B, Moore M A S, Clarkson B D 1978 Improved biochemical assay for terminal deoxynucleotidyl transferase in human blood cells: results in 89 adult patients with lymphoid leukemias and malignant lymphomas in leukemic phase. Leukemia Research 2: 57–69

24 Oken M M, Sarin P S, Gallo R C, Johnson G T, Gormus B J, Rydell R E, Kaplan M E 1978 Terminal transferase levels in chronic myelogenous leukemia in blast crisis and in remission. Leukemia Research 2: 173–180

25 Penit C, Brouet J-C, Rouget P 1977 Terminal deoxynucleotidyl transferase in acute lymphoblastic leukemias and chronic T cell proliferations. Leukemia Research 1: 345–350

26 Ross D D, Wiernik P H, Sarin P S, Whang-Peng J 1979 Loss of terminal deoxynucleotidyl transferase (TdT) activity as a predictor of emergence of resistance to chemotherapy in a case of chronic myelogenous leukemia in blast crisis. Cancer 44: 1566–1570

27 Saffhill R, Dexter T M, Muldal S, Testa N G, Jones P M, Joseph A 1976 Terminal deoxynucleotidyl transferase in a case of Ph′ positive infant chronic myelogenous leukaemia. British Journal of Cancer 33: 664–667

28 Sarin P S 1977 Terminal transferase as a biological marker for human leukemia. Recent Advances in Cancer Research 1: 131–138

29 Sarin P S, Anderson P N, Gallo R C 1976 Terminal deoxynucleotidyl transferase activities in human blood leukocytes and lymphoblast cell lines: high levels in lymphoblast cell lines and in blast cells of some patients with chronic myelogenous leukemia in acute phase. Blood 47: 11–20

30 Srivastava B I S, Khan S A, Henderson E S 1976 High terminal deoxynucleotidyl transferase activity in acute myelogenous leukemia. Cancer Research 36: 3847–3850

31 Srivastava B I S, Khan S A, Minowada J, Gomez G A, Rakowski I 1977 Terminal deoxynucleotidyl transferase activity in blastic phase of chronic myelogenous leukemia. Cancer Research 37: 3612–3618

32 Stass S A, Veach S, Pasquale S M, Shumacher H R, Keneklis T P, Bollum F J 1978 Terminal-deoxynucleotidyl-transferase positive acute lymphoblastic leukemia with Auer rods. Lancet i: 1042–1043

33 Wiernik P H, Edwards L S, Sarin P S (in press) Marrow terminal deoxynucleotidyl transferase activity in adult acute leukemia. Modern Trends in Human Leukemia III

34 Coleman M S 1977 Terminal deoxynucleotidyl transferase: characterization of extraction and assay conditions from human and calf tissue. Archives of Biochemistry Biophysics 182: 525–532

35 Coleman M S 1977 A critical comparison of commonly used procedures for the assay of terminal deoxynucleotidyl transferase in crude tissue extracts. Nucleic Acids Research 4: 4305–4312

36 Cassani G R, Bollum F J 1969 Oligodeoxythymidylate: polydeoxyadenylate and oligodeoxyadenylate: polydeoxythymidylate interactions. Biochemistry 8: 3928–3936

37 Chang L M S, Bollum F J 1971 Enzymatic synthesis of oligodeoxynucleotides. Biochemistry 10: 536–544

38 Chang L M S, Bollum F J 1970 Deoxynucleotide-polymerizing enzymes of calf thymus gland IV. Inhibition of terminal deoxynucleotidyl transferase by metal ligands. Proceedings of the National Academy of Sciences of the USA 65: 1041–1048

39 1972 Specifications and Criteria for Biochemical Compounds, 3rd edn (ISBN 0–309–01917–6) National Academy of Sciences, National Research Council: Washington, DC

40 Bollum F J 1966 Filter paper disk techniques for assaying radioactive macromolecules. In: Cantoni G L, Davies D R (eds) Procedures in Nucleic Acid Research vol I. Harper and Row, New York, pp 296–300

41 Bollum F J 1975 Antibody to terminal deoxynucleotidyl transferase. Proceedings of the National Academy of Sciences of the USA 72: 4119–4122

42 Kung P, Gottlieb P D, Baltimore D 1976 Terminal deoxynucleotidyl transferase. Serological studies and radioimmunoassay. Journal of Biological Chemistry 251: 2399–2404

43 Goldschneider I, Gregoire K, Barton R W, Bollum F J 1977 Demonstration of terminal deoxynucleotidyl transferase in thymocytes by immunofluorescence. Proceedings of the National Academy of Sciences of the USA 74: 734–738

44 Gregoire K E, Goldschneider I, Barton R W, Bollum F J 1977 Intracellular distribution of terminal deoxynucleotidyl transferase in rat bone marrow and thymus. Proceedings of the National Academy of Sciences of the USA, 74: 3993–3996

45 Hutton J J, Bollum F J 1978 Terminal transferase and DNA polymerases in leukemia. In: Ruddon W (ed) Biological markers of neoplasia: basic and applied aspects. Elsevier North Holland, Inc., New York, pp 569–579

46 Staas S A, Shumacher H K, Keneklis T P, Bollum F J 1979 Terminal deoxynucleotidyl transferase immunofluorescence on bone marrow smears; experience in 156 cases. American Journal of Clinical Pathology, 72: 898–903

47 Bollum F J 1979 Deoxynucleotide-polymerizing enzymes in mammalian cells: Immunofluorescence. In: Chandra P (ed) Antiviral Mechanisms for Control of Neoplasia. Plenum Press, New York, pp 587–601

48 Bollum F J, Brown M 1979 A high molecular weight form of terminal deoxynucleotidyl transferase. Nature 278: 191–192

8

The Clonal Culture *in vitro* of Human Leukemic Cells

Donald Metcalf

INTRODUCTION

This chapter will be restricted to a discussion of methods developed in the last 10 years for the primary culture of leukemic cells in semisolid cultures. The reader is no doubt aware that a number of continuously propagable culture lines of human leukemic cells exist and may wonder why such lines will not be discussed. The establishment of continuous cell lines often involves major cell selection during initiation of the cultures and secondary mutations are common when cell lines proliferate continuously *in vitro*. Because of this, continuous lines of leukemic cells can offer little reliable information on the nature of leukemia or the changes actually present in leukemic cells as they exist in a patient. Liquid culture systems for hemopoietic cells have many uses but changes in the number or differentiation of a particular cell type in cultures of mixed hemopoietic populations are difficult to interpret. Cell input and output can be monitored well enough but liquid cultures are 'black boxes' that do not permit events such as proliferation or differentiation to be related to individual cells or their progeny.

Progress in recent years in understanding the cellular events in normal or leukemic hemopoiesis has come almost entirely from the application of semisolid culture technics in which the progeny of individual cells can be identified because they remain in a fixed location as a colony or cluster of cells. By means of this technology, most of the various hemopoietic ancestral cells can now be enumerated and characterized (see review by Metcalf[1]) and the same cultures have proved to be very sensitive bioassay systems for the detection and analysis of regulatory factors controlling both normal and leukemic hemopoiesis. Based on this newer information, it is now possible to perform fairly selective liquid cultures for certain cell types. These liquid cultures certainly have some uses, but semisolid cultures remain the most reliable method for the characterization of normal and leukemic populations sampled directly from the human subject.

A SHORT HISTORY OF SEMISOLID CLONING

The first semisolid culture technics were introduced in 1966 with the simultaneous demonstration by Bradley and Metcalf[2] and Ichikawa et al[3] that colonies of normal mouse neutrophilic granulocytes and/or macrophages could be grown in semisolid agar cultures of mouse hemopoietic cells. Such colonies were shown to be clones produced by the proliferation and differentiation of the specific precursor cells (progenitor or colony-forming cells) of this double hemopoietic family. Most mouse granulocyte-macrophage colony-forming cells (GM-CFC or CFU-C) were shown to be bi-potential and capable of giving rise to both polymorphs and monocyte-macrophages.[1,4] The proliferation of such colonies was shown to depend absolutely on the presence in the culture medium of an adequate concentration of a specific glycoprotein, granulocyte-macrophage colony stimulating factor (GM-CSF) (termed CSA or MGI by other workers), high concentrations favoring neutrophil formation and low concentrations monocyte-macrophage formation.[1]

In subsequent studies, it was shown that mouse myeloid or myelomonocytic leukemic cells could be grown in the same type of agar culture, and again colony formation and differentiation of the leukemic colony cells were found to depend on stimulation by GM-CSF.[5,6,7]

The agar culture system was adapted by Pike and Robinson[8] to permit the clonal growth *in vitro* of colonies of human granulocytes and monocyte-macrophages. Much of the initial work with this system was performed using underlayers of peripheral blood cells to stimulate colony formation and analysis showed that the monocytes in the underlayer released the CSF necessary for stimulation of colony formation.[9,10,11] Media conditioned by peripheral blood cells were also found to be able to stimulate colony formation[12] and again the active cells producing the CSF were shown to be monocytes.[9]

It was pointed out by Chervenick and Boggs[13] that this type of human marrow culture also developed colonies of eosinophils and these have since been analyzed by morphological and histological studies.[14–17]

During this work, it was demonstrated that colonies or clusters of granulocyte-macrophage cells could regularly be grown from the marrow or blood of patients with acute or chronic myeloid leukemia and the neoplastic nature of the cells was confirmed by karyological examination of the proliferating cells.

Stephenson et al[18] introduced a semisolid culture technic based on plasma clots and the use of erythropoietin that permitted the clonal proliferation of relatively mature erythroid precursors (colony-forming units, erythroid; CFU-E). Following improvements in the media and the use of higher concentrations of erythropoietin, these cultures also supported the growth of large, often multicentric, erythroid colonies originating from the most ancestral progenitor cells in the erythropoietic series, the so-called burst colony-forming units, erythroid (BFU-E).[19] Both technics have now been modified to permit the growth of corresponding cells from human marrow and peripheral blood.[20]

Mitogen-stimulated mouse lymphoid cells have been shown to be capable of synthesizing the specific factors required to stimulate the formation of colonies of mouse eosinophil, megakaryocyte and erythroid cells. Using medium conditioned by such cells, Metcalf and co-workers developed cloning technics for mouse eosinophils,[21] megakaryocytes[22] and pure and mixed erythroid colonies.[23] Recently, a method has been described for cloning mixed human colonies,[24] based on the observation of McLeod et al[25] that impure preparations of erythropoietin also contain a factor able to stimulate the proliferation of the megakaryocyte precursors.

These developments have made it possible to clonally analyze all the major

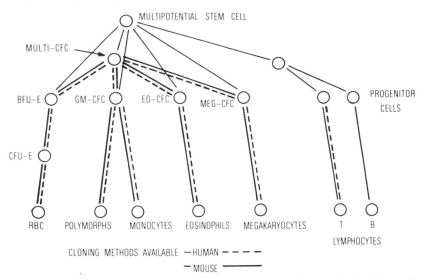

Fig. 8.1 Diagram showing the various hemopoietic precursor populations. Broken lines indicate the populations in human hemopoietic tissue whose proliferation and differentiation can now be analyzed clonally *in vitro* using semisolid culture technics.

hemopoietic populations in semisolid cultures using cells taken directly from the animal or patient. These are summarized in Figure 8.1.

The situation with lymphoid cells is less satisfactory. Good cloning technics exist for the culture of normal mouse B-lymphocytes[26] and normal human T-lymphocytes[27,28] but not vice-versa. Some continuously propagable lines of mouse and human leukemic lymphoid cells can be cloned in agar and EBV-transformed human B-lymphocytes also can readily be cloned in agar.[29] Furthermore, human myeloma cells can now be cloned in agar[30] using technics based on the cloning of mouse myeloma cells.[31] However, attempts to culture mouse or human T- or B-lymphoid leukemic cells taken directly from the animal or patient so far have been unsuccessful and no method yet exists to study these leukemias *in vitro* comparable with those routinely available for the myeloid leukemias. The present review will, of necessity, be concerned mainly with methods for the analysis of myeloid leukemic cells and the information these technics have produced.

TECHNICAL PROCEDURES

GENERAL CONSIDERATIONS

For convenience, semisolid cultures are usually performed in 35 mm plastic petri dishes although the methods are equally applicable to the growth of cells in larger dishes, tubes, capillary tubes or microtiter trays. In essence, the cultures involve adding a dispersed suspension of marrow or peripheral blood cells to culture medium containing an agent that will produce either a firm gel or a highly viscous solution. Three agents are used commonly to produce this semisolid state—agar, plasma clot or methylcellulose. Methylcellulose, which produces merely a highly viscous solution, has the theoretical advantages of allowing colonies to be harvested more readily than from genuine semisolid cultures. However, in practice, it is very difficult to ensure that only a single colony is harvested from such material. Furthermore, the cells settle continuously during the culture period and the growing colonies and clusters tend to form a carpet over the bottom of the culture dish. While this does not interfere with colony counting it makes the identification and enumeration of clusters impossible. As shall be shown later, this is of critical importance in the analysis of cultures from patients with acute myeloid leukemia (AML). Use of methylcellulose is not recommended, therefore, in studies on preleukemic or leukemic patients. Plasma gel cultures are also unsatisfactory because their rubbery consistency essentially prevents the harvesting of growing colonies or clusters. For these reasons, it is strongly recommended that all semisolid cultures be performed using soft agar (final concentration 0.3 per cent) with which no scoring problems arise and from which colonies or clusters can readily be harvested for further study.

As discussed in more detail elsewhere[1] there are three requirements for successful semisolid cultures of hemopoietic cells: use of a satisfactory batch of serum in the medium; proper incubating conditions and use of an adequate concentration of the specific stimulus required to stimulate the proliferation of the cells under study. The latter question will be discussed in more detail shortly but first some general comments on serum and incubators.

1. Serum

While it has been possible to grow granulocyte-macrophage colonies in serum-free, fully characterized, culture medium,[32] this requires high levels of technical expertise and most semisolid cultures are performed routinely using a relatively high concentration of 15 to 20 per cent serum. As is true for all tissue cultures, the nature of this serum is of critical importance. 'Bad' batches of serum will support neither survival nor proliferation of cells and 'good' batches will support colony formation with varying degrees of efficiency. Analysis of this phenomenon has revealed a more serious situation than previously suspected. Progenitor (colony-forming) cells are an heterogeneous population and, where a 'fair' batch of serum supports some colony formation, the situation is commonly that colony formation by some subsets of progenitors is supported but not colony formation by others. It is essential, therefore, that the very best serum be used in cultures if all subsets of progenitor cells are to be analyzed satisfactorily.

Choice of a 'good' serum batch can only be made by trial and error—that is by tests using normal marrow cells. It should be emphasized that the properties of the serum which are good for one type of culture are not necessarily the same required for other types of cultures. Thus the serum may support good PHA-stimulated proliferation of human lymphocytes in liquid cultures, but be useless for the culture of human GM colonies. Even a serum supporting relatively good colony formation may be poor when eosinophil or erythroid colony formation is considered.

In general, fetal calf serum is satisfactory for human hemopoietic cultures (final concentration 20 per cent), or a combination of 15 per cent fetal calf serum and 5 per cent horse serum may be better. Preheating sera to 56°C for 30 minutes is often used to inactivate complement but in most cases this has little influence on the performance of the serum. Most suppliers of serum allow pretesting of batches before a definitive purchase is made. Fetal calf serum retains its activity best when stored at 4°C but as the activity of serum falls progressively on storage it is unwise to purchase in advance more than is sufficient for 6 months' work. It is preferable to avoid excessive millipore filtering of media, sera or stimulatory preparations since the filters release cytotoxic material and/or inactivate proteins in low concentrations. Since sera are supplied prefiltered, such sera can be added without refiltration to filtered batches of serum-free culture medium immediately before use.

Unsatisfactory serum is the most common cause of poor cultures and this must always be excluded when difficulties arise with semisolid cultures.

2. Incubating conditions

Semisolid cultures are usually incubated at 37°C in a fully humidified atmosphere of 10 per cent CO_2 in air. It has been shown recently that incubation in 10 per cent CO_2 and only 5 per cent oxygen produces better and more sustained colony growth.[33] Although the latter gas mixture is more expensive, its use for special purposes may be worthwhile.

On continued incubation, petri dish cultures tend to dry out, a process resulting in inhibition of colony formation, because of the large surface area of a 35 mm culture dish in proportion to the standard 1 ml volume of the culture. This is of special importance for human GM cultures which must be kept for 2 weeks. Drying out can be avoided by a number of procedures: (a) use of a 2 ml volume in the culture dish; (b) reduction of the gas flow rate to less than 2 l per minute; and (c) use of a water bath in the bottom of the incubator through which the gas mixture enters the incubator via a scintered glass filter.

A fully humidified incubator should show condensed water on the glass door and the lids of the petri dishes. If such condensation is not present, the door seal should be checked and possibly filter paper introduced into the water bath and taped to the back wall of the incubator to increase the moist surface area. Water jacketed incubators keep a more uniform temperature than incubators with solid insulation but the water level in the jacket must be constantly checked. If the water level falls, cultures on the top trays and on the edges of trays will dry out.

A continuous gas flow is not essential for semisolid cultures and a more cumbersome but quite satisfactory method is to culture the dishes in a gas-tight plastic box that is re-gassed every time the box is opened.

As petri dish lids fit loosely and are essentially open to liquid droplets in the atmosphere of the incubator, under no conditions should antifungal or antibacterial agents of any type be put in the water bath. Water baths regularly become contaminated and while this does not necessarily cause problems with contamination of cultures, eventually the quality of colony formation diminishes. This can be avoided by thorough washing of the incubator with soap and water every 2 to 3 months.

For the same general reasons, use of incubators with a fan for circulating the atmosphere within the incubator should be avoided as this causes frequent contamination of the cultures.

The final common problem of incubators is maintenance of a satisfactory pH as indicated by the yellow-salmon pink color of the phenol red indicator in the culture medium. Where incubator doors are opened at regular intervals throughout the working day, the pH of the incubator is usually alkaline (red color in the medium). This requires the use of an incubator, e.g. a National incubator, possessing a valve which is used to pulse pure CO_2 through the incubator for 45 to 60 seconds after each occasion on which the door is opened.

GENERAL CULTURE TECHNICS

The technics for culturing normal and leukemic granulocyte-monocyte (GM) colonies in agar and the problems of scoring and interpreting these cultures will be described in detail. Space limitations prevent a detailed discussion of special semisolid technics for erythroid and lymphoid cells but references to key papers will be provided at the end of this section.

1. Collection of cells

Marrow aspirates, preferably less than 2 ml in volume to avoid excessive hemo-dilution, are collected in 1000 Units of preservative-free heparin. These aspirates are added to 5 ml of single strength culture medium and a dispersed cell suspension prepared by pipetting. It is important that no cell clumps be allowed to remain in the cultured cell suspension and visible bone or undispersed cell clumps should be allowed to settle, the supernatant cell suspension then being transferred to another tube. Viable cell counts are performed using eosin and if undispersed cell clumps are seen in the counting chamber, the suspension should be redispersed.

Contaminating red cells do not interfere with the growth of GM colonies and in fact improve cell growth.[34] If excessive numbers of red cells in the culture dishes impede visibility during colony scoring, these can be lysed by the addition of 0.5 ml of 3 per cent acetic acid immediately prior to counting.

Marrow cell suspensions should be washed by centrifugation through culture medium or buffered saline to remove inhibitory substances and/or damaged cells as this process has been shown to increase colony numbers.[35] It has been shown that high concentrations of polymorphs are inhibitory for GM colony formation, particularly in culture systems depending on endogenous production of GM-CSF (e.g. by feeder layers).[34, 36] Such cells can be removed by prefractionation of the marrow cell suspension, e.g. by the removal of the denser polymorphs as a pellet by centrifugation of the cells in bovine serum albumin of density 1.070 g/ml.[37] However, this procedure is unnecessary if a preformed source of GM-CSF is used in the cultures, e.g. by the use of placental or WBC conditioned medium. In general, prefractionation of a cell suspension to be cultured is undesirable since the properties of colony- and cluster-forming cells in an abnormal marrow cannot be predicted and loss of such cells during fractionation procedures can introduce unnecessary complexities into the interpretation of the culture data.

Peripheral blood cells can be collected for culture in preservative-free heparin and the buffy coat cells removed and washed by centrifugation, using similar methods to those used for marrow cells.

2. Preparation of cultures

Semisolid cultures are prepared by mixing equal volumes of double strength medium (held at room temperature) and 0.6 per cent agar (boiled for 2 minutes, then held at 37°C) then adding the required number of cells for culture. One or 2 ml volumes of this cell suspension in agar medium are then pipetted into 35 mm petri dishes containing the GM-CSF source, either in the form of 0.1 to 0.2 ml of conditioned medium or an underlayer of peripheral blood cells. The cell suspension is mixed thoroughly by circular movement of the culture dish and the cultures allowed to gel. These are then incubated without further delay in a fully humidified atmosphere of 10 per cent CO_2 in air.

A satisfactory formula for the double strength medium is: Dulbecco's Modified Eagle's HG-16 Instant Tissue Culture Powder (Grand Island Biological Company, New York) 10 g; 390 ml double glass distilled water; 3 ml L-asparagine (6.7 mg/ml—final concentration in medium 20 μg/ml); 1.5 ml DEAE dextran (50 mg/ml—final concentration in medium 75 μg/ml) (Pharmacia, Sweden, molecular weight $= 500\,000$); 0.575 ml penicillin (2×10^5 Units/ml); 0.375 ml streptomycin (200 mg/ml); 4.9 g NaH CO_3; 200 ml fetal calf serum and 50 ml horse serum.

The double strength medium is millipore filtered before the addition of the fetal calf and horse serum. This medium can be stored at 4°C for up to 14 days, the appropriate volume of serum being added at the time of preparation of cultures.

Human marrow and peripheral blood contain cells (probably monocytes) that can produce GM-CSF *in vitro*. If high cell concentrations are cultured, apparently GM-CSF-independent colony formation can occur. This can be a problem if experiments are designed to investigate, for example, the dependency or autonomy of leukemic cells with respect to stimulation by GM-CSF. Analysis of this phenomenon has shown that the 'spontaneous' colony formation is in fact due to the elaboration of GM-CSF within the culture dish by adherent cells (probably mainly monocytes) in the cultured marrow or peripheral blood population.[9] Because of this, many laboratories remove adherent cells prior to culture by allowing the cells to adhere to petri dishes[38] or by carbonyl iron adherence with removal of the adherent cells using a magnet.[39] Such non-adherent (NA) marrow or peripheral blood cells exhibit minimal spontaneous cell proliferation and are used widely. However, for the general reasons mentioned above on the potential dangers of pre-fractionation, the use of a preliminary adherence fractionation is probably undesirable particularly where cultures are being used simply to enumerate and characterize colony- or cluster-forming cells.

Spontaneous colony formation is markedly dependent on cell concentration and usually only becomes evident if more than 100 000 per ml are cultured.[9]

A useful procedure for minimizing this phenomenon is therefore simply to culture 50 000 to 100 000 cells per ml rather than the conventionally used 2×10^5 cells/ml. A more important reason for choosing to culture only 50 000 to 100 000 marrow cells per dish is that this cell number produces 'comfortable' numbers of discrete colonies to count in a single dish (20 to 150). Use of higher cell concentrations can lead to colony confluence and serious underestimates of colony numbers. For peripheral blood cells, the frequency of colony-forming cells is so low that higher numbers of cells can be cultured, e.g. 200 000 per ml.

It is important not to adhere inflexibly to the above cell concentrations. If it is suspected that either a high frequency of colony- or cluster-forming cells might be present, e.g. in chronic myeloid leukemic (CML) or a regenerating marrow, much lower cell numbers can, and should, be cultured, e.g. 10 000/ml. In cultures of acute myeloid leukemia (AML) cells where it is important to perform cluster counts, it may be necessary to culture even lower cell concentrations, e.g. 1000 per ml otherwise cluster crowding may make accurate counting impossible, obscure the assessment of cluster size or even lead to the formation of pseudo-colonies. Many published studies have used routinely 2×10^5 cells or more per ml regardless of the type of marrow being cultured and the data produced from cultures of AML cells are quite meaningless because of overcrowding.

3. Provision of a colony stimulating factor

The proliferation of GM and eosinophil colonies in the above type of culture depends absolutely on the continuous presence of an adequate concentration of two specific regulatory factors—GM-CSF for the granulocyte-monocyte cells and EO-CSF for the eosinophil cells. This may be achieved by one of two methods: (a) the use of underlayers of peripheral blood cells, or (b) adding 0.1 or 0.2 ml of a conditioned medium containing adequate concentrations of both factors.

Where underlayers of peripheral blood WBC are used to stimulate colony formation, peripheral blood is collected from normal donors or Rhesus monkeys using preservative-free heparin. After removal and washing of the buffy coat by centrifugation, 1 to 2×10^6 cells/ml are added to an equal volume mixture of the above double strength medium and 1.0 per cent agar to give a more rigid underlayer with a final agar concentration of 0.5 per cent.[40]

Underlayers may be stored in a CO_2 incubator for up to 7 to 14 days before use but colony stimulating activity falls progressively on storage. Cell separation studies have shown that in underlayers the material with colony stimulating activity is produced by the monocytes. Polymorphs in the peripheral blood from most donors and patients exhibit an inhibitory effect on GM-CSF production by release of inhibitory macromolecules. For this reason, many laboratories now prefractionate peripheral blood cells by centrifugation through bovine serum albumin (density 1.070 g/ml osmolarity 270 mOsm).[37] The polymorphs, being more dense, are pelleted through the bovine serum albumin and the supernatant mononuclear cells are used to prepare the underlayers.

Peripheral blood WBC are able to produce conditioned medium with satisfactory colony stimulating activity (1 to 50×10^6 cells/ml are cultured for up to

7 days),[12,40–42] and it has also been shown that addition of phytohemagglutinin to cultures of peripheral blood cells can result in the production of medium with high colony stimulating activity by mitogen-stimulated lymphocytes.[43–45] However, this type of conditioned medium can be extremely variable in its colony stimulating activity.

A more satisfactory method for producing a human-active GM-CSF and EO-CSF is to incubate fragments of human placental tissue.[46,47] Human placentas are stored at 4°C and used within 12 h delivery. The outer membranes are removed and the placental tissues cut in 5 mm^3 pieces. After being rinsed three times in Eisen's Balanced Salt Solution, 6 pieces are placed in each flat-sided tissue culture bottle containing 20 ml of RPMI-1640 (Gibco, Grand Island, New York) with 5 per cent fetal calf serum. The bottles are incubated for 7 d at 37°C in a fully humidified atmosphere of 10 per cent CO_2 in air. The conditioned medium is harvested then centrifuged at 10 000 g for 20 min to remove debris and stored at $-15°C$. Crude placental conditioned medium often contains inhibitory material. A preparation with increased colony stimulating activity can be prepared by preliminary calcium phosphate gel absorption of the placental conditioned medium, followed by gel filtration on a Sephadex column. Such preparations, after concentration by ultrafiltration, are capable of delivering a supramaximal stimulus for granulocyte-monocyte and eosinophil colony formation without evidence of high-dose inhibition.[47]

SCORING OF CULTURES

An Olympus dissection microscope at $\times 35$ for colonies and $\times 40$ for clusters is used to score cultures. The mirror is tilted to give semi-indirect lighting, counting white colonies against a brown or black background.

Most workers have adopted the convention that human colonies are discrete aggregates of 40 or more cells and clusters are aggregates of 3 to 39 cells. The reader is cautioned to note carefully the criteria used by individual authors as some use quite different (less satisfactory) criteria and the results cannot be compared directly with those of most workers.

Scoring of agar cultures is *not* a task to be delegated to a technician. Technicians usually lack sufficient awareness of the potential information present in the culture dish to be sufficiently observant and maintain their concentration. Moreover, no two human cultures are exactly alike and important new information or abnormalities in cultures from a particular patient are easily missed if scoring is treated as a low level mechanical procedure.

Underlayer- and conditioned medium-stimulated human cultures of the above type develop eosinophil as well as neutrophil-monocyte (GM) colonies. At 10 days of incubation, 20 to 30 per cent of colonies are composed of eosinophils.[13,16,17] Almost all published data on 'GM' colonies have made no attempt to separately count eosinophil and neutrophil-macrophage colonies. However, methods now exist for performing differential colony counts and the frequency of GM and eosinophil colonies should always be recorded separately.[17,45]

In the simplest procedure, a fine Pasteur pipette is used to pick off 45 intact sequential colonies with a small amount of surrounding agar, using a gentle scooping-sucking action. Each colony is deposited on a microscope slide previously marked into 15 squares using a diamond pencil. The colonies are allowed to dry, fixed with 100 per cent methanol for 10 min, then stained for 2 h with a solution of Luxol fast blue MBS (0.1 per cent w/v Luxol fast blue MBS (G.T. Gurr, High Wycombe, Bucks) dissolved in 70 per cent ethanol saturated with urea). Slides are washed in running water for 2 h then counterstained with Harris' hematoxylin. Slides are rinsed with water, allowed to dry, then coverslips mounted using DPX. These stained colonies are typed at $\times 100$ or $\times 400$. Differential counts are particularly easy for human colonies because of the bright apple green color of the eosinophil cytoplasm (either uniform green or large green granules) and the hematoxylin counterstain is sufficient to permit subclassification of GM colonies into neutrophil, monocytic or neutrophil-monocytic types.

It should be emphasized that colony counts from marrow cultures give an estimate of the frequency, *not* the total number of GM or eosinophil progenitor cells. Where peripheral blood is cultured, the data can be converted to absolute numbers per ml. Colony- and cluster-forming cell levels in peripheral blood are extremely low in comparison with those in the marrow and all marrow samples are potentially diluted by an unknown volume of peripheral blood. This will always raise difficulties in interpretation of data on the frequency of normal or leukemic colony- or cluster-forming cells in cultured specimens. If aspirate volumes are restricted to 1 to 2 ml and aspirates are obtained without difficulty, the data from normal marrow vary from 20 to 150 GM-CFC/10^5 cells[35] and this degree of variability is tolerable where major disturbances in GM-CFC levels are being sought, e.g. in AML or CML etc.

PROBLEMS IN THE INTERPRETATION OF AGAR CULTURES

1. Variability in culture efficiency

Because there is considerable intrinsic variability in the responsiveness of GM-CFCs to stimulation by GM-CSF, it is essential to use supra-plateau concentrations of GM-CSF to ensure that all GM-CFC are stimulated to proliferate and thereby detected. It is probably preferable to use a stable liquid source of GM-CSF where these conditions can be guaranteed. Use of suboptimal stimuli can give rise to quite misleading information regarding the properties of GM-CFC if only the most readily stimulated cells are detected.

This problem is of special importance in cultures of AML or preleukemic cells. The implications of cultures containing only clusters is of great importance, both diagnostically and prognostically. Furthermore, the exact size of clusters is also of importance. Extremely misleading data will be obtained if poor culture conditions lead to the formation only of clusters instead of colonies or the formation of small clusters instead of medium sized or large clusters.

To minimize this problem of variability it is essential always to culture control marrow suspensions in which normal colony-forming cells are present. Ideally, such control cultures can also be used to standardize colony numbers grown from an unknown marrow specimen so that the results obtained in one experiment can validly be added to, or compared with, results obtained on other occasions. Where laboratories have facilities for, and experience with, liquid nitrogen storage of cells, replicate ampules of a single specimen of normal marrow or even a CML marrow can be used as a standard.

2. Special problems with underlayer-stimulated cultures

While cultures stimulated by underlayers usually exhibit more rapid and sustained colony growth than cultures stimulated by placental conditioned medium, underlayer-stimulated cultures have a number of special problems. Different batches of underlayers vary in their colony stimulating activity and this activity declines on storage. Furthermore, contamination of underlayers on storage is common. Often the underlayer cells themselves exhibit colony formation that is not always readily discriminated from colony formation in the upper layer of cultured marrow cells and many underlayers are so opaque because of residual cell debris that the scoring of clusters is difficult.

3. Time of scoring of cultures

It is routine with cultures of animal marrow cells to use 7 d as the incubation interval before scoring and a number of workers also have used this convenient end point for scoring human cultures. However, human colonies grow more slowly than animal colonies and many investigators delay scoring cultures until 14 to 21 d. Major discrepancies exist in the literature because of the use of these differing timepoints. For example, in cultures of some AML cells, large clusters present at 7 d and scored as such by one investigator may continue slow growth and be scored as colonies by another investigator scoring at 14 d.

The events occurring in a human culture are extremely complex and in fact no one timepoint is entirely satisfactory: (a) cluster numbers are maximal early in the culture period (3 to 5 d) then may decrease due to dispersion and/or disintegration; (b) with high concentrations of GM-CSF, higher cluster numbers will develop but their premature dispersion leads to lower cluster counts when such cultures are scored at 10 to 14 d than in cultures containing low GM-CSF concentrations; (c) eosinophil colonies exhibit an initial growth lag. No eosinophil colonies are present at day 7 and colony numbers are maximal at 2 to 3 weeks; (d) subpopulations of GM-CFC exist that form colonies characteristically dispersing and/or dying between day 7 and 14 of incubation. For this reason cultures at day 7 and 14 do not detect the same GM-CFCs.[48]

In this laboratory, as a compromise, duplicate sets of cultures are scored at 7 and 14 d, eosinophil colony counts being performed only at day 14. Each investigator needs to consider carefully his own requirements. For example with AML cultures, if it is desired to follow the classification of Moore et al[49] or Spitzer et al,[50] cultures must be scored at 7 d. If other classifications are being followed, the incubation period should be matched to that used by the original investigator.

SPECIAL PROCEDURES PRIOR TO CULTURE

To characterize the nature of cells proliferating in agar cultures it is now common to use a variety of separative or preliminary procedures on the marrow or peripheral blood poulation prior to culture.

Leukemic colony- and cluster-forming cells are characterized by their abnormally light buoyant density.[51] An estimate of the proportion of cells of abnormally light buoyant density can be obtained by centrifuging the cells through bovine serum albumin of density 1.062 g/ml, a higher than normal proportion of leukemic cells remaining in suspension.[51] To fully characterize the density profile of proliferating cells it is necessary to fractionate the cells in a continuous density gradient, culturing and analyzing each fraction. It is important *not* to use a discontinuous gradient for this purpose as artefacts occur at the interfaces of the density regions.

A striking feature of hemopoietic precursor cells of any one type is their heterogeneity in cell volume. A very useful procedure for analyzing subpopulations of normal or leukemic progenitor cells is to separate them on the basis of cell volume using a simple sedimentation chamber (velocity sedimentation separation). Details of this procedure have been published elsewhere.[48,52,53]

Removal of adherent (GM-CSF-producing) cells from marrow specimens by adherence separation has been described earlier, but adherence separation can also be used to fractionate and characterize hemopoietic subpopulations in an analytical manner. Details of this technic are described elsewhere.[54]

Newer methods of cell fractionation using affinity chromatography lectin columns[55] or fluorescence-activated cell sorters have yet to be applied to the fractionation of leukemic populations but are proving extremely powerful tools and an extensive literature based on these technics can be anticipated in the near future.

For a number of purposes it has proved valuable to be able to estimate, or selectively kill, the fraction of normal or leukemic cells in the S-phase of the cell cycle. Two methods are available for pretreating human cells in S-phase by preincubation of the cells *in vitro* either with high concentrations of ^{3}HTdR,[56] or more simply, with hydroxyurea.[57] After washing, the cells are cultured and the proportion of cells in S-phase calculated from the percentage reduction in colony or cluster numbers compared with control cultures.

CULTURE TECHNICS FOR OTHER CELL TYPES

This review is restricted to a discussion of the behavior *in vitro* of myeloid leukemic cells but, for completeness, references will be given for procedures for culturing other neoplastic and normal hemopoietic cells.

Methods for the clonal culture of human erythropoietic cells have been published by Teppeman et al,[20] human megakaryocytic by Vainchenker et al[24] and human T-lymphocytes by Rozenszajn et al[27] and Claesson et al.[28]

Methods for the clonal culture of human myeloma cells have been published by Hamburger and Salmon.[30,58]

Special procedures for obtaining colony formation in agar cultures by acute myeloid leukemic cells using stimulation by phytohemagglutinin or phyto-hemagglutinin-stimulated conditioned medium have been described by Dicke et al[59,60] and Minden et al.[61]

CULTURE OF CELLS FROM PATIENTS WITH CHRONIC MYELOID LEUKEMIA (CML)

When agar cultures of bone marrow or peripheral blood cells from a patient with untreated CML are stimulated, either by white cell underlayers or con-ditioned media, a very uniform and quite spectacular culture pattern is observed. The general pattern of size and shape of cluster and colony formation appears normal enough—what is abnormal is the extremely high frequency of colonies and clusters. While the frequency of colony-forming cells in cultures of marrow cells is markedly elevated above normal ($230/10^5$ cells for 27 such patients versus $28/10^5$ for normal subjects) in one study in this laboratory,[62] the differences are even more striking in the case of peripheral blood—$510/10^5$ cells versus $0.2/10^5$ cells in normal blood, in the same study. It should be noted from these figures that in CML the frequency of granulocytic precursors in the blood actu-ally exceeds the elevated levels in the marrow, a combination unique to CML.

Unlike the situation with acute myeloid leukemic cells to be discussed below, cells from patients with CML grow uniformly well in culture and there is re-markably good agreement between the findings of various groups on the ele-vated frequency of colony-forming cells in CML.[42,51,63-67]

It should be noted that in the majority of published studies, no effort was made to record separately the frequency of neutrophil and/or monocyte colonies (GM) versus the frequency of eosinophil colonies. In studies performed on cultures after only 1 week of incubation the data do in fact refer only to GM colonies since eosinophil colonies only become apparent in the second week of incubation. More recent studies on cultures examined after 2 weeks of incuba-tion have indicated a near-normal ratio of eosinophil to GM colonies and it can thus be concluded that in CML there is a corresponding massive increase also in the total number of eosinophil progenitor cells.[17,68]

GM colonies grown from CML patients increase in size at a normal rate and exhibit the heterogeneity of size and general shape characteristic of normal GM colonies. This heterogeneity is a matter of some interest since it is character-istic of many established leukemic cell lines when cloned in agar that they pro-duce remarkably uniform colonies.[1] The apparent normality of CML colonies is further emphasized when the colony populations are examined morphologic-ally. The various colonies contain granulocytic and/or monocytic cells that appear to differentiate in a normal pattern, maturation of colonies resulting in the production of what appear to be normal polymorphs, monocytes or macrophages.

Further evidence of the normality of CML colonies was obtained from an analysis of their dependency on CSF-containing material for continued prolifera-tion. As is true for cultures of normal marrow cells, if sufficiently high concentra-tions of CML cells are cultured, spontaneous colony formation occurs.[40] How-ever, if endogenous CSF-producing cells are removed by preliminary density fractionation or adherent separation, the colony-forming cells are quite unable to proliferate in the absence of an exogenous source of CSF.[40] Furthermore, on exposure *in vitro* to CSF, non-cycling CML colony-forming cells enter S phase within 3 h as is the case for normal cells.[69] While a detailed analysis of the dose–response curves of CML cells after stimulation by CSF suggested that they may be slightly hyporesponsive to stimulation compared with normal cells,[70] this study re-emphasized the absolute dependency of CML cells on GM-CSF for every cell division.

Although the growth of CML cells has many resemblances to that of normal marrow cells, analysis has revealed that a number of differences do exist:

1. Karyotypic analysis of dividing CML colony cells has revealed the presence of the Ph^1 chromosome[63, 71–73]
2. When CML cells are fractionated in continuous gradients of bovine serum albumin, an abnormally high proportion of the colony-forming cells is found to be of lighter buoyant density than 1.062 g/ml.[51,67] This proportion (up to 70 to 90 per cent in individual patients, versus 5 per cent for normal marrow) is always higher in the blood than the marrow[67]
3. A lower proportion of CML colony-forming cells is in the S phase of the cell cycle than normal (less than 10 per cent versus 30 per cent for normal cells).[51] Fluctuations have been reported in the proportion of CML colony-forming cells in cycle, according to whether or not a leukocytosis was developing in the patient[74] or whether the patient was responding to therapy or in relapse[67]
4. The ratio of clusters to colonies is slightly lower than normal and there is some tendency for the early appearance of monocytes in mixed colonies grown from CML cells[51]
5. CML colony-forming cells sediment as a single peak with a modal sedimentation velocity of 7 to 9 mm/h in contrast to the double peak of colony-forming cells observed with normal marrow[48] (Dresch, C. and Johnson, G. R., unpublished data).

The abnormally light buoyant density characteristic of most CML colony-forming cells has permitted the morphological identification of these cells. In at least some patients, light density fractions of CML blood or marrow were found to contain up to 100 per cent of cells identifiable on morphological grounds as 'myeloblasts.'[51,62,68] When such populations were cultured *in vitro*, up to 100 per cent of the cells formed colonies or clusters.[1,62,68] This indicates that at least some of the colony-forming cells in CML must have the morphology of myeloblasts. The findings do not exclude the possibility that some CML colony-forming cells may have a different morphology although this must be considered unlikely.

Following initiation of myleran therapy, there is a dramatic fall in progenitor cell levels in the blood, preceding and of relatively greater magnitude than the fall in peripheral blood white cell levels.[62] While a similar fall also occurs in marrow levels, in most patients these levels remain somewhat higher than normal in the stable phase of the disease.

As assessed from the behavior in culture of marrow and blood cells from CML patients, this disease can be regarded as one in which there is a massive enlargement of the progenitor cell compartment of the neutrophil-monocyte series and also of the eosinophil series. Little information exists on the spleen content of progenitor cells but this seems likely to be as greatly elevated above normal as is true of the progenitor cell content of the peripheral blood. Although agar culture of CML cells has revealed some characteristic abnormalities in these cells, has supported the clonal origin of these cells and has shown that the CML clone remains dependent on GM-CSF, there are a number of questions that have not been resolved. Are the numerous eosinophil progenitors present in these patients also members of the Ph[1] clone? To what degree are the colony-forming cells in the population capable of self-replication? Are they in fact the stem cells of the leukemic clone?

The most crucial question of course is whether CML is really a neoplastic disease. The ability of cells to produce differentiating progeny as is true for CML cells does not by itself exclude CML as a neoplastic disease. The cells in many tumors are often capable of reasonable differentiation. The fundamental property of a neoplastic population is its capacity for progressive proliferation (population enlargement) without restraint by the body. On this question, the answers so far obtained *in vitro* are equivocal. The massive enlargement of the ancestral population certainly appears to be progressive prior to reduction therapy and the patients would eventually die as those with any malignant neoplasm. Despite this, the colony-forming cells remain completely responsive to regulator control. One possible explanation of this paradox is that the colony-forming cells in CML are not the genuine stem cells of the clone but are the progeny of such stem cells. The stem cells are in fact multipotential and generate other hemopoietic populations known to be part of the Ph[1] clone. It may be that the stem cell population does increase progressively with time and it may not be subject to any significant limitation or regulation by the body. The *in vitro* observations would then be explained if the GM progenitor (colony-forming) cells generated by these stem cells did exhibit responsiveness to control systems in terms both of proliferation and the ability to form cells able to differentiate to mature end cells. There is urgent need for further analysis of these questions *in vitro*, in particular for studies on the nature of other hemopoietic populations known to be members of the Ph[1] clone, i.e. the erythroid, mega-karyocytic and B-lymphoid populations.

It is generally held that when CML terminates in acute transformation, the abnormal populations displacing the original CML clone are derived from mutant cells arising in the CML population. Although there is evidence that in some patients the acutely transformed population is lymphoid in nature, in the majority the abnormal cells appear to be members of the neutrophil-monocyte series.

The results from agar cloning of such transformed populations have been unsatisfactory to resolve this problem since in some cases the cells fail to proliferate *in vitro* and cannot therefore be characterized either as being GM in nature or as being responsive to GM-CSF.

In most patients progressing to acute transformation, a progressive fall occurs in the frequency of colony-forming cells with a progressive rise in the ratio of clusters to colonies.[51,62,67,75] In one third of patients, the acutely transformed population is capable only of forming clusters with an upper size limit of either 20 or 40 cells, a growth pattern characteristic of AML cells (see below).[75] In contrast to the behavior of CML cells *in vitro*, there are clearly evident abnormalities in differentiation in the colony and cluster cells grown from most transformed patients.[51,62] The cluster- and colony-forming cells in these patients exhibit the abnormally light buoyant density of corresponding CML cells and their cell cycle status is usually abnormal.[51,62,67] As with CML cells, the proliferation of acutely transformed cells *in vitro* appears to remain wholly dependent on GM-CSF.

As shall be discussed below, there is a correlation between the *in vitro* growth pattern of AML cells and the probability of entering a remission following chemotherapy. This type of correlation is seen also in the growth pattern in acute transformation—patients whose cells form only small clusters have a relatively higher probability of entering remission than do patients whose cells form large clusters or an abnormally high ratio of clusters to colonies.[75]

It has been observed that the growth patterns characteristic of acute transformation are seen 2 to 6 m before transformation is diagnosed using clinical parameters.[51,62,75] Agar cultures of this type therefore appear to have a useful role in monitoring the progress of patients with chronic myeloid leukemia.

The resemblance between the growth patterns *in vitro* of most patients with acute transformation and those from patients with AML supports the conclusion that transformed populations are in fact GM in nature, not lymphoid. A similar conclusion has been reached from *in vitro* culture studies using PHA stimulation of the cultures. As shall be described below, it is possible, using PHA, to stimulate some cells in AML to form colonies of leukemic cells *in vitro*.[59,60] The same phenomenon has been observed with acutely transformed populations but not with CML populations.[76] Indeed, using these special cultures, it seems possible to detect the emergence of transformed clones by their ability to form colonies in PHA-stimulated cultures with no added GM-CSF. Such colony-forming cells are detectable 2 to 6 m before transformation is diagnosed by conventional morphological examination.

CULTURE OF CELLS FROM PATIENTS WITH ACUTE MYELOID LEUKEMIA (AML)

The culture patterns in agar of bone marrow or peripheral blood cells from untreated patients with AML are also very characteristic. Such cultures either completely lack colonies or exhibit greatly reduced numbers of normal colonies; the cultured cells either proliferate to form clusters of various sizes or, less commonly, fail to proliferate.

In a study of 127 patients with untreated AML,[48] one of four culture patterns was exhibited by marrow or peripheral blood cells: (1) the cultures showed no colony or cluster formation and contained no living cells; where cells were from patients with monocytic leukemia such cultures often contained numerous single surviving monocytic cells (12 per cent of patients); (2) the cultures exhibited no colonies but varying numbers of clusters of 3 to 20 cells in size (47 per cent of patients); (3) the cultures exhibited no colonies but varying numbers of clusters of up to 40 cells in size (24 per cent of patients); or (4) some colonies or clusters developed but often an abnormally high ratio of clusters to colonies was present (17 per cent of patients). Comparable results have been reported.[49,77,78]

Some laboratories (e.g.[12,79,80]) have reported culture data in which 20 cells was used as the minimum size for classification of a clone as a colony. From the above description, it will be realized that this method of classification raises unnecessary problems in interpretation of the culture data and seems unwise.

The presence of large numbers of cluster-forming cells in the blood is almost diagnostic of AML. In some patients with myeloproliferative disorders in a pre-leukemic phase, cultures of marrow may also exhibit large numbers of clusters. However, cultures of the blood from such patients usually do not exhibit large numbers of clusters and in fact may have elevated numbers of colony-forming cells.[62,81]

It is important to emphasize that the data on which the above descriptions are based were collected after 7 d of incubation. In cultures maintained for longer intervals, clusters formed by leukemic cells from some patients can continue to increase in size and exceed the minimum size limit for colonies. Thus in some publications where cultures are scored at 14 or 21 d, colony formation by AML cells is described. Furthermore, if cultures are re-fed, leukemic clusters can often increase in size to become colonies[82] and the ability to grow colonies from leukemic cells can be of importance for special purposes. However, in routine cultures it seems counter productive to extend the culture period until some leukemic cells form colonies since a simple parameter for distinguishing normal from leukemic cells (i.e. colony versus cluster) is lost. Late scoring of cultures becomes particularly confusing if the patient is in partial remission when it can become impossible to decide without extensive examination which colonies are normal and which leukemic. The observation of colony formation *in vitro* by AML cells is a useful property to have documented since it indicates that AML cells really have a more sustained capacity for proliferation *in vitro* than might be assumed from the cluster formation seen after 7 d of incubation. However, having established this proposition, it appears far simpler in practice to work with 7 d cultures where the differences between leukemic and normal are most clearly evident.

Comparison of culture patterns *in vitro* with the morphological subtype of leukemia has indicated that there is no correlation between these parameters and the type of AML. For example, acute myeloblastic, promyelocytic or monocytic cells can proliferate in any one of the above four patterns.[48]

It has also been observed that there can be extreme variation from 10 to 40 000 in the absolute number of clusters developing per 10^5 cultured cells, even between patients with similar percentages of blast cells in the marrow or blood.[51,83] Classification of culture patterns into one or other of the above four categories can be made regardless of the actual numbers of clusters present. The significance of the extreme variability in the apparent frequency of cluster-forming cells per 10^5 cells or per 10^5 blast cells is difficult to assess. While cluster-forming cells in AML clearly are some type of more ancestral cell within the leukemic population, from work to be discussed later it is a little improbable that they are leukemic stem cells in the usually accepted meaning of this word, i.e. a cell capable of self-generation and generating the entire leukemic population. At the present time it seems more reasonable to assume that the variability may be merely an *in vitro* artefact based on differing metabolic requirements of different leukemic populations *in vitro* than to postulate extreme differences in kinetics or population hierarchies.

The leukemic nature of the clusters and colonies developing in AML cultures has been confirmed by comparing the karyotype of the dividing cells in such aggregates with karyotypes performed directly on the leukemic tissues. Where marker chromosomes were present in the patient these were also present in the cells dividing in agar culture.[71, 72, 82, 84]

Fractionation of leukemic populations using buoyant density separation indicated that the proliferating cells were of abnormally light buoyant density (50 to 60 per cent of the cells were less than 1.062 g/ml) and abnormally low proportions were cycling as assessed by *in vitro* exposure of the cells to high concentrations of tritiated thymidine.[51]

In favorable specimens where the majority of cells were myeloblasts and a very high proportion of cultured cells proliferated *in vitro*, analysis of density-separated fractions indicated that the cluster-forming cells had the morphology of myeloblasts.[51, 62] This conclusion may be equally true for other AML patients but the data need to be interpreted with caution since not all 'myeloblasts' may be cluster- or colony-forming cells and certainly there is no numerical correlation between the frequency of cells proliferating *in vitro* and the percentage of cells identified morphologically as 'myeloblasts.'[51, 85]

While this type of GM-CSF-stimulated agar culture has proved to have a number of useful applications in the analysis of AML leukemic cells, several deficiencies prevent the more extensive application of this type of culture: (1) the cultures do not support the *selective* culture of leukemic cells since both leukemic and normal cells are GM-CSF-dependent and will grow in the cultures; (2) AML cells usually grow as clusters similar in size and shape to normal GM clusters. This makes it extremely difficult to detect whether a few residual AML cluster-forming cells are persisting in a regenerating remission marrow; (3) the cultures do not detect the genuine stem cells in the leukemic populations and certainly do not detect the multipotential leukemic stem cells which presumably are present.

Several recent reports suggest that it may be possible to modify semisolid cultures to overcome some of these problems. If AML cells are preincubated with PHA, then cultured in agar containing PHA but no added GM-CSF, colonies can develop that appear to be composed of myeloid leukemic cells.[59, 60] It remains to be determined whether this proliferation is genuinely CSF-independent or whether CSF is generated endogenously in the cultures. The latter possibility does almost certainly occur because of the known capacity of lectins to stimulate CSF production by lymphocytes, but the level of resulting CSF production in a PHA-stimulated AML culture has yet to be determined. This PHA culture system appears to be very useful in demonstrating the presence of residual leukemic cells in treated AML patients[60] and in detecting the early stages of transformation in CML patients.[76]

This technic often has two methodological problems. PHA can induce a marked agglutination of the cultured cells in the preliminary liquid culture step. Unless great care is exercised to ensure adequate redispersion of these aggregates during the subsequent preparation of the semisolid cultures, pseudo-colonies will be present in the cultures. Even if these contain proliferating cells, the significance of such 'colonies' is of course quite different from that of true colonies. The second problem arises from the fact that PHA stimulation procedures are essentially the same as those used to obtain colony formation in agar by normal T-lymphocytes.[27,28] The general morphological appearance of leukemic AML and normal T-lymphocyte colonies is similar and the two types of colony cannot be readily discriminated from one another by simple inspection. Careful morphological examination of the cells in individual colonies may permit some of the leukemic colonies to be identified because of their content of immature granulocytes[59] and T-lymphocyte colony cells can be identified because of their capacity to form rosettes with sheep red cells.[27,28] Neither procedure lends itself to the simple enumeration of leukemic or normal colonies in a culture dish and for this reason it is probably preferable prior to culture to remove all T-lymphocytes by rosetting with sheep red cells, thus eliminating or minimizing subsequent T-lymphocyte colony formation.[121]

The second procedure for growing colonies from AML populations has been described by Minden et al.[61] This involves stimulation of AML peripheral blood cultures by PHA-stimulated leukocyte conditioned medium. With this system, small numbers of leukemic colonies composed of blast cells have been grown from AML peripheral blood. Use of cell cycle agents has indicated that these colony-forming cells are in active cell cycle (as distinct from the more slowly proliferating general population of leukemic blast cells) and it has been suggested that these colony-forming cells may be the true stem cells of the leukemic population.[61] It has yet to be reported whether such colonies contain erythroid or megakaryocytic cells as might be expected if they were derived from the multipotential stem cells of the leukemic clone. Unless such conditioned media are fractionated to remove residual PHA, it can be anticipated that such cultures will also exhibit the two problems seen with the direct PHA stimulation—cell agglutination with pseudo-colony formation and the parallel formation of normal T-lymphocyte colonies. Indeed the latter type of colony has been reported in such cultures.[61]

While it appears that both these newer methods offer interesting possibilities for exploring the biology of AML and detecting residual AML cells, both appear in need of standardization and improvement and neither may yet be able to provide the badly needed technic for detecting multipotential leukemic stem cells.

Some discrepancies exist in the literature on the question of whether the cells in clusters and colonies generated *in vitro* by AML cells exhibit normal differentiation. There are some reports of normal differentiation, usually in colonies grown from leukemic patients.[42] As discussed above, there must always be some reservation concerning the nature of 'colonies' grown from AML patients, particularly if the patients had undergone therapy, since an unknown proportion of such colonies may in fact be derived from regenerating normal cells. Where the morphology of cluster cells has been examined in 7 d cultures of AML cells most workers have noted that the cells exhibit abnormalities in differentiation.[49,51,62] The most common of these are maturation arrest at the myelocyte or promyelocyte stage but, in about one quarter of cases, cluster cells exhibited qualitative abnormalities in nuclear morphology, nuclear versus cytoplasmic differentiation or degenerative changes.[48] Where Auer rods were present in the leukemic cells *in vivo* these were also seen in cluster cells grown *in vitro*.

The question of the capacity of AML cells to differentiate normally *in vitro* is not a trivial issue since it has profound implications for the nature of acute leukemia and indeed for the attempted therapy of the disease. In one well-analyzed myeloid leukemia (the M1 leukemia) it has been demonstrated that relatively stable sub-clones exist in the leukemic population that are capable of essentially normal differentiation when stimulated by GM-CSF (D+ clones).[7] If agar cultures of these myeloblast clones are stimulated by GM-CSF, the cells proliferate to form colonies of progeny cells that not only exhibit the morphology of apparently normal polymorphs or macrophages but also develop a variety of normal membrane and special cytoplasmic proteins. Of greater importance is the fact that, on retransplantation to syngeneic animals, such populations can be shown to have lost their leukemogenicity—that is, their capacity for progressive proliferation and killing the grafted animals.[7] Even with the M1 tumor there are however other sub-clones (D− clones) that can be stimulated to proliferate by GM-CSF but fail to differentiate and remain capable of indefinite proliferation. In another mouse myelomonocytic leukemic model, the WEHI-3 tumor, only a minority of the colony-forming cells appears capable of generating progeny cells that differentiate to nondividing polymorphs or macrophages and while these cells develop some markers and functional activities shown by normal cells of this type, maturation is usually neither complete nor qualitatively normal[5,86] (Metcalf, D., unpublished data).

It must be emphasized that the extensive literature on the M1 and WEHI-3 leukemias in fact relates to the progeny of only two leukemic cells—one originally giving rise to the M1 leukemia and the other to the WEHI-3 tumor. Attempts to grow many other mouse myeloid leukemias *in vitro* have failed. The mouse data must therefore be interpreted with considerable caution as not necessarily being applicable to the leukemic clones present in different AML patients. There may indeed be AML patients with M1 or WEHI-3 type leukemias but equally many leukemic clones may be quite unable to differentiate normally when stimulated by GM-CSF. The real situation in human AML has not yet been documented sufficiently carefully to provide precise information on this question and these data are in urgent need of collection. The initial evidence of continuing abnormal differentiation in most AML cells grown *in vitro* strongly suggests that the dominant leukemic subclones in most patients are of the D-type, and may possess sufficiently severe genetic derangement that they are unlikely ever to be able to exhibit normal differentiation, regardless of the culture conditions.

At the present time cells from possibly a thousand cases of AML have been cultured in agar in various centers and in at least one respect have been shown to exhibit remarkable uniformity. In not a single instance has autonomous proliferation *in vitro* been reported, all proliferating cells being dependent absolutely on stimulation by GM-CSF-containing material.[1,70] Unlike the dependency-autonomy situation in other types of cancer, no progression to autonomy with respect to GM-CSF has been observed as the disease evolves in individual patients and the leukemic population remains dependent until death of the patient. Preliminary data suggest that the dose–response curves of AML cells to stimulation by GM-CSF may not be entirely normal[70] but dependency is absolute.

The practical implications of these questions concern the understanding of what happens during the remarkable phenomenon of remission induction in acute leukemia in which an apparently normal hemopoietic population replaces the pre-existing leukemic population. Are these apparently normal cells the progeny of the leukemic clone, or are they the progeny of normal stem cells that were previously suppressed by the leukemic population?

In patients with karyotypic markers in the leukemic population, studies have indicated that during remission the proliferating marrow cells exhibit a normal karyotype.[87] This suggests strongly that remission is indeed associated with the re-emergence of suppressed normal populations. Do the *in vitro* culture data support this conclusion? Can leukemic cells in fact suppress the proliferation of normal cells and what are the *in vitro* behavior and properties of cells in remission marrow?

Early in the work using agar cultures a number of groups investigated what happens when mixtures of normal and leukemic cells are co-cultured. The initial results failed to document convincing suppression of normal GM-colony formation.[51,77,88] It was noted, however, that where the percentage of blasts in an AML marrow exceeded 20 per cent only subnormal numbers of GM colonies could be grown.[89] A number of studies followed in which significant suppression of proliferation by normal colony cells was observed in mixed cultures of normal and leukemic cells.[90,91] More recent studies have confirmed the occurrence of this suppression and have shown that a high molecular weight factor can be obtained from leukemic but not normal cells which can suppress colony formation and force normal GM-CFC into a non-cycling state.[92,93] Suppression of normal populations *in vivo* is no doubt a much more complex process, presumably also involving suppression in the stem cell compartment and probably interference with the production of regulatory factors by local stromal cells within the marrow. In this context it is of interest that two groups have observed that where stromal production of GM-CSF is normal in marrow or blood populations taken from AML patients in relapse, the probability of them entering remission following chemotherapy is higher than in patients where the capacity to produce GM-CSF is depressed.[80,94]

The *in vitro* data, therefore, support the likelihood that leukemic cells can suppress normal populations by a variety of competitive interactions and would favor the alternative that in remission normal populations regain proliferative ascendency over the leukemic clone.

Direct evidence for the return of normal granulopoietic populations during remission has been obtained from an analysis of the *in vitro* growth patterns of remission marrow samples. When remission marrow cells are cultured, a normal pattern of colony and cluster formation is observed with often an increased frequency of both cluster- and colony-forming cells.[51,89,78] Early return of colony-forming cells following chemotherapy has in fact been shown to be correlated with a high probability of successful remission induction.[78,80] Analysis of such colonies has shown that granulocyte-macrophage and eosinophil colonies are present in normal proportions,[17] that colony cells exhibit normal differentiation,[51,62] that the colony cells exhibit a normal karyotype[72] and that the colony-forming cells have a normal buoyant density and cell cycle status.[51,62] Marrow cells also exhibit a normal capacity to produce CSF.[51,94]

By all these criteria, the granulopoietic populations in most bone marrows in remission are of normal origin. Two qualifications need to be made to this conclusion: (1) in a few patients, the growth pattern in remission cultures continues to exhibit abnormalities similar to those seen in cultures of preleukemic marrow, suggesting that in these patients the re-emergent cells are of preleukemic rather than normal type;[78] and (2) it has been reported that reverse transcriptase of the type found in leukemic cells is present in remission marrow but not in normal marrow cells.[96] The significance of this latter observation remains to be determined but just as in the lymphoid cells of a young AKR mouse, insertion of leukemia virus genome into the chromosome does not necessarily mean that the cells behave phenotypically as leukemic cells,[97] so all hemopoietic cells in a leukemic patient might exhibit viral 'footprints' regardless of whether the population behaves functionally as a normal or leukemic population.

The *in vitro* data strongly support the conclusion that in AML two populations coexist on a competitive basis—normal clones and a leukemic clone. In relapse, the leukemic clone is dominant and in remission the reverse is true. The conclusion does not eliminate completely the possibility that in some patients the leukemic population might also be capable of improved differentiation during remission. However, from the existing data, the latter could not be a quantitatively important source of mature cells and is unlikely in most patients to be the origin of the normal hemopoietic population during remission.

An interesting correlation has been demonstrated between the initial growth pattern of AML cells in culture and the probability of response to chemotherapy, assessed by the occurrence of a remission.[48,49] This correlation varies somewhat according to the time and method of scoring the cultures but can be summarized as follows: (1) patients whose cells fail to proliferate *in vitro* or form small clusters after 7 d of incubation have a better remission rate than patients whose cells either fail to grow or form large clusters. This correlation is seen regardless of the age of the patient; (2) patients whose cells form colonies have a better prospect of remission if such colony-forming cells are of normal buoyant density (? residual normal population), are present in low frequency and/or the ratio of clusters to colonies is normal; (3) patients whose cells form a high frequency of clusters or colonies per 10^5 cells have lower remission rates than patients whose cells form only small numbers of clusters or colonies.[48,49]

As mentioned earlier, appearance of colony-forming cells early after the initiation of chemotherapy has also been observed to correlate with a high probability of remission induction.[95]

It is not clear why these correlations exist between growth patterns and remission inducibility. The ability of proliferating AML cells *in vitro* to form clusters of only limited size may reflect a genuine restriction in the capacity of such cells for extended proliferation but this apparent restriction could well be a misleading *in vitro* artefact consequent on the use of suboptimal media. This reservation finds some support in the observation by Park et al[82] that, if cultures are re-fed, clusters can continue to proliferate and generate large colonies. Similar comments could be made regarding the apparent frequency of cluster- or colony-forming cells in an AML population. On the other hand, the favorable prognosis associated with the initial presence of normal colony-forming cells may be due to the cultures identifying patients in whom the leukemic clone never achieved total dominance over normal granulopoietic populations. In such patients it could be anticipated that a competitive rebound of normal populations could occur more readily following chemotherapy than in patients lacking detectable precursor cells.

Whatever the basis for the observed correlations, initial agar cultures of pretreatment AML patients are, in addition to age, an important prognostic factor in assessing the likelihood of remission induction. The ability to identify poor risk patients has little practical importance at present but should alternative forms of treatment develop, e.g. immunotherapy, bone marrow transplantation or regulator therapy, the identification of such poor risk patients could become an important factor in determining the early use of alternative therapy.

ROLE OF GM-CSF IN MYELOID LEUKEMIA DEVELOPMENT

It is well established from studies on carcinogenesis that prolonged imbalance in regulator control systems resulting in chronic excess stimulation of target cell populations ultimately can lead to, or permit, the emergence of cancer clones in the stimulated populations.[98]

Transfer of this concept to the problem of myeloid leukemia development leads to the conclusion that GM-CSF is likely to be involved both in the emergence of the leukemic clone and its progressive proliferation. *In vitro* data indicate clearly that all myeloid leukemic populations in man are GM-CSF-dependent. This makes it likely that the proliferation of leukemic cells *in vivo* is also completely GM-CSF-dependent and, if so, GM-CSF would represent an essential cofactor in leukemogenesis. However, GM-CSF has a second action on myeloid cells—that of forcing or permitting differentiation to post-mitotic end cells. Observation of the behavior of CML cells *in vitro* and of the two mouse myeloid leukemia models (M1 and WEHI-3) has indicated that GM-CSF has a comparable action on myeloid leukemic cells, leading to the formation of morphologically mature cells. Tests on these differentiated mouse leukemic populations have shown that they exhibit a restricted or no capacity for producing leukemia on transplantation to syngeneic recipients.[7]

The influence of GM-CSF on the *progressive* proliferation of a leukemic clone is therefore likely to be quite complex and to depend heavily on whether the clone is capable of differentiation under the action of GM-CSF (D+ clone) or is only partially responsive or unresponsive (D− clone).

Recent experiments in this laboratory have given a clear indication of the complexities possible in the relationships between GM-CSF and leukemic cells. Starting with a cloned line of WEHI-3 cells some members of which were capable of differentiation, others not, it was possible to produce individual subclones in which virtually all or none of the members of the subclone were capable of differentiation. The original cloned WEHI-3 leukemic cells have been maintained in continuous *in vitro* culture for more than 5 years in the absence of added CSF, although the situation is complex because the leukemic cells themselves are able of synthesizing significant concentrations of GM-CSF.[5] For whatever reason, the proliferation of WEHI-3 colonies in agar is now almost independent of GM-CSF, but the *differentiation* of the leukemic cells remains GM-CSF-dependent.

As a consequence of these current properties of the WEHI-3 primary clone, serial recloning of agar colonies of WEHI-3 cells has shown that while individual subclones can be forced to differentiate to extinction as proliferating cell populations, other clones can continue to generate so many undifferentiated progeny that the total content of clonogenic cells continues to increase exponentially even when the cells are grown in the continuous presence of GM-CSF.

It remains to be determined what exact situation is present in emerging myeloid leukemic clones in man. All 'successful' leukemic clones (i.e. clones capable of producing progressive leukemia) in man appear to be growth-dependent on GM-CSF. In theory therefore, removal of GM-CSF should uniformly arrest the progressive proliferation of the leukemic clone. However, this is not a practicable option since normal GM populations are also GM-CSF-dependent and a GM-CSF-depleted patient would be defenseless against bacterial infections.

Although CML clones appear to respond uniformly to the differentiating effects of GM-CSF, the situation could well be similar to the above WEHI-3 model, where despite the impressive induction of differentiation, expanding numbers of leukemic stem cells develop. Increase of GM-CSF concentrations in such a patient would not appear to be able to suppress the leukemic population.

The situation in many potentially preleukemic subjects is even less certain. It may be that in many such persons, leukemic clones arise that are wholly responsive to the differentiating effects of GM-CSF and the clones are extinguished by regulator action. Those subjects in whom a progressively proliferating clone emerges and causes clinical disease could in fact be a small minority of persons in whom leukemic clones are initiated.

Several observations suggest that an ability to produce high GM-CSF levels may commonly prevent or suppress temporarily the progressive proliferation of emerging leukemic clones. It has been observed in patients with myeloproliferative disorders that are potentially leukemic that a capacity of bone marrow or peripheral blood cells to produce high levels of GM-CSF *in vitro* is associated with a relatively low frequency of leukemia development.[99] Similarly, a correlation has been observed in AML patients between the capacity to produce

GM-CSF and the likelihood of entering a sustained remission following chemotherapy.[80,94]

On the other hand, indirect evidence from mice suggests strongly that GM-CSF is necessary for the emergence of myeloid leukemic populations. Whole-body irradiation leads to the activation of latent leukemogenic viruses[100] and in Rf mice causes the development of myeloid leukemia. However, irradiation of germfree Rf mice does not lead to myeloid leukemia development, although such mice will subsequently develop leukemia if conventionalized, i.e. infected with microorganisms.[101] Parallel studies have shown that whole-body irradiation elevates serum GM-CSF levels[102,103] but not in germfree mice.[104] Irradiated germfree mice, exposed subsequently to Gram-negative organisms, will develop elevated GM-CSF levels,[105] due presumably to endotoxin-mediated stimulation of GM-CSF production.[106,107] These observations suggest strongly that GM-CSF is a necessary cofactor in the emergence of viral-altered granulopoietic cells as leukemic populations.

From the above discussion it is clear that precise information is needed regarding GM-CSF levels in serum and tissues prior to and during AML development. While this information should in theory be readily available by use of agar cultures of marrow cells as the bioassay system, considerable difficulties exist. GM-CSF is produced in many, perhaps all, tissues.[1] While GM-CSF levels can be monitored in the serum and urine, these do not necessarily give an accurate picture of the levels impinging on target granulopoietic cells in the marrow. Studies in mice have shown that bone marrow stromal production of GM-CSF is an important process that selectively fluctuates during hemopoietic regeneration without comparable detectable fluctuations in GM-CSF levels in the serum or other tissues.[108,109] In addition, the ability of a tissue to produce GM-CSF *in vitro* may not accurately reflect the activity of that tissue *in vivo*. Most studies to date have sought to determine GM-CSF levels in the serum and urine and GM-CSF production by peripheral blood or marrow cells as a first approach to this problem.

A technical problem has also complicated the bioassay of human GM-CSF levels. Initial studies on GM-CSF levels were performed using mouse marrow target cells on the basis that uniform populations of target cells are available from inbred mice and that mouse cells respond to stimulation by human GM-CSF.[110,111] However, other workers objected that the use of target cells from a foreign species might produce misleading estimates of GM-CSF levels and indeed parallel assays of human sera on mouse and human target cells produced discordant estimates.[112,113] Subsequent studies have shown that the ability of human serum to stimulate colony formation in cultures of unfractionated human marrow cells in largely due to an indirect action of the serum in promoting production of GM-CSF by the marrow cells in the culture dish itself.[114,115] This promoting factor is not GM-CSF and presumably for this reason, anti-GM-CSF sera do not completely suppress colony formation in 'serum-stimulated' human cultures, unlike the situation in mouse cultures where essentially no endogenous GM-CSF production occurs.[113] More recent studies have employed non-adherent human marrow cells as the assay system but the data obtained are not yet very extensive.

With the above reservations concerning the validity of some of the published data, the existing information can be summarized as follows:

1. Mouse marrow assays

In an early study, urine CSF levels were reported to be low or absent in the majority of AML patients prior to treatment or in relapse, levels returning to normal after remission induction.[116] In other studies serum and urine GM-CSF levels were found to be elevated for varying periods in most patients with AML and CML often, but not exclusively, during episodes of secondary infection.[111] Serum and urine GM-CSF levels were also often elevated in patients with myeloproliferative disorders, GM-CSF levels being exceptionally high in the serum of patients with CML or myelofibrosis.[1,117] No differences were observed in GM-CSF levels in relapse versus remission AML patients, excluding the frequent periods during which relapse patients were suffering apparent infections.

Level of serum inhibitors to GM-CSF were abnormally low or absent in one half of patients with AML and in patients with CML in acute transformation.[111]

Using dog marrow cells as the bioassay system, cyclic fluctuations in plasma GM-CSF levels were reported in a patient with CML associated with cyclic fluctuations in peripheral white cell levels.[118]

2. Human marrow assays

Production of GM-CSF by human peripheral blood cells was abnormally low in AML patients who subsequently exhibited poor responses to therapy[80] or in myeloproliferative patients who subsequently progressed to AML.[94] Marrow stromal production of GM-CSF was subnormal in the same two groups of patients.

Serum capacity to stimulate colony formation was claimed to be higher than normal in patients with CML or chronic lymphoid leukemia but to be normal or subnormal in the serum of patients with AML.[119] This was not confirmed in other studies. Mangalik and Robinson[120] found that the addition of AML sera to cultures of normal or leukemic marrow did not alter the number of colonies stimulated by standard peripheral blood underlayers. Serum levels of GM-CSF were found to be highly variable in patients with myeloid leukemia.[112,113]

Initial reports suggested that the peripheral blood cells from patients with AML had a decreased capacity to stimulate GM colony formation.[38,77] However, other studies reported that in some cases colony stimulating activity was normal.[40,80,122,123] The basis for this variability may well depend on the morphological subtype of leukemia involved and on the level of monocytes in the peripheral blood. The capacity of peripheral blood cells to produce GM-CSF or act as feeder layers has been found to vary in a predictable fashion in leukemic patients according to the presence or absence of monocytes in the peripheral blood. Where blood monocytes were low, e.g. in acute myeloblastic leukemia, low activity was found whereas in acute monocytic leukemia, activity was often high.[124,125] However, in one other study no correlation was observed between the capacity of peripheral blood cells to stimulate colony formation and their content of monocytes.[80] It is unclear from the present data how frequently the leukemic cells themselves are a significant source of GM-CSF.

The capacity of peripheral blood cells from leukemic patients to stimulate colony formation was relatively resistant to chemotherapy and was not significantly depressed by chemotherapy, in contrast to the sharp fall in colony-forming cell levels.[80] In AML patients with full clinical remission following chemotherapy, the colony stimulating activity of peripheral blood cells was found to be normal.[40,51,77]

From the above review of published data it is not possible to present a simple summary statement regarding GM-CSF levels in patients prior to or following leukemia development. However, despite the inconsistencies in the present data, it is evident that abnormal levels of GM-CSF are often present and the role played by this regulator in myeloid leukemia development is in urgent need of more detailed investigation.

CONCLUSIONS

The introduction of semisolid culture technics has revolutionized cellular hematology and has led not only to the identification and enumeration of the various types of hemopoietic precursor cells but also to the characterization of at least some of the humoral regulators controlling proliferation and differentiation in hemopoietic cells.

The impact of semisolid culture technology has been equally dramatic on the analysis of the nature of myeloid leukemia. The present cloning methods offer substantial improvements in the capacity to diagnose and monitor responses to therapy in myeloid leukemia. Of major importance has been the discovery that myeloid leukemic populations remain dependent on regulator control, offering the future possibility of more sophisticated control measures for suppressing the proliferation of leukemic populations.

Acknowledgments

The work from the author's laboratory referred to in this review was supported by grants from the Anti-Cancer Council of Victoria, The National Health and Medical Research Council, Canberra and The National Cancer Institute, Bethesda.

REFERENCES

1 Metcalf D 1977 Hemopoietic Colonies: In Vitro Cloning of Normal and Leukemic Cells. Springer-Verlag, Berlin
2 Bradley T R, Metcalf D 1966 The growth of mouse bone marrow cells in vitro. Australian Journal of Experimental Biology and Medical Science 44: 287–300
3 Ichikawa Y, Pluznik D H, Sachs L 1966 In vitro control of the development of macrophage and granulocyte colonies. Proceedings of the National Academy of Sciences (USA) 56: 488–495
4 Moore M A S, Williams N, Metcalf D 1972 Purification and characterisation of the in vitro colony forming cells in monkey hemopoietic tissue. Journal of Cellular Physiology 79: 283–292

5 Metcalf D, Moore M A S, Warner N L 1969 Colony formation in vitro by myelomonocytic leukemic cells. Journal of the National Cancer Institute 43: 983–1001

6 Ichikawa Y 1964 Differentiation of a cell line of myeloid leukemia. Journal of Cellular Physiology 74: 223–234

7 Sachs L 1978 Control of normal cell differentiation and the phenotypic reversion of malignancy in myeloid leukemia. Nature 274: 535–539

8 Pike B, Robinson W A 1970 Human bone marrow colony growth in agar gel. Journal of Cellular Physiology 76: 77–84

9 Moore M A S, Williams N 1972 Physical separation of colony stimulating from in vitro colony-forming cells in hemopoietic tissue. Journal of Cellular Physiology 80: 195–206

10 Golde D W, Cline M J 1972 Identification of the colony-stimulating cell in human peripheral blood. Journal of Clinical Investigation 52: 2981–2983

11 Chervenick P A, Lo Buglio A F 1972 Human blood monocytes: Stimulation of granulocyte and mononuclear formation in vitro. Science 178: 164–166

12 Iscove N N, Senn J S, Till J E, McCulloch E A 1971 Colony formation by normal and leukemic human marrow cells in culture. Effect of conditioned medium from human leukocytes. Blood 37: 1–5

13 Chervenick P A, Boggs D R 1971 In vitro growth of granulocytic and mononuclear colonies from blood of normal individuals. Blood 37: 131–135

14 Shoham D, Ben David E, Rozenszajn L A 1974 Cytochemical and morphological identification of macrophages and eosinophils in tissue cultures of normal human bone marrow. Blood 44: 221–233

15 Parmley R T, Ogawa M, Spicer S G, Wright N J 1976 Ultrastructure and cytochemistry of human bone marrow granulocytes in culture. Experimental Hematology 4: 75–89

16 Dao C, Metcalf D, Bilski-Pasquier G 1977 Eosinophil and neutrophil colony-forming cells in culture. Blood 50: 833–839

17 Dresch C, Johnson G R, Metcalf D 1977 Eosinophil colony formation in semisolid cultures of human bone marrow cells. Blood 49: 835–844

18 Stephenson J R, Axelrad A A, McLeod D L, Shreeve M M 1971 Induction of colonies of hemoglobin-synthesizing cells by erythropoietin in vitro. Proceedings of the National Academy of Sciences (USA) 68: 1542–1546

19 Heath D S, Axelrad A A, McLeod D L, Shreeve M M 1976 Separation of the erythropoietin-responsive progenitors BFU-E and CFU-E in mouse marrow by unit gravity sedimentation. Blood 47: 777–792

20 Tepperman A D, Curtis J E, McCulloch E A 1974 Erythropoietic colonies in cultures of human marrow. Blood 44: 659–669

21 Metcalf D, Parker J, Chester H M, Kincade P M 1974 Formation of eosinophilic-like granulocytic colonies by mouse bone marrow cells in vitro. Journal of Cellular Physiology 84: 275–290

22 Metcalf D, MacDonald H R, Odartchenko N, Sordat B 1975 Growth of mouse megakaryocyte colonies in vitro. Proceedings of the National Academy of Sciences (USA) 72: 1744–1748

23 Johnson G R, Metcalf D 1977 Pure and mixed erythroid colony formation in vitro stimulated by spleen conditioned medium with no detectable erythropoietin. Proceedings of the National Academy of Sciences (USA) 74: 3879–3882

24 Fauser A A, Messner H A 1978 Granuloerythropoietic colonies in human bone marrow, peripheral blood and cord blood. Blood 52: 1243–1248

25 McLeod D L, Shreeve M M, Axelrad A A 1976 Induction of megakaryocyte colonies with platelet formation in vitro. Nature 261: 492–494

26 Metcalf D, Nossal G J V, Warner N L, Miller J F A P, Mandel T E, Layton J E, Gutman G A 1975 Growth of B-lymphocyte colonies in vitro. Journal of Experimental Medicine 142: 1534–1549

27 Rozenszajn L A, Shoham D, Kalechman I 1975 Clonal proliferation of PHA-stimulated human lymphocytes in soft agar culture. Immunology 29: 1041–1055

28 Claesson M H, Rodger M B, Johnson G R, Whittingham S, Metcalf D 1977 Colony formation by human T lymphocytes in agar medium. Clinical and Experimental Immunology 28: 526–534

29 Yamamoto N, Hinuma Y 1976 Clonal transformation of human leukocytes by Epstein-Barr virus in soft agar. International Journal of Cancer 17: 191–196

30 Hamburger A W, Salmon S E 1977 Primary bioassay of human myeloma stem cells. Journal of Clinical Investigation 60: 846–854

31 Metcalf D 1974 The serum factor stimulating colony formation in vitro by murine

plasmacytoma cells. Response to antigens and mineral oil. Journal of Immunology 113: 235–243

32 Guilbert L J, Iscove N N 1976 Partial replacement of serum by selenite, transferrin, albumin and lecithin in haemopoietic cell cultures. Nature 263: 594–595

33 Bradley T R, Hodgson G S, Rosendaal M 1978 The effect of oxygen tension on hemopoietic and fibroblast cell proliferation in vitro. Journal of Cellular Physiology 97: 517–522

34 Heit W, Kern P, Kubanek B, Heimpel H 1974 Some factors influencing granulocyte colony formation in vitro by human white blood cells. Blood 44: 511–515

35 Entringer M A, Robinson W A, Kurnick J E 1977 Colony growth of normal human bone marrow in agar gel. Experimental Hematology 5: 125–135

36 Broxmeyer H E, Moore M A S, Ralph P 1977 Cell-free granulocyte colony inhibiting activity derived from human polymorphonuclear neutrophils. Experimental Hematology 5: 87–102

37 Broxmeyer H E, Baker F L, Galbraith P R 1976 In vitro regulation of granulopoiesis in human leukemia. Application of an assay for colony-inhibiting cells. Blood 47: 389–402

38 Messner H A, Till J E, McCulloch E A 1973 Interacting cell populations affecting granulopoietic colony formation by normal and leukemic human marrow cells. Blood 42: 701–710

39 Lundgren G, Zukoski Ch F, Moller G 1968 Differential effects of human granulocytes and lymphocytes on human fibroblasts in vitro. Clinical and Experimental Immunology 3: 817–836

40 Moore M A S, Williams N, Metcalf D 1973 In vitro colony formation by normal and leukemic human hemopoietic cells. Interactions between colony-forming and colony-stimulating cells. Journal of the National Cancer Institute 50: 591–602

41 Chervenick P A, Boggs D R 1970 Bone marrow colonies. Stimulation in vitro by supernatant from incubated human blood cells. Science 169: 691–692

42 Paran M, Sachs L, Barak Y, Resnitsky P 1970 In vitro induction of granulocyte differentiation in hematopoietic cells from leukemic and non-leukemic patients. Proceedings of the National Academy of Science (USA) 67: 1542–1549

43 Cline M J, Golde D W 1974 Production of colony-stimulating activity by human lymphocytes. Nature 248: 703–704

44 Prival J T, Paran M, Gallo R C, Wu A M 1974 Colony-stimulating factors in cultures of human peripheral blood cells. Journal of the National Cancer Institute 53: 1583–1588

45 Shah R G, Caporale L H, Moore M A S 1977 Characterization of colony-stimulating activity produced by human monocytes and phytohemagglutinin-stimulated lymphocytes. Blood 50: 811–821

46 Burgess A W, Wilson E, Metcalf D 1977 Stimulation by human placental conditioned medium of hemopoietic colony formation by human marrow cells. Blood 49: 573–583

47 Nicola N A, Metcalf D, Johnson G R, Burgess A W 1978 Preparation of colony stimulating factors from human placental conditioned medium. Leukemia Research 2: 313–320

48 Johnson G R, Dresch C, Metcalf D 1977 Heterogeneity in human neutrophil, macrophage and eosinophil progenitor cells demonstrated by velocity sedimentation separation. Blood 50: 823–831

49 Moore M A S, Spitzer G, Williams N, Metcalf D, Buckley J 1974 Agar culture studies in 127 cases of untreated acute leukemia: The prognostic value of reclassification of leukemia according to in vitro growth characteristics. Blood 44: 1–18

50 Spitzer G, Dicke K A, Gehan E A, Smith T, McCredie K B, Barlogie B, Freireich E J 1976 A simplified in vitro classification for prognosis in adult acute leukemia: The application of in vitro results in remission—predictive models. Blood 48: 795–807

51 Moore M A S, Williams N, Metcalf D 1973 In vitro colony formation by normal and leukemic human hematopoietic cells. Characterisation of the colony-forming cells. Journal of the National Cancer Institute 50: 603–623

52 Miller R G, Phillips R A 1969 Separation of cells by velocity sedimentation. Journal of Cellular Physiology 73: 191–201

53 Metcalf D, MacDonald H R 1975 Heterogeneity of in vitro colony- and cluster-forming cells in the mouse marrow. Segregation by velocity sedimentation. Journal of Cellular Physiology 85: 643–654

54 Metcalf D, Moore M A S, Shortman K 1971 Adherence column and buoyant density separation of bone marrow stem cells and more differentiated cells. Journal of Cellular Physiology 78: 441–450

55 Nicola N A, Burgess A W, Metcalf D, Battye F L 1978 Separation of mouse bone marrow

cells using wheat germ agglutinin affinity chromatography. Australian Journal of Experimental Biology and Medical Science 56: 663–679

56 Iscove N N, Till J E, McCulloch E A 1970 The proliferative states of mouse granulopoietic progenitor cells. Proceedings of the Society of Experimental Biology 134: 33–36

57 Sinclair W K 1967 Hydroxyurea. Effects on Chinese hamster cells grown in culture. Cancer Research 27: 297–308

58 Salmon S E, Hamburger A W, Soehnlen B, Durie B G M, Alberts D S, Moon T E 1978 Quantitation of differential sensitivity of human tumor stem cells to anti-cancer drugs. New England Journal of Medicine 298: 1321–1327

59 Dicke K A, Spitzer G, Ahearn M J 1976 Colony formation in vitro by leukaemic cells in acute myelogenous leukemia with phytohaemagglutinin as stimulating factor. Nature 259: 129–130

60 Dicke K A, Spitzer G, Cork A, Ahearn M J 1976 In vitro colony growth of acute myelogenous leukemia. Blood Cells 2: 125–137

61 Minden M D, Till J E, McCulloch E A 1978 Proliferative state of blast cell progenitors in acute myeloblastic leukemia (AML). Blood 52: 592–600

62 Moore M A S 1975 In vitro studies in the myeloid leukemias. In: Cleton F J, Crowther D, Malpas J B (eds) Advances in Acute Leukemia North-Holland, Amsterdam, pp 161–227

63 Shadduck R K, Nankin H R 1971 Cellular origin of granulocytic colonies in chronic myeloid leukemia. Lancet ii: 1097–1098

64 Brown C H, Carbone P P 1971 In vitro growth of normal and leukemic human bone marrow. Journal of the National Cancer Institute 46: 989–1000

65 Goldman J M, Th'ng K H, Lowenthal R M 1974 In vitro colony-forming cells and colony stimulating activity in chronic granulocytic leukaemia. British Journal of Cancer 30: 1–12

66 Moberg C, Olofsson T, Olsson I 1974 Granulopoiesis in chronic myeloid leukaemia. I. In vitro cloning of blood and bone marrow cells in agar culture. Scandinavian Journal of Haematology 12: 381–390

67 Berthier R, Douady F, Holland D 1977 Cellular factors regulating granulopoiesis in myeloid leukemia. Blood Cells 3: 461–474

68 Metcalf D, Johnson G R, Kolber S, Dresch C 1978 Clonal analysis of chronic myeloid leukemic cells using agar cultures. In: Bentvelson P (ed) Advances in Comparative Leukemia Research 1977. Elsevier/North-Holland Biomedical Press, Amsterdam, pp 307–310

69 Moore M A S, Williams N 1973 Functional, morphologic and kinetic analysis of the granulocyte-macrophage progenitor cell. In: Robinson W A (ed) Hemopoiesis in Culture. DHEW Publication No. 74–205. Washington, pp 17–27

70 Metcalf D, Moore M A S, Sheridan J W, Spitzer G 1974 Responsiveness of human granulocytic leukemic cells to colony stimulating factor. Blood 43: 847–859

71 Duttera M J, Whang-Peng J, Bull J M L, Carbone P P 1972 Cytogenetically abnormal cells in vitro in acute leukaemia. Lancet i: 715–718

72 Moore M A S, Metcalf D 1978 Cytogenetic analysis of human acute and chronic myeloid leukemic cells cloned in agar culture. International Journal of Cancer 11: 143–152

73 Aye M T, Till J E, McCulloch E A 1973 Cytological studies of granulopoietic colonies from two patients with chronic myelogenous leukemia. Experimental Hematology 1: 115–118

74 Olofsson T, Olsson I 1976 Granulopoiesis in chronic myeloid leukemia. II. Serial cloning of blood and bone marrow cells in agar culture. Blood 48: 351–360

75 Moore M A S 1975 Marrow culture—a new approach to classification of leukemias. In: Bessis B, Brecher G (eds) Unclassifiable leukemias. Springer-Verlag, Berlin, pp 149–158

76 Spitzer G, Schwartz M A, Dicke K A, Trujillo J M, McCredie K B 1976 Significance of PHA-induced clonogenic cells in chronic myeloid leukemia and early acute myeloid leukemia. Blood Cells 2: 149–159

77 Greenberg P L, Nichols W, Schrier S L 1971 Granulopoiesis in acute myeloid leukemia and preleukemia. New England Journal of Medicine 284: 1225–1232

78 Vincent P C, Sutherland R, Bradley M, Lind D, Gunz F W 1977 Marrow culture studies in adult acute leukemia at presentation and during remission. Blood 49: 903–912

79 Senn J S, McCulloch E A, Till J E 1967 Comparison of colony-forming ability of normal and leukaemic human marrow in cell culture. Lancet ii: 597–598

80 Hornsten P, Granstrom M, Wahren B, Gharton G 1977 Prognostic value of colony-stimulating and colony-forming cells in peripheral blood in acute non-lymphoblastic leukemia. Acta Medica Scandinavica 201; 405–410

81 Moore M A S, Spitzer G R 1974 In vitro studies in the myeloproliferative disorders. In: Lindahl-Kiessling K, Osoba D (eds) Lymphocyte recognition and effector mechanisms. Academic Press, New York, pp 431–437

82 Park C H, Savin M A, Hoogstraten B, Amare M, Hathaway P 1977 Improved growth of in vitro colonies in human acute leukemia with the feeding culture method. Cancer Research 37: 4595–4601

83 Till J E, Lan S, Buick R N, Sousan P, Curtis J E, McCulloch E A 1978 Approaches to the evaluation of human hemopoietic stem cell function. In: Clarkson B, Marks P A, Till J E (eds) Differentiation of normal and neoplastic hematopoietic cells. Cold Spring Harbor Laboratory, New York, pp 81–92

84 Aye M T, Till J E, McCulloch E A 1974 Cytological studies of colonies in culture derived from the peripheral blood of cells of two patients with acute leukemia. Experimental Hematology 2: 362–371

85 McCulloch E A, Buick R N, Minden M D, Izaguirre C A 1978 Differentiation programmes underlying cellular heterogeneity in the myeloblastic leukemias of man. In: Golde D W, Cline M J, Metcalf D, Fox C F (eds) Hematopoietic Cell Differentiation. Academic Press, New York, pp 317–333

86 Cline M J, Metcalf D 1972 Cellular differentiation in a murine myelomonocytic leukemia. Blood 39: 771–777

87 Rowley J D 1978 The cytogenetics of acute leukemia. Clinics in Haematology 7: 385–406

88 Robinson W A, Kurnick J E and Pike B L 1971 Colony growth of human leukemic peripheral blood cells in vitro. Blood 38: 500–508

89 Bull J M, Duttera M J, Stashick E D, Northrup J, Henderson E, Carbone P P 1973 Serial in vitro marrow culture in acute myelomonocytic leukemia. Blood 42: 679–686

90 Morris T C M, McNeill T A, Bridges J M 1975 Inhibition of normal human in vitro colony forming cells by cells from leukaemic patients. British Journal of Cancer 31: 641–648

91 Chiyoda S, Mizoguchi H, Kosaka K, Takaku F, Miura Y 1975 Influence of leukaemic cells on the colony formation of human bone marrow cells in vitro. British Journal of Cancer 31: 355–358

92 Chiyoda S, Mizoguchi H, Asano S, Takaku F, Miura Y 1976 Influence of leukaemic cells on the colony formation of human bone marrow cells in vitro. II. Suppressive effects of leukaemic cell extracts. British Journal of Cancer 33: 379–384

93 Broxmeyer H E, Jacobsen N, Kurland J, Mendelsohn N, Moore M A S 1978 In vitro suppression of normal granulocytic stem cells by inhibitory activity derived from human leukemic cells. Journal of the National Cancer Institute 60: 497–511

94 Greenberg P, Mura B 1978 Microenvironmental influences on granulopoiesis in acute myeloid leukemia. In: Clarkson B, Marks P A, Till J E (eds) Differentiation of Normal and Neoplastic Hematopoietic Cells. Cold Spring Harbor Laboratory, New York, pp 405–409

95 Spitzer G, Dicke K A, McCredie K B, Barlogie B 1977 The early detection of remission in acute myelogenous leukaemia by in vitro cultures. British Journal of Haematology 35: 411–418

96 Mak T W, Aye M T, Messner H A, Sheinin R, Till J E, McCulloch E A 1974 Reverse transcriptase activity. Increase in marrow cultures from leukemic patients in relapse and remission. British Journal of Cancer 29: 433–437

97 Rowe W P 1973 Genetic factors in the natural history of murine leukemia virus infection. Cancer Research 33: 3061–3068

98 Furth J 1953 Conditioned and autonomous neoplasms. Cancer Research 13: 477–492

99 Dicke K A, Lowenberg B 1975 In vitro analysis of pancytopenia. Its relevance to the clinic. In: Fliedner T M, Perry S (eds) Advances in Biosciences 14. Permagon Press, Vieweg. pp 259–270

100 Kaplan H S 1967 On the natural history of the murine leukemias. Cancer Research 27: 1325–1340

101 Upton A C, Jenkins V K, Walberg H E, Tyndall R L, Conklin J W, Wald N 1966 Observations on viral, chemical and radiation-induced myeloid and lymphoid leukemias in RF mice. Journal of the National Cancer Institute. Monograph 22: 329–345

102 Hall B M 1969 The effects of whole-body irradiation on serum colony-stimulating factor and in vitro colony-forming cells in the marrow. British Journal of Haematology. 17: 553–561

103 Morley A A, Rickard K A, Howard D, Stohlman F 1971 Studies on the regulation of granulopoiesis. VI. Possible humoral regulation. Blood 37: 14–22

104 Morley A A, Quesenberry P J, Bealmear P, Stohlman F, Wilson R 1972 Serum colony stimulating factor levels in irradiated germfree and conventional CFW mice. Proceedings of the Society of Experimental Biology New York 140: 478–480

105 Chang C F, Pollard M 1973 Effects of microbial flora on levels of colony stimulating factor in serum of irradiated CFW mice. Proceedings of the Society of Experimental Biology New York 144: 177–180

106 Metcalf D 1971 Acute antigen-induced elevation of serum colony stimulating factor (CSF) levels. Immunology 21: 427–436
107 Quesenberry P J, Morley A, Stohlman F, Rickard K, Howard D, Smith M 1972 Effect of endotoxin on granulopoiesis and colony stimulating factor. New England Journal of Medicine 286: 227–232
108 Chan S H, Metcalf D 1972 Local production of colony stimulating factor within the bone marrow. Role of non-hematopoietic cells. Blood 40: 646–653
109 Chan S H, Metcalf D 1973 Local and systemic control of granulocytic and macrophage progenitor cell regeneration after irradiation. Cell Tissue Kinetics 6: 185–197
110 Foster R, Metcalf D, Robinson W A, Bradley T R 1968 Bone marrow colony stimulating activity in human sera. British Journal of Haematology 15: 147–159
111 Metcalf D, Chan S H, Gunz F W, Vincent P, Ravich R B M 1971 Colony stimulating factor and inhibitor levels in acute granulocytic leukemia. Blood 38: 143–152
112 Lind D E, Bradley M L, Gunz F W, Vincent P C 1974 The non-equivalence of mouse and human marrow culture in assay of granulopoietic stimulating factors. Journal of Cellular Physiology 83: 35–42
113 Metcalf D 1974 Stimulation by human urine or plasma of granulopoiesis by human marrow cells in agar. Experimental Hematology 2: 157–173
114 Furusawa S, Komatsu H, Saito K, Enokihara H, Hirose K, Shishido H 1978 Effect of normal human serum on granulocyte colony formation by human bone marrow cells. Journal of Laboratory and Clinical Medicine 91: 377–386
115 Knudtzon S 1974 Growth stimulation of normal bone marrow cells in agar culture by human serum. Scandinavian Journal of Haematology 12: 298–306
116 Robinson W A, Pike B L 1970 Leukopoietic activity in human urine. The granulocytic leukemias. New England Journal of Medicine 282: 1291–1297
117 Metcalf D, Moore M A S 1975 Growth and responsiveness of human granulocytic leukemic cells in vitro. In: Ito Y, Dutcher R M (eds) Comparative Leukemia Research 1973 University of Tokyo Press, Tokyo/Karger Basel, pp 235–241
118 Chikkappa G, Bomer G, Burlington H, Chanana A D, Cronkite E P, Ohl S, Pavelec M, Robertson J S 1976 Periodic oscillations of blood leukocytes, platelets and reticulocytes in a patient with chronic myelocytic leukemia. Blood 47: 1023–1030
119 Mintz U, Sachs L 1973 Differences in inducing activity for human bone marrow colonies in normal serum and serum from patients with leukemia. Blood 42: 331–339
120 Mangalik A, Robinson W A 1972 The effect of serum from patients with acute granulocytic leukemia on granulocyte colony formation in vitro: A search for inhibitors. Proceedings of the Society of Experimental Medicine 141: 515–518
121 Lowenberg B, Hagemeijer A 1977 Colony formation of human acute myeloid leukemic cells in vitro. In: Bentvelsen P, Hilgers J, Yohn D S (eds) Advances in Comparative Leukemia Research 1977. Elsevier/North-Holland, Amsterdam, pp 274–277
122 Aye M T, Till J E, McCulloch E A 1975 Interacting populations affecting proliferation of leukemic cells in culture. Blood 45: 485–493
123 Granstrom M, Gahrton G 1974 Colony-forming and colony-stimulating cells in relation to prognosis in leukemia. Acta Medica Scandinavica 196: 221–226
124 Golde D W, Rothman B, Cline M J 1974 Production of colony-stimulating factor by malignant leukocytes. Blood 43: 749–756
125 Goldman J M, Th'ng K H, Catovsky D, Galton D A G 1973 Production of colony-stimulating factor by leukemic leukocytes. Blood 47: 381–388

9
Glucocorticoid Receptors

Gerald R. Crabtree   Kendall A. Smith   Allan Munck

INTRODUCTION

Glucocorticoids are used in the treatment of virtually all lymphoid malignancies and are included in several chemotherapy protocols for adult and childhood non-lymphocytic leukemia. Several early studies in which glucocorticoids were used alone indicated that some cases of acute lymphocytic leukemia (ALL) and perhaps 50 per cent of non-Hodgkin's lymphomas are insensitive to glucocorticoids.[1-10] Furthermore, it is known that among patients with non-lymphocytic leukemia, there are some whose disease is accelerated by glucocorticoid treatment.[11] These findings, and the toxic side effects of steroid therapy, have prompted several investigators to look for methods of predicting clinical response to glucocorticoids.

The success of estrogen receptor determinations in predicting response to hormonal manipulation in breast cancer suggested that an analogous correlation would be found with hematopoietic malignancies and glucocorticoid receptors. Initial investigations in which glucocorticoid receptors were measured by means of cytosol assays of the type developed for estrogen receptors showed that white blood cells from patients with acute myelocytic leukemia,[12,13] ALL which was unresponsive to chemotherapy,[14,15] chronic lymphocytic leukemia,[13] and lymphocytes from normal humans[14,15] contained few or no receptors. On the other hand, cells from patients with untreated ALL[13,14,15] contained large numbers of glucocorticoid receptors.

Subsequent studies with whole cell assays of the type to be described in this chapter, however, have cast serious doubt on the validity of cytosol assays. These studies show that cells from virtually all patients and normal individuals have significant numbers of receptors.[16-27] Such correlations as may emerge between receptor levels and response are therefore unlikely to be of a simple all-or-none type. This chapter describes those properties of glucocorticoid receptors that are important for the assay of these substances in malignant and normal cells, and details a general technic for measurement of glucocorticoid receptors.

PRINCIPLES OF MEASURING GLUCOCORTICOID RECEPTORS

A general definition of a receptor R is that it is a molecule or group of molecules that interacts with a hormone H through specific binding sites to form a hormone-receptor complex HR, which, in turn, mediates the events in the cell that ultimately are amplified into physiologically recognizable effects of the hormone.[28]

At present, all assays of glucocorticoid receptors determine the amount of tritium-labeled glucocorticoid that is bound under various conditions to the specific binding sites. What is measured, therefore, is hormone binding sites, not receptor molecules or receptor proteins for which immunoassays will no doubt eventually become available. Binding of glucocorticoids to these sites can be represented by the simple reaction:

$$H + R \rightleftharpoons HR$$

For such a reaction the association constant K_a, which gives a direct measure of affinity, is equal to the ratio of the concentration of reactants at equilibrium:

$$K_a = \frac{[HR]}{[H][R]}$$

Brackets indicate concentrations, and [R] is the concentration of free binding sites. The dissociation constant

$$K_d = \frac{[H][R]}{[HR]}$$

is the reciprocal of the association constant. For the simple reaction above it has units of concentration, and is equal to the concentration [H] of hormone for which [HR]=[R] or half the sites are occupied.[28]

In common with other steroid hormones, glucocorticoids at physiological temperatures seem to penetrate rapidly into cells. There they react first with apparently free receptors to form so-called 'cytoplasmic' hormone-receptors complexes that undergo a temperature-sensitive 'activation' and become bound partly to the nuclei.[29, 30] Biological effects are thought to be initiated by stimulation in the nuclei of synthesis of specific mRNA.[29] The ability of a cell to respond to a hormone is assumed to require the formation of nuclear complexes. Intact cells incubated at physiologic temperatures to a steady state with hormone will therefore have receptor-bound hormone associated with both cytoplasmic and nuclear-bound complexes. When the cells are broken, and separated into cytosol and nuclear fractions by centrifugation, the cytoplasmic complexes are found in the cytosol and the nuclear complexes in the nuclear fraction.[31-33] The procedures described subsequently are designed to measure separately hormone bound in the cytoplasmic and nuclear complexes. Because the activation step takes place very slowly at low temperatures (0 to 3°C), in normal cells incubated with hormone at low temperature the predominant complex found is cytoplasmic. When such cells are warmed, there is rapid formation of nuclear complexes. This procedure is used to study cytoplasmic-to-nuclear translocation.[21, 31-33]

Despite the complicated and as yet poorly understood receptor transformations that take place in intact cells, steady-state hormone binding to receptors in intact cells, whether measured with unbroken cells[34] or as cytoplasmic and nuclear complexes separately, is reasonably well described by the simple equations given above. With cortisol the dissociation constants K_d that have been found are generally around 10 to 50 nmol/l. With dexamethasone, the steroid commonly used for measuring glucocorticoid receptors, the K_d is around 1 to 10 nmol/l.[29]

In addition to binding to glucocorticoid receptors with high affinity and stereospecificity,[28] glucocorticoids participate in at least two other forms of binding that can complicate receptor assays. One of these is nonspecific—low-affinity (or nonsaturable) binding to sites that appear to be present in almost unlimited amounts.[28] It is intrinsic to every assay and can be corrected for by methods described later. The other is binding to proteins such as 'transcortin' or corticosteroid-binding globulin (CBG). CBG is present in plasma and possibly in cells, and appears as a contaminant in many cell and tissue preparations.[29] Cortisol binds to CBG with about the same dissociation constant with which it binds to glucocorticoid receptors, but fortunately synthetic steroids such as dexamethasone do not bind significantly to human CBG.

There are several reasons, in addition to its low affinity for CBG, for using dexamethasone in preference to cortisol for measuring glucocorticoid receptors.[29] One is that dexamethasone binds more tightly to glucocorticoid receptors and dissociates more slowly than cortisol. A second is that it cross-reacts less with mineralocorticoid receptors. A third is that it is less susceptible to metabolic inactivation.

In what are commonly referred to as equilibrium methods, cells or supernatants prepared from cells are incubated with several different concentrations of free labeled hormone. The total number of binding sites is estimated by extrapolation to infinite hormone concentration, at which all sites would be occupied.[28]

Common methods of analysis of the data obtained from equilibrium binding studies such as those described in this chapter, make the assumption that an equilibrium exists between bound and free hormone at the time as the measurements are made.

MEASUREMENT OF GLUCOCORTICOID RECEPTORS IN INTACT CELLS

Outline of methods[28, 32]

To measure cytoplasmic and nuclear glucocorticoid receptors (see below) cells in suspension are incubated with 10 different concentrations of dexamethasone (9α-fluoro-16α-methyl-11β,17,21-trihydroxypregna-1,4-diene-3,20-dione) for 30 min at 37°C. This time and temperature allow equilibration of the steroid between free and receptor-bound forms. To measure steroid bound in the nucleus, nuclei are obtained by hypotonic lysis using a 1:60 dilution into 1.5 mmol/l $MgCl_2$. A 'cytosol' fraction assumed to contain cytoplasmic complexes is obtained from the supernatant after hypotonic lysis using a 1:6 dilution into 1.5 mmol $MgCl$ containing dextran-coated charcoal. The dextran-coated charcoal adsorbs free steroid while leaving protein-bound steroid in the supernatant. Steroid bound in these fractions is then analyzed into receptor-bound and nonspecifically-bound steroid by assuming that receptor binding is saturable and nonspecific binding is not saturable. The numbers of receptor sites in the cell suspension is determined by extrapolation from the number of receptor sites occupied by (^{3}H)dexamethasone at the different free steroid concentrations to the number which would be occupied at an infinite concentration. A Scatchard plot may be used to facilitate the extrapolation. This number is then converted to the number of nuclear and cytoplasmic receptor sites per cell.

The simplified single-point assay (see below) uses the same incubation conditions described above, except that only a single near-saturating concentration of (^{3}H) dexamethasone is used. Non-saturable bound hormone is determined from the (^{3}H) dexamethasone bound during a parallel incubation with a saturating concentration of unlabeled dexamethasone. The molecules of (^{3}H) dexamethasone bound to cytoplasm and nuclei, after subtraction of the nonsaturably bound hormone are used to calculate the number of sites per cell in the cytoplasm and nucleus that are occupied by hormone. These values are extrapolated to infinite hormone concentration to estimate the total number of receptor sites per cell.

Translocation of the steroid-receptor complex from cytoplasmic to nuclear form (see below) is studied by measuring cytoplasmic and nuclear binding after incubation with (^{3}H)dexamethasone at 3°C for 120 min and again after incubation at 37°C for 30 min. At low temperature most of the steroid is generally in the cytoplasmic fraction, while at 37°C most will be bound to the nuclei if translocation has taken place. The long incubation at 3°C is necessary because equilibration is much slower at low temperatures; in fact even 120 min is probably not sufficient for complete equilibration, but it is usually adequate for demonstrating translocation.

Materials and equipment

For clarity this list includes the specific items and sources we employ, but undoubtably there are others that would be satisfactory:

1. (^{3}H)dexamethasone, (6,7-^{3}H(N)) mol wt 392.5 35–50 Ci/mmol (New England Nuclear, Boston, Mass, USA)
2. Dexamethasone (Steraloid, Inc, Wilton, NH, USA)
3. RPMI 1640 (Roswell Park Memorial Institute medium 1640) with 25 mmol/l HEPES (4(2-hydroxyethyl)-1-piperazine ethanesulfonic acid) buffer (Grand Island Biological Company, Grand Island, NY, USA)
4. Polypropylene tubes, 1.5 ml (Brinkman Instruments, Inc., Westbury, NY, USA)
5. Ficoll (Pharmacia, Piscataway, NJ, USA)
6. Hypaque (Winthrop Laboratories, New York)
7. Dextran, clinical grade (Sigma, St Louis, MO, USA)
8. Charcoal, Norit A (Fisher Scientific, Pittsburg, PA, USA)
9. Biofluor, liquid scintillation fluid (New England Nuclear, Boston, Mass, USA)
10. Brinkmann Centrifuge Model 72 (Brinkmann Instruments, Westbury, NY, USA)
11. Cytocentrifuge, Shannon-Elliot (Shannon Southern Instruments, Sewickley, PA, USA)

12. Liquid scintillation Counter, Model 3390, refrigerated (Packard Instruments, Downer's Grove, Ill., USA).

Reagents and solutions

1. (^3H)dexamethasone stock solution (0.5 µmol/l)
The manufacturer's solution is diluted in triple distilled benzene to 2 µmol/l. Twenty µl of this solution is evaporated in a glass container that can be capped. The steroid is redissolved immediately in 80 µl of RPMI 1640 with 25 mmol/l HEPES buffer by leaving at 37°C for 30 min or room temperature for several hours. The solution should be kept at 3°C and discarded after 1 week or if it becomes cloudy.

2. Dexamethasone stock solutions (20 µmol/l)
A 0.2 mmol/l solution in ethanol is prepared. Dexamethasone will require several hours at 37°C to go into solution. This stock solution may be kept for 2 months at 3°C. For the assays, 20 µl of the stock ethanol solution is evaporated to dryness and dissolved in 200 µl of RPMI 1640 with 25 mmol/l HEPES buffer. This solution should be kept at 3°C and discarded after 1 week or if it becomes cloudy.

3. $MgCl_2$ solution in water (1.5 mmol/l)

4. Dextran-coated charcoal in 1.5 mmol/l $MgCl_2$[32]
The suspension is prepared by adding 0.1 g of charcoal and 0.01 g dextran to a 10 ml graduated cylinder, bringing to 10 ml with 1.5 mmol/l $MgCl_2$ and shaking. After allowing 24 h at 3°C to sediment the large charcoal particles, the supernatant is aspirated and replaced by an equal volume of 1.5 mmol/l $MgCl_2$. The suspension must be shaken well before using. It can be stored at 3°C for 1 month.

5. Ficoll-Hypaque[35]
Ten parts by vol. of 33.9 per cent (v/v) Hypaque (N methyl-3,5,diacetamido 2,4,6-triiodobenzoate) are mixed with 24 parts of 11 per cent (w/v) Ficoll and mixed thoroughly. The resulting solution should have a density of 1.080 g/ml.

Assay of nuclear and cytoplasmic glucocorticoid receptors

1. Preparation of cell suspensions
Cells are obtained from peripheral blood anticoagulated with heparin (10 units/ml). The vol of blood required varies with the leukocyte and differential cell count. Table 9.1 gives an estimate of the amount of blood necessary for an assay.

With lymph nodes or other solid tissues a cell suspension can be prepared by gently teasing the tissue apart using forceps and needles. In dealing with malignant tissue, excessive fibrous tissue will occassionally prevent one from obtaining a viable cell suspension. In general about 0.1 to 0.5 g of lymphoid tissue are necessary for the assay.

White blood cells are separated from red blood cells and platelets using a discontinuous density gradient of Ficoll-Hypaque.[35] Heparinized blood is diluted 1:3 in saline at room temperature and 30 ml carefully layered over 8 ml

Table 9.1

Peripheral leukocyte count (cells $\times 10^9/l^a$)	Vol. of blood required (ml)
2–5	100
5–10	50
10–50	20
>50	10

[a] Assuming that the cells to be studied make up most of the peripheral white cells.

of Ficoll-Hypaque, without disturbing the interface between the cell suspension and Ficoll-Hypaque, in 50 ml clear centrifuge tubes. The tubes are centrifuged at 200 g for 45 min at room temperature and the cells at the interface with Ficoll-Hypaque are washed twice in 50 ml of phosphate-buffered saline (pH 7.4) at room temperature with centrifugation at 200 g for 10 min between washes.

Removal of most of the endogenous steroid is accomplished by incubating the cells in RPMI 1640 with 25 mmol/l HEPES buffer at 37°C for 30 min at approximately 10^6 cells per ml.

When all of the materials have been assembled to carry out the assay the above cell suspension is centrifuged to a pellet and resuspended in RPMI 1640 with 25 mmol/l HEPES buffer to 1 to 2×10^8 cells/ml. Cell counts, cytocrits (volume of packed cells) viabilities and cytocentrifuge slides are prepared. This suspension should be used immediately.

2. Incubation of cells with dexamethasone
Incubations are carried out in 1.5 ml polypropylene tubes. With the (^{3}H)dexamethasone stock solution a series of ten 1:2 dilutions of (^{3}H)dexamethasone are prepared in duplicate 20 μl aliquots with concentrations from 0.4 μmol/l to 0.8 nmol/l. For measurement of nonsaturable binding a solution of RPMI 1640 with 20 nmol/l (^{3}H)dexamethasone plus 2 μmol/l unlabeled dexamethasone is prepared. Aliquots (20 μl) are placed in each of four 1.5 ml polypropylene tubes. One of the duplicate sets of tubes (each including 2 tubes for determining nonsaturable-bound steroid) is numbered 1 to 12 and is used for measuring nuclear binding; the other, numbered 13 to 24, is used for cytoplasmic binding.

The incubation is initiated by adding 20 μl of cell suspension to each of the 24 tubes. The tubes are placed in a 37°C water bath and incubated with gentle shaking (60 oscillations per minute) for 30 min.

3. Measurement of free concentrations of dexamethasone
After the incubation the tubes are centrifuged for 2 min at 12 000 g, and 20 μl of each supernatant are removed and placed in a scintillation vial with 5 ml of Biofluor for liquid scintillation counting.

4. Measurement of nuclear receptor sites
The tubes containing the centrifuged cell suspensions are cooled to 3°C. With one of the duplicate sets of tubes (labeled 1 to 12) the cells are broken by adding 1.2 ml of 1.5 mmol/l MgCl$_2$ at 3°C. The contents are vigorously mixed and left at 3°C for 30 min to complete lysis. The tubes are then centrifuged at 12 000 g

for 4 min. The supernatants are carefully aspirated and discarded without disturbing the nuclear pellets or leaving excessive supernatant. The tips of the tubes containing the nuclear pellet are cut off and placed in 5 ml of Biofluor for liquid scintillation counting.

5. *Measurement of cytoplasmic receptor sites* (steps 4 and 5 can be done concurrently)
With the second set of 12 tubes (numbered 13 to 24), the cells are broken by adding 100 μl of 1.5 mmol/l $MgCl_2$ containing dextran-coated charcoal. The contents are vigorously mixed and left at 3°C for 30 min to complete lysis. The tubes are then centrifuged at 12 000 g for 4 min, and 100 μl of the supernatant carefully removed (with care not to contaminate the supernatant with charcoal), and placed in 5 ml of Biofluor for liquid scintillation counting.

Table 9.2 Binding of (^{3}H)dexamethasone to human lymphoblasts.
The data listed are those used for the Scatchard plot in Fig. 9.1. The terms (H), (T), (HN), and (HR) are defined in the text.

Tube	(H)	(T)	Nuclei ($\alpha = .003$) (HN)	(HR)	(T)/(H)	(HR)/(H)	Tube	(H)	(T)	Cytoplasmic ($\alpha = $) (HN)	(HR)	(T)/(R)	(HR)/(H)
1	33894	312	203	109	.009	.003	13						
2	22723	241	136	105	.010	.005	14						
3	14384	176	86	90	.012	.006	15						
4	9704	148	58	90	.015	.009	16						
5	5759	102	35	67	.018	.012	17						
6	3810	82	23	59	.022	.015	18						
7	1913	47	12	35	.024	.018	19						
8	942	25	6	19	.026	.020	20						
9	508	15	3	12	.031	.024	21						
10	251	9	2	7	.036	.027	22						
11	7168	43	43	0	.006	0	23						
12	7410	44	44	0	.006	0	24						

6. *Calculation of the dissociation constant (K_d) and number of receptor sites per cell (R_o)*
To avoid confusion and minimize errors in calculations we have found it useful to tabulate the data as indicated in Table 9.2. In addition, we have given data for an actual determination (Table 9.2, nuclei, and Fig. 9.1). The following abbreviations are used:

(H)   The concentration of free dexamethasone in cpm per 20 μl of the supernatant from the incubation mixture.

(T)   total (^{3}H)dexamethasone bound to the cells in cpm per 20 μl of the original cell suspension (or 40 μl of the final incubation mixture)

(HN)   (^{3}H)dexamethasone nonsaturably-bound to the cells in cpm per 20 μl of the original cell suspension.

(HR)   (^{3}H)dexamethasone bound to the receptor in cpm per 20 μl of the original cell suspension

α The fraction of free hormone nonsaturably-bound in the incubation mixture. The dimensions are cpm (^{3}H)dexamethasone nonsaturably-bound per 20 μl of the original cell suspension (or 40 μl of incubation mixture) divided by the cpm (^{3}H)dexamethasone per 20 μl of the supernatant from the incubation mixture.

The cpm of (^{3}H)dexamethasone per 20 μl of supernatant from each of the tubes is corrected for background and entered in Table 9.2 under (H).

The cpm of (^{3}H)dexamethasone bound (T) (after subtracting background) for the 100 μl cytoplasmic samples are corrected to the full vol. of 120 μl by multiplying by 1.2. This gives the cytoplasmic-bound steroid in cpm per 20 μl of the original cell suspension. The values for the nuclear pellets will be the total cpm (^{3}H)dexamethasone bound per 20 μl of the original cell suspension and do not require correction other than subtraction of background. These data are entered in Table 9.2 under the column headed (T).

Each of the values for both cytoplasmic and nuclear-bound steroid must be corrected for nonsaturable binding at the same concentration. This is done by first determining the fraction of free hormone nonsaturably-bound (α)[28] to the cells as follows: $\alpha = Bns/Fns$ where Bns is the cpm (^{3}H)dexamethasone bound per 20 μl of the original cell suspension in tubes containing an excess of unlabeled dexamethasone (tubes 11, 12, 23 and 24). Fns is the cpm (^{3}H)dexamethasone per 20 μl of supernatant from the same tubes.

The nonsaturably-bound hormone (HN) at each free concentration (H) is then calculated as follows:[28] $(HN) = \alpha(H)$, and the values for (HN) entered in Table 9.2.

After calculating the nonsaturable-bound (^{3}H)dexamethasone (HN) for each tube containing a different free concentration of (^{3}H)dexamethasone, the receptor-bound dexamethasone (HR) is calculated as: $(HR) = (T) - (HN)$, and (HR) for each tube entered in Table 9.2. (T)/(H) and (HR)/(H) are calculated and entered in Table 9.2 under the appropriate column. Note that the values for α, (H), (T), (HN), and (HR) must be determined for both cytoplasmic and nuclear assays.

To obtain estimates of the number of receptor sites in the cell suspension and the affinity of these sites the data can be analyzed by Scatchard analysis.[28, 36] This method linearizes the binding data to allow accurate extrapolation to the total number of receptor sites occupied at an infinite free hormone concentration. The Scatchard plot is prepared as indicated in Fig. 9.1 by plotting the bound hormone concentration in cpm per 20 μl of the original cell suspension ((T) in Table 9.2 and Bound in Fig. 9.1) against the ratio of bound (T) to free (H) hormone concentration ((T)/(H) in Table 9.2, and Bound/Free in Fig. 9.1). For the example depicted in Fig. 9.1 this gave the curved line indicated by the closed circles for the nuclear bound hormone at 37°C. On the same sheet of graph paper (HR) is plotted against (HR)/(H), where (HR) is used for bound and (H) for free. For the example in Fig. 9.1 this gave the straight line indicated by the open circles.

It is also worthwhile presenting the value for α, which will represent a straight line parallel to the X axis, as indicated in Fig. 9.1 by the dashed line. At high free hormone concentrations the line through the values for (T) vs (T)/(H) should approach α (Fig. 9.1).

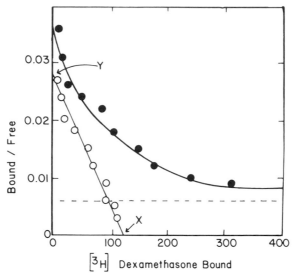

Fig. 9.1 Scatchard plot of the binding of (^{3}H)dexamethasone to nuclei of human lymphoblasts. Data are from Table 9.2. Cells were incubated with dexamethasone and nuclei obtained by hypotonic lysis as described in the text. The closed circles represent the results using the total nuclear-bound hormone (T in Table 9.2) as bound. The proportion of the free hormone concentration nonsaturable bound to the nuclei (α) is indicated by the dashed line. The results for the receptor-bound hormone (HR in Table 9.2) is indicated by the open circles and is calculated by subtracting the nonsaturable bound hormone as indicated in the text. Bound (^{3}H)dexamethasone is in cpm per 20 μl of the original cell suspension (or per 40 μl of the incubation mixture) while free (^{3}H)dexamethasone is in cpm per 20 μl of the supernatant from the incubation mixture. The original cell suspension contained 1.07×10^8 cells per ml, the specific activity of the dexamethasone was 33 000 Ci/mole, and the counting efficiency 0.47 cpm/dpm. Using the equations on this page, it can be calculated that there are 930 receptor sites per cell nucleus with a K_d of 6.35 nmol/l.

A line is drawn through the points obtained by plotting (HR)/(R) vs (HR) to intersect the x and y axes at X and Y (Fig. 9.1) respectively. The value of (HR) at the intersection on the axis (Fig. 9.1, X) will give the concentration of the hormone-receptor complex per 20 μl of the original cell suspension when the receptor is fully occupied. This is converted to receptor sites per cell (R$_o$) in the cytoplasm or nucleus as follows:

$$R_o = (X)(50/E)(1/C)(1/2.22 \times 10^{12})(6.023 \times 10^{23}/S) = 1.36 \times 10^{13}(X)/(E)(C)(S)$$

where: E is efficiency (cpm/dpm)
50 is a conversion factor to ml
C is the cell count (cells per ml) in the original suspension
2.22×10^{12} is the number of dpm per Ci
6.023×10^{23} is Avogadro's number (molecule per mol)
S is the specific activity in Ci/mol.

The dissociation constant (K_d) of the binding sites for dexamethasone is determined from the slope of the line (Fig. 9.1, X/Y):

$$K_d = (X/Y)(50\,000/E)(1/2.22 \times 10^{12})(1/S)$$
$$= 2.3 \times 10^{-8}(X)/(Y)(S)(E)$$

where K_d has the dimension of mol/l, and slope (X/Y) the dimensions of cpm per 20 μl of cell suspension and 50 000 is the correction factor from 20 μl to liters. The remainder of the terms are defined above.

Abbreviated single point assay

1. Incubation of cell suspensions with dexamethasone

Aliquots (80 μl) of the cell suspension prepared (see above) are added to 1.5 ml polypropylene tubes containing either 10 μl (^{3}H)dexamethasone (0.5 μmol/l) plus 10 μl of RPMI 1640 or 10 μl (^{3}H)dexamethasone (0.5 μmol/l) plus 10 μl of unlabeled dexamethasone (20 μmol/l) which have been well mixed prior to the addition of the cells. This will usually give a free concentration of (^{3}H)dexamethasone between 40 and 50 nmol/l depending on the amount bound by the cells.

The tubes are placed in a pre-warmed 37°C water bath and incubated with gentle shaking (60 oscillations per min) for 30 min. They are then cooled to 3°C.

2. Measurement of cytoplasmic and nuclear binding

Duplicate 20 μl aliquots are removed from both tubes and used to measure nuclear and cytoplasmic binding by adding them to 1.2 ml of 1.5 mmol/l $MgCl_2$ (p. 257) and 100 μl of $MgCl_2$ with dextran-coated charcoal (p. 258).

3. Measurement of [H], the concentration of free hormone

The cell suspensions left in the tubes are centrifuged at 12 000 $\times g$ for 3 min. With calibrated glass pipettes (not vacuum displacement pipettes) duplicate 5 μl aliquots of the supernatants are placed in scintillation fluid and counted. The cpm per 5 μl (h) are converted to free hormone concentration [H] (in mol/l) as follows:

$$[H] = (h)(2 \times 10^5)(1/E)(1/2.22 \times 10^{12})(1/S) = (9 \times 10^{-8})(h)/(E)(S)$$

where 2×10^5 converts (h) from cpm/5 μl to cpm/l, and other terms are defined on p. 220. [H] should generally be above 3×10^{-8} mol/l.

4. Calculation of R_o, the number of receptor sites per cell

As outlined on p. 259, the cpm of bound (^{3}H)dexamethasone in the cytoplasmic samples are multiplied by 1.2 to convert to cpm bound per 20 μl cell suspension (nuclear cpm require no conversion), values of α are computed and used to determine (HR) for the cytoplasmic and nuclear assays. R_o is then calculated from the formula

$$R_o = (HR)(5/4)(50/E)(1/C)(1/2.22 \times 10^{12})(6.023 \times 10^{23}/S)(1 + 10^{-8}/[H])$$
$$= 1.7 \times 10^{13}(HR)(1 + 10^{-8}/[H])/(E)(C)(S).$$

Here 5/4 corrects for the dilution of 80 μl cell suspension by 20 μl dexamethasone solution, [H] is defined above and the other terms on p. 260. The term $(1 + 10^{-8}/[H])$ extrapolates binding at hormone concentration [H] to saturating (infinite) concentration. It arises from the equation

$$[HR] = K_a R_o[H]/(1 + Ka[H]) = R_o[H]/(K_d + [H])$$

which gives the concentration of receptor-bound hormone [HR] as a function of [H] for the reaction on p. 253[28]. From this equation it follows that $R_o =$ [HR] $(1 + K_d/[H])$. With 10^{-8} mol/l as a reasonable estimate for K_d (see p. 267) we obtain $R_o =$ [HR] $(1 + 10^{-8}/[H])$. If [H] is around 3×10^{-8} mol/l as recommended, $(1 + 10^{-8}/[H])$ is 1.33. The lower [H] is the larger this term becomes the less reliable the extrapolation.

5. Calculation of total receptor sites per cell
The total number of receptor sites per cell is obtained by adding the cytoplasmic and nuclear receptor sites.

Cytoplasmic to nuclear translocation of the hormone-receptor complex

1. Cell suspension
Prepared as above (p. 256) and cooled to 3°C.

2. Dexamethasone solutions
Two solutions are prepared, one containing 20 μl of (^{3}H)dexamethasone (0.5 μmol/l plus 20 μl of RPMI 1640, the other, for measurement of nonsaturable binding, containing 20 μl of unlabeled dexamethasone (20 μmol/l).

3. Incubation at 3°C
The 3°C incubation is initiated after adding 160 μl of cooled cell suspension to the two tubes containing either labeled dexamethasone alone or a combination of labeled and unlabeled dexamethasone. The solutions are thoroughly mixed and incubated with gentle shaking (60 oscillations per min) for 120 min at 3°C. Twenty μl aliquots are removed in duplicate for measurement of nuclear- and cytoplasmic-bound hormone as described on pp. 257 and 258.

4. Incubation at 37°C
The two tubes containing the remaining cell suspension are transferred to a 37°C water bath. Here they are incubated for 30 min with gentle shaking (60 oscillations per min). At the end of the incubation 20 μl aliquots are removed for measurement of nuclear and cytoplasmic bound hormone as described on pp. 257 and 258.

5. Measurement of the concentrations of free (^{3}H)dexamethasone
This is done as described above.

6. Calculations
The data in cpm are converted to cpm bound per 20 μl of cell suspension and the number of nuclear and cytoplasmic receptor sites per cell at 3°C and 37°C calculated as indicated in page 261. These data may be conveniently displayed as in Fig. 9.2.

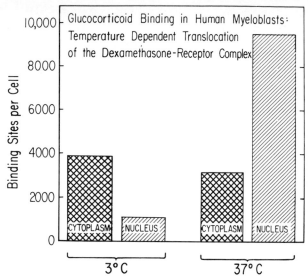

Fig. 9.2 Dexamethasone binding to human myeloblasts; temperature-dependent translocation of the hormone-receptor complex. Cytoplasmic and nuclear binding were assayed after a 2 h incubation at 3°C (data on left) and after a 30 min incubation at 37°C (data on right) as described on page 262. The apparent increase in the number of total receptor sites at 37°C results from the failure of complete association between hormone and receptor at 3°C. At 37°C this reaction comes closer to equilibrium.

PRACTICAL ASPECTS OF MEASURING GLUCOCORTICOID RECEPTORS IN MALIGNANT CELLS

The cell suspension

The results calculated in the assays described above are the mean number of binding sites per cell. With non-homogeneous cell populations such results are likely to be misleading. Thus is is important to assess the homogeneity of the cell suspension. For this reason we have routinely done differential cell counts on Wright stained cytocentrifuge preparations, and have excluded results in cases with more than 30 per cent contaminating cells by morphologic criteria. Additional tests of homogeneity which we have found useful include determining the proportion of cells bearing surface immunoglobulin, Fc or complement receptors or forming rosettes with sheep red blood cells. The latter methods are applicable to lymphoid cells and allow the recognition of morphologically identical but functionally different cell types.

In addition it is essential that some test of viability be performed on the cell suspension prior to assay of glucocorticoid receptors. Although Trypan blue exclusion probably over-estimates viability, it is convenient and is one of the only methods applicable to non-dividing cells. We have found that cells which are non-viable by Trypan blue exclusion have no detectable glucocorticoid receptors. Thus, the mean number of receptor sites per cell should be corrected for non-viable cells. Furthermore, cell suspensions containing large numbers of non-viable cells should not be used for assay of receptors. We exclude results from cell suspensions containing fewer than 80 per cent viable cells.

The cell suspension used in the above assays contains a very high concentration of cells (1–2×10^8/ml). Since metabolites will accumulate rapidly in such a cell suspension it is essential to carry out the assay as quickly as possible after the suspension is prepared. The incubation at 37°C should not be prolonged for more than 40 min.

The culture medium used for assay of glucocorticoid receptors should not include fetal calf serum which may itself contain steroid hormones, and the cells should be adequately washed at room temperature to remove as much endogenous hormone as possible. Any remaining cortisol present in the medium will compete with the labeled dexamethasone used in the assay and give inaccurate results. This problem is particularly difficult when studying cells from patients currently receiving treatment with glucocorticoids. In these cases it is important that the cells be incubated at 37°C for 30 min prior to assaying for receptors, to allow dissociation of endogenous glucocorticoid from the receptors. The possibility that this incubation may not be adequate to allow the complete dissociation of steroid is suggested by studies we have done on patients receiving treatment with glucocorticoids. Glucocorticoid receptor levels have consistently dropped during treatment with dexamethasone or prednisolone compared to pretreatment levels (see below: Interpretation of results). Although there are other possible explanations for the decrease in receptor levels, incomplete removal of the steroid prior to the assay may account for part of the problem.

Incubation conditions

The time and temperature of incubation should be sufficient to allow an equilibrium (or at least a steady state) to be achieved at each concentration of free hormone. This should be checked for the incubation conditions used in each laboratory. Since the incubations containing the lowest concentrations of free hormone will be the slowest to come to equilibrium,[28] these should be tested with particular care.

The concentrations of radiolabeled hormone used in the incubation should extend from approximately $K_d/10$ to $K_d \times 10$. For dexamethasone this will give a range of 1 nmol/l to 100 nmol/l.

Lysis of cells to obtain nuclei and cytosol

Variability in susceptibility to osmotic lysis among human leukemia cells requires that this part of the assay should be carefully monitored if the values for cytoplasmic and nuclear receptor sites and translocation are to be meaningful.

Osmotic lysis may be monitored in several ways. Electronmicroscopy, a method we have applied to rat thymus cells,[31] allows morphological examination of the nuclei to determine if they are intact and free of contamination by cytoplasmic organelle. The adequacy of lysis may also be checked by the release of intracellular proteins after hypotonic dilution. Using ^{51}Cr to label cellular proteins we have found that 75 to 100 per cent of the maximal-releasable ^{51}Cr (determined by freeze-thawing the cells in distilled water) is released within 30 min of a 1:6 dilution in 1.5 mmol/l $MgCl_2$ at 3° C. The release of the glucocorticoid receptor may be used in a similar way to determine the adequacy of lysis. After a 3 to 4 h incubation at 0°C the majority of receptor sites should be found in the supernatant of a 1:6 dilution in 1.5 mmol/l $MgCl_2$ containing dextran-coated charcoal. If most of the receptor sites are in the nuclear pellet, the possibility that the cells did not release their cytoplasmic contents should be considered. The release of cytoplasmic enzymes such as lactic acid dehydrogenase may also be used to assess cell lysis.

Finally, the adequacy of lysis may be checked morphologically by inspection of the cells following hypotonic dilution on a precooled microscopic stage with Trypan blue. During this procedure the cells should not be allowed to warm, since they will lyse more easily at higher temperatures. Lysed cells should stain with Trypan blue and have no cytoplasm attached to the nuclei, which should be intact and not fragmented.

Occassionally, we have been unable to lyse cells by one of the above criteria and have used freezing in a dry ice acetone bath followed by thawing and a 1:6 or 1:60 dilution in 1.5 mmol/l $MgCl_2$ at 3°C to complete the lysis. While this freeze-thaw method results in complete lysis, it reduces the amount of nuclear-bound hormone receptor complex in rat thymus cells and human lymphocytes and for this reason we have been reluctant to use the freeze-thaw technic.

Evaluation of data

The technic most commonly used to calculate the affinity and number of binding sites is visual inspection of a Scatchard plot, drawing a straight line through the points obtained following correction for nonsaturable binding. While this simple method is satisfactory in most cases, more objective methods of analysis of the binding data have been described in detail.[37,38] The choice of these methods is largely dependent on the availability of computer facilities and one's familiarity with these methods of evaluating data. In any case the computer-generated estimates should be checked by inspection of the Scatchard plot.

Use of a single concentration of steroid to estimate receptor number

This abbreviated and more convenient assay assumes that most of the receptors are occupied at the concentration of dexamethasone used in the assay. For this reason it is important that the concentration of hormone be carefully controlled if results are to be reproducible. Calculation of the number of glucocorticoid receptor sites using this method assumes that the affinity of binding does not vary among the individuals studied. Although this may not be completely accurate[24] we have found good correspondence between the values obtained using the single-point assay and those obtained from the 10-point binding study.

Use of stored cells

In general we have noted only a moderate reduction in the number of binding sites, and no change in affinity, after preservation in liquid nitrogen using controlled rate freezing[39] and providing that the cells were viable after storage. However, mature human granulocytes or chronic myelocytic leukemia cells do not survive storage well.

Incubation of human leukemia or lymphoma cells at $1-3 \times 10^6$ cells per ml at 25 to 37°C for 24 h in RPMI 1640 with 25 mmol/l HEPES buffer and fetal calf serum has little effect on receptor number or affinity, again provided that the cells are viable at the time of assay.

If assays are to be carried out routinely on stored or shipped cells, it is important to test the effect of such procedures in advance.

INTERPRETATION OF RESULTS

Although two studies have indicated that glucocorticoid receptors levels may be useful guides in the treatment of leukemia and lymphoma,[23,40] it is not possible at present to give levels which will indicate a favourable response to treatment. Since the level of glucocorticoid receptors varies among the different hematologic malignancies[19,21,23,25] results will probably have to be interpreted in relation to the disease being studied. In addition, variations in technics between laboratories may necessitate individual laboratory standards.

Results from patients receiving glucocorticoids should be interpreted with caution. In 9 of 11 patients with a variety of hematologic malignancies, we have found a drop in receptor levels during treatment compared to values before treatment. For the group of 11 patients treatment levels averaged 58 ± 14 per cent of pre-treatment levels.

Table 9.3 Glucocorticoid receptors in various normal and malignant cells

Cells	Subjects	R_o	K_d nmol/l	%N	CTN
Normal human lymphocytes[21]	10	3300(840–6720)	8	70	4/4
Normal human granulocytes	1	2100	ND	ND	ND
Normal human monocytes[41]	1	9000	13	ND	ND
Peripheral lymphoblasts from patients with ALL[21]	6	4600(900–7071)	12	65	6/6
Peripheral lymphocytes from patients with CLL[21]	12	2100(400–4620)	9	81	9/11
Lymph node cells from patients with lymphoma[21]	6	1700(477–2690)	10	70	6/6
Blasts from patients with ANLL[25]	23	4800(1260–13230)	15	65	12/12
Blasts from patients with CML in blast crisis[21]	4	5000(2610–6300)	13	60	3/3
Rat thymus cells	5	3600(2100–5100)	9	73	6/6
Rat lymph node cells[42]	13	1970(1100–2300)	5	78	5/5
MOLT cell line	—	4400	14	ND	ND
HL-60 cell line	—	1500	11	55	ND
CEM C7 cell line	—	9500	6	60	ND
MOPC 21 (subline 574 and 582)	—	0	—	—	—

R_0, mean number of nuclear binding sites per cell, ranges are in parentheses
K_d, mean dissociation constant, for the number of cases listed under 'Subjects'
%N, mean percentage of total receptors bound to the nucleus at 37°C
CNT, cytoplasmic-to-nuclear translocation, scored positive if cells which had been incubated with 10 nmol/l desamethasone at 3°C showed an increase in the ratio of cytoplasmic to nuclear binding when warmed to 37°C
ALL, acute lymphocytic leukemia
CLL, chronic lymphocytic leukemia
ANLL, acute non-lymphocytic leukemia
CML, chronic myelogenous leukemia
HL-60, a human granulocytic cell line[43]
CEM-C7 and MOLT are human lymphoid cell lines
MOPC 21 (Sublines 574 and 582)[44] are tissue culture lines derived from the original solid tumor MOPC 21
ND, not done

RESULTS

Table 9.3 lists our results for a variety of different tissues and cultured cell lines and is intended primarily as a source of expected results with the technics described above. All of the cells we have studied contain measurable numbers of glucocorticoid receptors with the exception of red blood cells, platelets and a few cultured cell lines. The large variation in receptor number within each of the patient categories in Table 9.3 to some degree results from grouping various subtypes of leukemia and lymphoma under the same category. Recently different levels of glucocorticoid receptors have been noted among subclasses of ALL[19,23] and acute non-lymphocytic leukemia.[25] Furthermore, preliminary evidence indicates that the cells of malignancies responding to chemotherapy have higher levels of receptors than those not responding.[23,40]

The dissociation constant (K_d) of the receptors for dexamethasone varies by a factor of approximately 10 among the different individuals listed in Table 9.3. The median value of 10 nmol/l is similar to that reported by of other investigators.[16,18-20] This value corresponds to physiologic concentrations of glucocorticoids, indicating that the receptors would be partly occupied at physiologic levels of hormone.

Translocation of the hormone-receptor complex to the nucleus occurs to some degree with nearly all cells (Table 9.3, last column). The percentage of total receptors present in the nucleus at 37°C has varied in our results from as little as 27 per cent to over 90 per cent, with a median of approximately 75 per cent.

Acknowledgments

This work was supported in part by Research Grants CA17323, and AM03535, from the National Institutes of Health, US Public Health Services.

We wish to thank Drs Robert Gallo, Steven Collins and Robert Gallagher of the National Cancer Institute for the HL-60 cell line, and Dr Olive Pettengill of Dartmouth Medical School for the sublines 574 and 584 of the original MOPC 21 cell line.

REFERENCES

1 Burningham R A, Restrepo A, Pugh R P, Brown E B, Schlossman S F, Khuri D D, Lessner H E, Harrington W J 1964 Weekly high dosage glucocorticoid treatment of lymphocytic leukemias and lymphomas. New England Journal of Medicine 270: 1160–1166
2 Southwest Cancer Chemotherapy Study Group 1962 Studies of ACTH, hydrocordisone and 6 mercaptopurine in the treatment of children with acute leukemia. Journal of Pediatrics 61: 693–701
3 Ezdinli E Z, Stutzman L, Aungst C W, Firat D 1969 Corticosteroid therapy for lymphoma and chronic lymphocytic leukemia. Cancer 23: 900–909
4 Cline M J 1973 Adrenal steroids in the treatment of malignant hematologic disease. In: Azarnoff D L (ed) Medical Clinics of North America Vol 57 No 5. Saunders, 1203–1209
5 Vietti T J, Sullivan M P, Berry D H, Haddy T B, Haggard M E, Blattner R J 1965 The response of acute childhood leukemia to an initial and a second course of prednisone. Journal of Pediatrics 66: 18–26
6 Leikin S L, Brubaker C A, Hartmann J R, Murphy M L, Wolff J A, Perrin E 1968 Varying prednisone dosage in remission induction of previously untreated childhood leukemia. Cancer 21: 346–351

7 Wolff J A, Brubaker C A, Murphy M L, Pierce M I, Severo N 1967, Prednisone therapy of acute childhood leukemia: prognosis and duration of response in 330 treated patients. Journal of Pediatrics 70: 626–631

8 Ranney H M, Gellhorn A 1957 The effect of massive prednisone and prednisolone therapy on acute leukemia and malignant lymphomas. American Journal of Medicine 23: 405–413

9 Granville N B, Rubio F, Asuman U, Schulman E, Dameshek W 1958 Treatment of acute leukemia in adults with massive doses of prednisone and prednisolone. New England Journal of Medicine 259: 207–213

10 Second Report to the Medical Research Council of the Working Party on the Evaluation of Different Methods of Therapy in Leukemia 1966 Treatment of acute leukemia in adults: Comparison of steroid and mercaptopurine therapy, alone and in conjunction. British Medical Journal 1: 1383–1389

11 Knospe W H, Conrad M E 1966 The danger of corticosteroids in acute granulocytic leukemia. Medical Clinics of North America 50: 1653–1668

12 Lippman M E, Perry S, Thompson E B 1975 Glucocorticoid binding proteins in myeloblasts of acute myelogenous leukemia. American Journal of Medicine 59: 224–227

13 Gailani S, Minowada J, Silvernail A, Nussbaum A, Kaiser N, Rosen F, Shimaoka K 1973 Specific glucocorticoid binding in human hemopoietic cell lines and neoplastic tissue. Cancer Research 33: 2653–2657

14 Lippman M E, Halterman R H, Leventhal B G, Perry S, Thompson E B 1973 Glucocorticoid-binding proteins in human acute lymphoblastic leukemic blast cells. Journal of Clinical Investigation 52: 1715–1725

15 Lippman M, Halterman R, Leventhal B, Thompson E B 1973 Glucocorticoid binding proteins in human leukemic lymphoblasts. Nature New Biology 242: 157–158

16 Homo F, Duval D, Meyer P 1975 Etude de la liaison de la dexamethasone tritiée dans les lymphocytes de sujets normaux et leucémiques. Compts Rendues de l'Academie de Science de Paris 280D: 1923–1926

17 Smith K A, Crabtree G R, Kennedy S J, Munck A 1977 Glucocorticoid receptors and glucocorticoid sensitivity of mitogen stimulated and unstimulated human lymphocytes. Nature 267: 523–526

18 Neifeld J P, Lippman M E, Tormey D C 1977 Steroid hormone receptors in normal human lymphocytes. Journal of Biological Chemistry 252: 2972–2977

19 Yarbro C S K, Lippman M E, Johnson G E, Leventhal B G 1977 Glucocorticoid receptors in subpopulations of childhood acute lymphocytic leukemia. Cancer Research 37: 2688–2695

20 Homo F, Duval D, Meyer P, Belas F, Debre P, Binet J L 1978 Chronic lymphatic leukemia: cellular effects of glucocorticoids in vitro. British Journal of Haematology 38: 491–499

21 Crabtree G R, Smith K A, Munck A 1978 Glucocorticoid receptors and sensitivity of isolated human leukemia and lymphoma cells. Cancer Research 38: 4268–4272

22 Duval D, Homo F 1978 Prognostic value of steroid receptor determination in leukemia. Cancer Research 38: 4263–4267

23 Lippman M E, Yarbro G K, Leventhal B G 1978 Clinical implications of glucocorticoid receptors in human leukemia. Cancer Research 38: 4251–4256

24 Crabtree G R, Smith K A, Munck A 1979 Glucocorticoid receptors and in vitro sensitivity of cells from patients with leukemia and lymphoma: a reassessment. In: Bell P A, Borthwick W M (eds) Glucocorticoid Action and Leukemia, Proceedings of 7th Tenovus Workshop, Alpha Omega Publisher, Cardiff, Wales, pp 191–204

25 Crabtree G R, Bloomfield C D, Smith K A, Peterson B A, McKenna R W, Gibbs G, Munck A 1980 Glucocorticoid receptors and in vitro sensitivity of leukemic blasts in acute non-lymphocytic leukemia. Cancer Treatment Reports, in press

26 Crabtree G R, Smith K A, Munck A 1979 Glucocorticoid receptors and sensitivity in cells from patients with leukemia and lymphoma. Results and methodologic considerations. In: Thompson E B, Lippman M E (eds) Steroid Receptors and the Management of Cancer, CRC Press, Inc, Cleveland, Ohio. Vol I, pp 81–97

27 Simonsson B 1976 Evidence for a glucocorticoid receptor in human leukocytes. Acta Physiologica Scandinavica 98: 131–135

28 Munck A 1976 General aspects of steroid hormone-receptor interactions. In: Pasqualini J R (ed) Receptors and Mechanism of Action of Steroid Hormones Part I. Marcel Dekker, Inc, New York, pp 1–40

29 Munck A, Leung K 1977 Glucocorticoid receptors and mechanisms of action. In: Pasqualini J R (ed) Receptors and Mechanism of Action of Steroid Hormones Part II. Marcel Dekker, Inc, New York, pp 311–397

30 Munck A, Foley R 1979 Activation of steroid hormone-receptor complexes in intact target cells in physiological conditions. Nature 278: 752–754

31 Wira C R, Munck A 1974 Glucocorticoid receptor complexes in rat thymus cells. Journal of Biological Chemistry 249: 5328–5336

32 Munck A, Wira C R 1975 Methods for assessing hormone-receptor kinetics with cells in suspension: receptor-bound and nonspecifically bound hormone; cytoplasmic-nuclear translocation. In: O'Malley F W, Hardman J G (eds) Methods in Enzymology, Vol 30 A. Academic Press, New York, pp 255–264

33 Munck A, Foley R 1976 Kinetics of glucocorticoid-receptor complexes in rat thymus cells. Journal of Steroid Biochemistry 7: 1117–1122

34 Munck A, Brinck-Johnsen T 1968 Specific and nonspecific physiochemical interactions of glucocorticoids and related steroids in rat thymus cells in vitro. Journal of Biological Chemistry 243: 5556–5565

35 Boyum A 1968 Separation of leukocytes from blood and bone marrow. Scandinavian Journal of Clinical Laboratory Investigation 21, Suppl 97: 51–76

36 Scatchard G 1949 The attractions of proteins for small molecules and ions. Annals of New York, Academy of Science 51: 660–672

37 Rodbard D, Feldman H A 1975 Theory of protein-ligand interaction. In: O'Malley B W, Hardman J G (eds) Methods in Enzymology, Vol. 36: Hormone Action Part A; Steroid Hormones. Academic Press, New York, pp 3–16

38 Reich J G, Wangermann G, Falck M, Rohde K 1972 A general strategy for parameter estimation from isosteric and allosteric-kinetic data and binding measurements. European Journal of Biochemistry 26: 368–379

39 Jewett M A S, Hansen J A, DuPont D 1976 Cryopreservation of lymphocytes. In: Rose M R, Friedman H (eds) Manual of Clinical Immunology, American Society of Microbiology, Washington, DC, pp 833–839

40 Bloomfield C D, Smith K A, Peterson B A, Hildebrandt L, Zaleskas J, Gajl-Peczalska K, Frizzera G, Munck A 1980 In-vitro glucocorticoid studies for predicting response to glucocorticoid therapy in adults with malignant lymphoma. The Lancet: 952–956

41 Werb Z, Foley R, Munck A 1978 Interaction of glucocorticoids with macrophages: Identification of glucocorticoid receptors in monocytes and macrophages. Journal of Experimental Medicine 22: 1684–1693

42 Crabtree G R, Munck A, Smith K A 1980 Glucocorticoids and lymphocytes. I. Increased glucocorticoid receptor levels in antigen-stimulated lymphocytes. The Journal of Immunology 124: 2430–2435

43 Collins S J, Gallo R C, Gallagher R E 1977 Continuous growth and differentiation of human myeloid leukemic cells in suspension culture. Nature 270: 347–349

44 Sorenson G D, Pettengill O S, Cate C C 1978 Loss of oncogenicity and concomitant increased immunogenicity of murine plasmacytoma cell lines. American Journal of Pathology 90: 565–581

Index

Note: Page numbers in italic type refer to illustrations